SIXTH EDITION

USMLE STEP 2

SECRETS

ELSEVIER

EDITORIAL REVIEW BOARD

SIXTH EDITION

USMLE STEP 2

SECRETS

TED O'CONNELL, MD, FAAFP
Program Director
Family Medicine Residency Program
Kaiser Permanente Napa-Solano, California
Associate Clinical Professor
Department of Community and Family Medicine
University of California, San Francisco School of Medicine
San Francisco, California

ELSEVIER

Elsevier
1600 John F. Kennedy Blvd.
Ste 1800
Philadelphia, PA 19103-2899

USMLE STEP 2 SECRETS,SIXTH EDITION   ISBN: 9780323824330
Copyright © 2022 by Elsevier, Inc. All rights reserved.

Notice

ISBN: 9780323824330

Content Strategist: James Merritt
Content Development Manager: Ellen Wurm-Cutter
Content Development Specialist: Casey Potter
Publishing Services Manager: Shereen Jameel
Project Manager: Nadhiya Sekar
Design Direction: Bridget Hoette

Printed in Canada

Last digit is the print number: 9   8   7   6   5   4   3   2   1

Working together
to grow libraries in
developing countries

www.elsevier.com • www.bookaid.org

To Nichole, Ryan, Sean, and Claire.
I love you.

CONTENTS

A list of errata for this book can be found at tedxoconnell.com, and at BookRevision.com.

I also welcome you to visit the website to submit errors, updates, or suggestions for this book.

Thank you for helping to ensure the accuracy and high quality of *USMLE Step 2 Secrets*.
— **TED O'CONNELL**

A NOTE FROM THE AUTHOR

On the USMLE examinations, and throughout medical education, associations are often made between disease processes and certain racial and ethnic groups or even socioeconomic status. These associations become linked with individual groups and can perpetuate stereotypes, misinformation, and racism. In essence, physicians in training are taught to link key words, phrases, and ideas for the purposes of making associations on examinations and in clinical contexts.

Associations made with certain terms or disease processes, without qualifications or explanation, can cause those of us in health care to believe that being part of a particular group causes one to have a predilection for health problems and disease process. The reasons a disease process is more prevalent in certain racial, ethnic, and socioeconomic groups may be due in large part to long-standing social inequities, health disparities, structural racism, oppression, adverse childhood experiences (ACEs), politics, environment, and likely many other factors. It is vitally important to remember that an increased prevalence should not be assumed to be intrinsically linked to being part of any particular group.

Because USMLE Step 2 Secrets is designed to help prepare you for success on the USMLE Step 2 exam, some of these keywords and linkages remain in this book out of necessity because the linkages are so prevalent on standardized exams. Despite this, I encourage you to consider the broader social issues outlined earlier and work within the health care system to call out and try to eliminate inappropriate associations between disease processes and individual groups of people. We owe it to our patients and to society to do this and to be better going forward.

Ted O'Connell, MD

SIXTH EDITION

USMLE STEP 2

SECRETS

ELSEVIER

100 TOP SECRETS

These secrets are 100 of the top board alerts. They summarize the concepts, principles, and most salient details that you should review before you take the Step 2 examination. Understanding of these Top Secrets will serve you well in your final review.

1. **Smoking** is the number-one cause of preventable morbidity and mortality in the United States (e.g., atherosclerosis, cancer, chronic obstructive pulmonary disease).
2. **Alcohol** is the number-two cause of preventable morbidity and mortality in the United States. More than half of accidental and intentional (e.g., murder and suicide) deaths involve alcohol. Alcohol is the number-one cause of preventable mental retardation (fetal alcohol syndrome); it also causes cancer and cirrhosis and is potentially fatal in withdrawal.
3. In **alcoholic hepatitis**, the classic ratio of aspartate aminotransferase to alanine aminotransferase is greater than or equal to 2:1, although both may be elevated.
4. **Vitamins:** give folate to reproductive-age women prior to conception and throughout pregnancy to prevent neural tube defects. Watch for pernicious anemia, and treat with vitamin B_{12} to prevent permanent neurologic deficits. Isoniazid causes pyridoxine (vitamin B_6) deficiency. Watch for Wernicke encephalopathy in those with alcohol use disorder and treat with thiamine to prevent Korsakoff dementia. Consider offering vitamin D supplementation to geriatric adults who are at increased risk of falls or have a history of recurrent falls.
5. **Minerals:** iron-deficiency anemia is the most common cause of anemia. Think of menstrual loss in reproductive-age women and of cancer in men and menopausal women if no other cause is obvious.
6. **Vitamin A** is a known teratogen. Counsel and treat reproductive-age women appropriately (e.g., take care in treating acne with the vitamin A analog isotretinoin).
7. Complications of **atherosclerosis** (e.g., myocardial infarction, heart failure, stroke, gangrene) are involved in roughly one-half of deaths in the United States. The primary risk factors for atherosclerosis are age/sex, family history, cigarette smoking, hypertension, diabetes mellitus, high low-density lipoprotein (LDL) cholesterol, and low high-density lipoprotein (HDL) cholesterol.
8. **Diabetes** leads to macrovascular and microvascular disease. Macrovascular disease includes coronary artery disease, stroke, and peripheral vascular disease (a leading cause of limb amputation). Microvascular disease includes retinopathy (a leading cause of blindness), nephropathy (a leading cause of end-stage renal failure), and peripheral neuropathy (sensory and autonomic). Diabetes also leads to an increased incidence of infections.
9. Although hypertension is often clinically silent, it can lead to end-organ damage such as chronic kidney disease, stroke, myocardial infarction, and heart failure. **Severe hypertension** can lead to acute problems (known as a hypertensive emergency): headaches, dizziness, blurry vision, papilledema, cerebral edema, altered mental status, seizures, intracerebral hemorrhage (classically in the basal ganglia), acute kidney injury/azotemia, angina, pulmonary edema, aortic dissection, myocardial infarction, and/or heart failure.
10. **Lifestyle modifications** (e.g., diet, exercise, weight loss, cessation of alcohol/tobacco use) may be able to treat the following disorders without the use of medications: hypertension, hyperlipidemia, diabetes, gastroesophageal reflux disease, insomnia, obesity, and sleep apnea.
11. **Arterial blood gas analysis:** in general, pH tells you the primary event (acidosis vs alkalosis), whereas carbon dioxide and bicarbonate values give you the cause (same direction as pH) and suggest any compensation present (opposite of pH).
12. **Exogenous causes of hyponatremia** to keep in mind: oxytocin, surgery, narcotics, inappropriate intravenous (IV) fluid administration, diuretics, and antiepileptic medications.
13. **Electrocardiogram (ECG) findings in electrolyte disturbances:** tall, tented T waves in hyperkalemia; loss of T waves/T-wave flattening and U waves in hypokalemia; QT prolongation in hypocalcemia; QT shortening in hypercalcemia.
14. **Shock:** first give the patient oxygen, start an IV line, and set up monitoring (pulse oximetry, ECG, frequent vital signs). Then give a fluid bolus (30 cc/kg of normal saline or lactated Ringer solution) if no signs of congestive heart failure (e.g., bibasilar rales) are present while you try to determine the cause, if unknown. If the patient is not responsive to fluids, start cardiac pressors.
15. **Virchow triad** of deep venous thrombosis: endothelial damage (e.g., surgery, trauma), venous stasis (e.g., immobilization, surgery, severe heart failure), and hypercoagulable state (e.g., malignancy, birth control pills, pregnancy, lupus anticoagulant, inherited deficiencies).
16. **Therapy for congestive heart failure:** diuretics (e.g., furosemide), angiotensin-converting enzyme inhibitors, and beta-blockers (for stable patients) are the mainstays of pharmacologic treatment. Be sure to screen for and address underlying atherosclerosis risk factors (e.g., smoking, hyperlipidemia). Most patients should be on antiplatelet therapy.

17. **Cor pulmonale:** right-sided heart enlargement, hypertrophy, or failure due to primary lung disease (usually chronic obstructive pulmonary disease). The most common cause of right-heart failure, however, is left-heart failure (not cor pulmonale).

18. In patients with **atrial fibrillation,** assess for an underlying cause with thyroid-stimulating hormone, electrolytes, urine drug screen, and echocardiogram. The main management issues are ventricular rate control (if needed, slow the rate with medications) and atrial clot formation/embolic disease (anticoagulation).

19. **Ventricular fibrillation** and pulseless ventricular tachycardia are treated with immediate defibrillation followed by epinephrine, vasopressin, amiodarone, and lidocaine as cardiopulmonary resuscitation (CPR) is initiated. If ventricular tachycardia with a pulse is present, treat with amiodarone and synchronized cardioversion.

20. **Obstructive vs. restrictive lung disease:** the FEV_1/FVC ratio is the most important parameter on pulmonary function testing to distinguish the two (FEV_1 may be the same). In obstructive lung disease, the FEV_1/FVC ratio is less than normal (<0.7). In restrictive disease, the FEV_1/FVC ratio is often normal.

21. The **most common type of esophageal cancer** in the United States is adenocarcinoma occurring as a result of longstanding reflux disease and the development of Barrett esophagus. Smoking and alcohol abuse contribute to the development of squamous cell carcinoma, the second most common histologic type of esophageal cancer.

22. All **gastric ulcers** must be biopsied or followed to resolution to exclude malignancy.

23. Testing a nasogastric tube aspirate for blood is the best initial test **to distinguish an upper from a lower gastrointestinal (GI) bleed**, although bright red blood via mouth or anus is a fairly reliable sign of a nearby bleeding source.

24. **Irritable bowel syndrome** is one of the most common causes of GI complaints. Physical exam and diagnostic studies are by definition negative; this is a diagnosis of exclusion. The classic patient is a young adult female with a chronic history of alternating constipation and diarrhea.

25. **Crohn disease vs ulcerative colitis**

	CROHN DISEASE	**ULCERATIVE COLITIS**
Place of origin	Distal ileum, proximal colon	Rectum
Thickness of pathology	Transmural	Mucosa/submucosa only
Progression	Irregular (skip lesions)	Proximal, continuous from rectum; no skipped areas
Location	From mouth to anus	Involves only colon, rarely extends to ileum
Bowel habit changes	Obstruction, abdominal pain	Bloody diarrhea
Classic lesions	Fistulas/abscesses, cobblestoning, string sign on barium x-ray	Pseudopolyps, lead-pipe colon on barium x-ray, toxic megacolon
Colon cancer risk	Slightly increased	Markedly increased
Surgery	No (may make worse)	Yes (proctocolectomy with ileoanal anastomosis)

26. All forms of **viral hepatitis** can present similarly in the acute stage; serology testing and history are needed to distinguish them. Hepatitis B, C, and D are transmitted parenterally and can lead to chronic infection, cirrhosis, and hepatocellular carcinoma.

27. **Hereditary hemochromatosis** is currently the most common known genetic disease in whites. The initial symptoms (fatigue, impotence) are nonspecific, but patients often have hepatomegaly, skin pigmentation changes ("bronze diabetes"), and diabetes. Initial tests include transferrin saturation (serum iron/total iron binding capacity) and ferritin level. Treat with phlebotomy after confirming the diagnosis with genetic testing and liver biopsy.

28. **Sequelae of liver failure:** coagulopathy (that cannot be fixed with vitamin K), thrombocytopenia, jaundice/hyperbilirubinemia, hypoalbuminemia, ascites, portal hypertension, hyperammonemia/encephalopathy, hypoglycemia, disseminated intravascular coagulation, and renal failure.

29. **Pancreatitis** is usually due to alcohol or gallstones. Patients present with abdominal pain, nausea/vomiting, and elevated amylase and lipase. Treat supportively and provide pain control. Complications include pseudocyst formation, infection/abscess, and adult respiratory distress syndrome.

30. **Jaundice/hyperbilirubinemia in neonates** is usually physiologic (only monitoring, follow-up lab tests, and possibly phototherapy are needed), but jaundice present at birth is always pathologic.

31. **Primary vs secondary endocrine disturbances.** In primary disorders (e.g., Graves disease, Hashimoto thyroiditis, or Addison disease) the gland malfunctions, but the pituitary or another gland and the central nervous system respond appropriately (e.g., thyroid-stimulating hormone, thyrotropin-releasing hormone, or adrenocorticotropic hormone elevates or depresses as expected in the setting of a malfunctioning gland). In secondary disorders (e.g., adrenocorticotropic hormone-secreting lung carcinoma, heart failure–induced hyperreninemia, renal failure–induced hyperparathyroidism), the gland itself is doing what it is told to do by other controlling forces (e.g., pituitary gland, hypothalamus, tumor, disease); they are the problem, not the gland itself.

32. **Corticosteroid side effects (aka Cushing syndrome):** weight gain, easy bruising, acne, hirsutism, emotional lability, depression, psychosis, menstrual changes, sexual dysfunction, insomnia, memory loss, buffalo hump, truncal and central obesity with wasting of extremities, round plethoric facies, purplish skin striae, weakness (especially of the proximal muscles), hypertension, peripheral edema, poor wound healing, glucose intolerance or diabetes, osteoporosis, and hypokalemic metabolic alkalosis (due to mineralocorticoid effects of certain corticosteroids). Growth can also be stunted in children.
33. **Osteoarthritis** is by far the most common cause of arthritis (≥75% of cases) and usually does not have hot, swollen joints or significant findings if arthrocentesis is performed.
34. Cancer incidence and mortality in the United States:

Overall Highest Incidence		Overall Highest Mortality Rate	
MALE	**FEMALE**	**MALE**	**FEMALE**
1. Prostate	1. Breast	1. Lung	1. Lung
2. Lung	2. Lung	2. Prostate	2. Breast
3. Colon	3. Colon	3. Colon	3. Colon

35. **Sequelae of lung cancer:** hemoptysis, Horner syndrome, superior vena cava syndrome, phrenic nerve involvement/diaphragmatic paralysis, hoarseness from recurrent laryngeal nerve involvement, and paraneoplastic syndromes (Cushing syndrome, syndrome of inappropriate antidiuretic hormone secretion, hypercalcemia, Eaton-Lambert syndrome).
36. **Bitemporal hemianopsia** (loss of peripheral vision in both eyes) is due to a space-occupying lesion pushing on the optic chiasm (classically a pituitary tumor) until proven otherwise. Order a computed tomography (CT) or magnetic resonance imaging (MRI) of the brain.
37. **Potential risks and side effects of estrogen therapy** (e.g., contraception, postmenopausal hormone replacement): endometrial cancer (with unopposed estrogen, therefore must be given with progesterone in patients with a uterus), hepatic adenomas, glucose intolerance/diabetes, deep venous thrombosis, pulmonary embolism, stroke, cholelithiasis, hypertension, endometrial bleeding, depression, weight gain, nausea/vomiting, headache, drug-drug interactions, teratogenesis, and aggravation of preexisting uterine leiomyomas (fibroids), breast fibroadenomas, migraines, and epilepsy. The risks of coronary artery disease and breast cancer may be increased with combined estrogen and progesterone therapy.
38. **ABCDE characteristics of a mole** that should make you suspicious of malignant transformation: **a**symmetry, **b**orders (irregular), **c**olor (change in color or multiple colors), **d**iameter (the bigger the lesion, the more likely that it is malignant), and **e**volution over time. Do an excisional biopsy of such moles and/or if a mole starts to itch or bleed.
39. **Bronchiolitis vs. croup vs. epiglottitis:**

	BRONCHIOLITIS	CROUP (ACUTE LARYNGOTRACHEITIS)	EPIGLOTTITIS
Child's age	0–18 mo	1–2 yr	2–5 yr
Common	Yes	Yes	No
Common cause(s)	Respiratory syncytial virus (≥75%), parainfluenza, influenza	Parainfluenza virus (50%–75% of cases), influenza	*Haemophilus influenzae* type b, *Staphylococcus* spp., *Streptococcus* spp.
Symptoms/signs	Initial viral upper respiratory infections symptoms followed by tachypnea and expiratory wheezing	Initial viral URI symptoms followed by "barking" cough, hoarseness, and inspiratory stridor	Rapid progression to high fever, toxicity, drooling, and respiratory distress
X-ray findings	Hyperinflation	Subglottic tracheal narrowing on frontal x-ray (steeple sign)	Swollen epiglottis on lateral neck x-ray (thumb sign)
Treatment	Generally supportive care with humidified oxygen and suctioning	Dexamethasone, nebulized racemic epinephrine, humidified oxygen	Prepare to establish an airway, antibiotics (e.g., third-generation cephalosporin and an antistaphylococcal agent active against MRSA such as vancomycin or clindamycin).

40. **Sequelae of group A streptococcal infection:** rheumatic fever, scarlet fever, and postinfectious glomerulonephritis. Only the first two can be prevented by treatment with antibiotics.

41. **Multiple sclerosis** should be suspected in any young adult with recurrent, varied neurologic symptoms/signs when no other causes are evident. Best diagnostic tests: MRI (most sensitive), lumbar puncture (elevated immunoglobulin G oligoclonal bands and myelin basic protein levels, mild elevation in lymphocytes and protein), and evoked potentials (slowed conduction through areas with damaged myelin).

42. For the **unconscious or delirious (encephalopathic) patient** in the emergency department with no history or signs of trauma: consider empiric treatment for hypoglycemia (glucose), opioid overdose (naloxone), and thiamine deficiency (thiamine should be given before glucose in suspected alcohol use disorder). Other commonly tested causes are alcohol, illicit or prescription drugs, diabetic ketoacidosis, stroke, epilepsy or postictal state, subarachnoid hemorrhage (e.g., aneurysm rupture), sepsis, electrolyte imbalance/metabolic causes, uremia, hepatic encephalopathy, and hypoxia.

43. **Delirium vs. dementia:**

	DELIRIUM	DEMENTIA
Onset	Acute and dramatic	Chronic and insidious
Common causes	Illness, toxin, withdrawal	Alzheimer disease, multiinfarct dementia, HIV/AIDS
Reversible	Usually	Usually not
Attention	Poor	Usually unaffected
Orientation	Impaired and fluctuating	Often normal but may be impaired
Arousal level	Fluctuates	Normal

44. **Always consider the possibility of pregnancy** (and order a pregnancy test to rule it out, unless pregnancy is an impossibility) in reproductive-age women before advising potentially teratogenic therapies or tests (e.g., antiepileptic drugs, x-ray, CT scan). Pregnancy is in the differential diagnosis of both primary and secondary amenorrhea.

45. **Anaphylaxis** is commonly caused by beestings, food allergy (especially peanuts and shellfish), medications (especially penicillins and sulfa drugs), or rubber glove allergy. Patients become agitated and flushed and shortly after exposure develop itching (urticaria), facial swelling (angioedema), and difficulty in breathing. Symptoms develop rapidly and dramatically in true anaphylaxis. Treat immediately by securing the airway (laryngeal edema may prevent intubation, in which case do a cricothyroidotomy, if needed), and give subcutaneous or IV epinephrine. Antihistamines and corticosteroids are not useful for immediate, severe reactions that involve the airway.

46. **Cancer screening in asymptomatic adults:**

CANCER	PROCEDURE	AGE TO BEGIN SCREENING	AGE TO STOP SCREENING	FREQUENCY
Breast	Mammography **Note:** *Clinical breast exam is no longer recommended.*	45 yr **Note:** *Interested patients may begin annual screening at age 40 yr.*	Life expectancy <10 yr. No age specified.	Annually (age 45–54 yr) Every 2 yr (age ≥55 yr)
Cervical	Pap smear only (age 21–29 yr) **or** Pap and HPV cotest (age 30–65 yr) **Note:** *HPV cotest only performed in age 21–29 yr if Pap is abnormal* **Note:** *A woman with prior total hysterectomy should not be screened unless she has other risk factors.*	21 yr regardless of sexual activity	65 yr **Note:** *Women with cervical precancer should continue screening for at least 20 more years, even if they pass age 65 yr.*	Every 3 yr (if screened by Pap only) Every 5 yr (if Pap and HPV cotest is used)

CANCER	PROCEDURE	AGE TO BEGIN SCREENING	AGE TO STOP SCREENING	FREQUENCY
Colorectal	Colonoscopy **or** Flexible sigmoidoscopy (FS) **or** CT colonography **or** Multitarget stool DNA test (mt-sDNA) **or** Guaiac-based fecal occult blood test (gFOBT **or** Fecal immunochemical test (FIT)	45 yr (qualified recommendation) **or** 50 yr (strong recommendation)	75 yr **or** Life expectancy <10 yr	Every 10 yr (colonoscopy) **or** Every 5 yr (FS or CT colonography) **or** Every 3 yr (mt-sDNA) **or** Annually (gFOBT or FIT)
Endometrial	Endometrial biopsy			Routine screening is not recommended unless the patient is symptomatic (e.g., unexplained vaginal bleeding)
Lung	Low-dose CT scan	55 yr **and** 30-pack-year smoking history **and** Currently smokes or quit within the last 15 yr	80 yr	Annually
Prostate	Prostate-specific antigen test (with or without DRE) *Note: Have a risk/benefit discussion with patients before screening. Shared decision making. Consider DRE for PSA between 2.5 and 4 ng/mL.*	50 yr *Note: Start screening at age 45 yr for all black men or men with a first-degree relative diagnosed before age 65 yr.* Start at age 40 yr for men at even higher risk (those with more than one first-degree relative with prostate cancer at an early age).	75 yr **or** Life expectancy <10 yr	PSA ≥2.5 ng/mL screened annually PSA <2.5 ng/mL screened every 2 yr

CT, Computed tomography; *DRE,* digital rectal exam; *HPV,* human papillomavirus; *Pap,* Papanicolaou.

47. Biostatistics calculations using a 2 × 2 table:

DISEASE	TEST NAME	FORMULA
Test or Exposure	Sensitivity	A/(A + C)
	Specificity	D/(B + D)
	PPV	A/(A + B)
	NPV	D/(C + D)
	Odds ratio	(A × D)/(B × C) [A/(A + B)] / [C/(C + D)]
	Relative risk	[A/(A + B)] − [C/(C + D)]
	Attributable risk	

48. The ***P*-value** reflects the likelihood of making a type I error or claiming an effect or difference where none existed (i.e., results were obtained by chance). When we reject the null hypothesis (i.e., the hypothesis of no difference) in a trial testing a new treatment, we are saying that the new treatment works. We use the *P*-value to express our confidence in the data.

49. **Side effects of antipsychotics:** acute dystonia (treat with antihistamines or anticholinergics), akathisia (beta-blocker may help), tardive dyskinesia (switching to newer agent may have benefit), parkinsonism (treat with antihistamines or anticholinergics), neuroleptic malignant syndrome, hyperprolactinemia (may cause breast discharge, menstrual dysfunction, and/or sexual dysfunction), and autonomic nervous system–related effects (e.g., anticholinergic, antihistamine, and alpha$_1$-receptor blockade).

50. Asking about **depression and suicidal thoughts**/intent is important in the right setting and does not cause people to commit suicide. Hospitalize psychiatric patients against their will if they are a danger to self or others or gravely disabled (unable to care for self).

51. **Drugs of abuse:** potentially fatal in withdrawal include alcohol, barbiturates, and benzodiazepines. Alcohol, cocaine, opiates, barbiturates, benzodiazepines, phencyclidine (PCP), and inhalants are potentially fatal in overdose.

52. **Pelvic inflammatory disease** is the most common preventable cause of infertility in the United States and the most likely cause of infertility in younger, normally menstruating women.

53. **Polycystic ovarian syndrome** is classically associated with women who are "heavy, hirsute, and [h]amenorrheic." It is the most common cause of dysfunctional uterine bleeding. Remember the increased risk of endometrial cancer due to unopposed estrogen.

54. **Fetal/neonatal macrosomia** is due to maternal diabetes until proven otherwise. Treat gestational/maternal diabetes by aiming for tight glucose control through diet, oral agents, or insulin.

55. **Low maternal serum alpha-fetoprotein causes:** Down syndrome, inaccurate dates (most common), and fetal demise. **High maternal serum alpha-fetoprotein** associated with neural tube defects, ventral wall defects (e.g., omphalocele, gastroschisis), inaccurate dates (most common), and multiple gestation. Measurement is generally obtained between 16 and 20 weeks of gestation.

56. Hypertension plus proteinuria in pregnancy equals **preeclampsia** until proven otherwise.

57. Positive pregnancy test (i.e., not a clinically apparent pregnancy) plus vaginal bleeding and abdominal pain equals **ectopic pregnancy** until proven otherwise. Order a pelvic ultrasound if the patient is stable.

58. **Decelerations during maternofetal monitoring:** *early* decelerations are normal and due to head compression. *Variable* decelerations are common and usually due to cord compression (turn the mother on her side, give oxygen and fluids, stop oxytocin, and consider amnioinfusion). *Late* decelerations are due to uteroplacental insufficiency and are the most worrisome pattern (turn the mother on her side, give oxygen and IV fluids, stop oxytocin, and measure fetal oxygen saturation or scalp pH). Prepare for prompt delivery.

59. Always perform an ultrasound before a pelvic exam in the setting of **third-trimester bleeding** (in case placenta previa is present).

60. **Uterine atony** is the most common cause of postpartum bleeding and is typically due to uterine overdistention (e.g., twins, polyhydramnios), prolonged labor, fibroids, and/or oxytocin usage. The risk is increased in multiparous women.

61. **Acute abdomen pathology localization by physical exam:**

AREA	ORGAN (CONDITIONS)
Right upper quadrant	Gallbladder/biliary (cholecystitis, cholangitis) or liver (abscess)
Left upper quadrant	Spleen (rupture with blunt trauma)
Right lower quadrant	Appendix (appendicitis), pelvic inflammatory disease
Left lower quadrant	Sigmoid colon (diverticulitis), pelvic inflammatory disease
Epigastric area	Stomach (peptic ulcer) or pancreas (pancreatitis)

62. The **"6 Ws" of postoperative fever:** water, wind, walk, wound, "wawa," and weird drugs. *Water* stands for urinary tract infection, *wind* for atelectasis or pneumonia, *walk* for deep venous thrombosis, *wound* for surgical wound infection, *"wawa"* for breast (usually relevant only in the postpartum state), and *weird drugs* for drug fever. In patients with daily fever spikes that do not respond to antibiotics, think about a postsurgical abscess. Order a CT scan to locate, then drain the abscess if one is present.

63. **ABCDEs of trauma** (follow in order if you are asked to choose): **a**irway, **b**reathing, **c**irculation, **d**isability, and **e**xposure.

64. **Six rapidly fatal thoracic injuries** that must be recognized and treated immediately:
    1. Airway obstruction (establish airway)
    2. Open pneumothorax (intubate, place chest tube at different site, and close defect on three sides)
    3. Tension pneumothorax (perform needle thoracentesis followed by chest tube)
    4. Cardiac tamponade (perform pericardiocentesis)
    5. Massive hemothorax (place chest tube to drain; thoracotomy if bleeding does not stop)
    6. Flail chest (consider intubation and positive pressure ventilation if oxygenation inadequate)

65. **Neonatal conjunctivitis** may be caused by chemical reaction (in the first 12–24 hours of giving drops for prophylaxis), gonorrhea (2–5 days after birth; usually prevented by prophylactic drops), and chlamydial infection (5–14 days after birth; often not prevented by prophylactic drops).

66. **Glaucoma** is usually (90%) due to the open-angle form, which is painless (no "attacks") and asymptomatic until irreversible vision loss (that starts in the periphery) occurs. Thus screening is important. Open-angle glaucoma is the most common cause of blindness in blacks.
67. **Uveitis** is often a marker for systemic conditions: juvenile rheumatoid arthritis, sarcoidosis, inflammatory bowel disease, ankylosing spondylitis, reactive arthritis, multiple sclerosis, psoriasis, or lupus. Photophobia, blurry vision, and eye pain are common complaints.
68. **Bilateral (though often asymmetric) painless gradual loss of vision** in older adults is usually due to cataracts, macular degeneration, or glaucoma, which can be distinguished on physical exam. Presbyopia is a normal part of aging and affects only near vision (i.e., accommodation).
69. **Compartment syndrome**, usually in the lower extremity after trauma or surgery, causes the "6 Ps":
    1. Pain (present on passive movement and often out of proportion to the injury)
    2. Paresthesias (numbness, tingling, decreased sensation)
    3. Pallor (or cyanosis)
    4. Pressure (firm feeling muscle compartment, elevated pressure reading)
    5. Paralysis (late, ominous sign)
    6. Pulselessness (very late, ominous sign); treat with fasciotomy to relieve compartment pressure and prevent permanent neurologic damage.
70. Peripheral nerve evaluation:

NERVE	NERVE ROOTS	MOTOR FUNCTION	SENSORY FUNCTION	CLINICAL SCENARIO
Radial	C5-T1	Wrist, thumb, and finger extension (watch for wrist drop)	Back of forearm, back of hand (first 3 digits)	Supracondylar humeral fracture with anterolateral displacement
Ulnar	C8-T1	Finger abduction (watch for "claw hand")	Front and back of last 2 digits	Elbow dislocation or fracture; supracondylar humeral fracture with posterior displacement
Median	C5-T1	Pronation of forearm, wrist flexion, thumb opposition	Palmar surface of hand (first 3.5 digits)	Carpal tunnel syndrome, humeral fracture, supracondylar humeral fracture with anteriomedial displacement (also consider brachial artery injury)
Axillary	C5-C6	Abduction and lateral rotation of arm	Lateral shoulder	Upper anterior humeral dislocation or fracture
Musculocutaneous	C5-C7	Flexion of the upper arm at the shoulder and elbow, supination of the forearm	Anterolateral forearm	Uncommon injury; penetrating trauma to the axilla
Peroneal	L4-S2	Dorsiflexion and eversion of foot (watch for foot drop)	Dorsal foot and lateral leg	Knee dislocation, fibula fracture

71. Pediatric hip disorders:

NAME	AGE	EPIDEMIOLOGY	SYMPTOMS/ SIGNS	TREATMENT
CHD	At birth	Female, firstborns, breech delivery	Barlow and Ortolani signs	Harness
LCPD	4–10 yr	Short male with delayed bone age	Knee, thigh, groin pain, limp	Orthoses
SCFE	9–13 yr	Overweight male adolescent	Knee, thigh, groin pain, limp	Surgical pinning

CHD, Congenital hip dysplasia; LCPD, Legg-Calvé-Perthes disease; SCFE, slipped capital femoral epiphysis.
Note: All of these conditions may present in an adult as arthritis of the hip.

72. **Avoid lumbar puncture** in a patient with acute head trauma or signs of increased intracranial pressure, coagulopathy, suspicion for intracranial hemorrhage, or suspicion for spinal epidural abscess. Do a lumbar tap only if you have a negative CT scan or MRI of the head in these settings. Otherwise, you may cause uncal herniation and death.
73. In children, 75% of **neck masses** are benign (e.g., lymphadenitis, thyroglossal duct cyst), but 75% of neck masses in adults are malignant (e.g., squamous cell carcinoma and/or metastases, lymphoma).
74. Manage symptomatic **carotid artery stenosis** of 70% to 99% with carotid endarterectomy; less than 50% with medical management (e.g., antihypertensive agents, statins, and antiplatelet therapy) and treatment of atherosclerosis risk factors. For stenosis between 50% and 69%, the data on management are less clear, and patient-specific factors affect the decision.
75. Pulsatile abdominal mass plus hypotension equals ruptured **abdominal aortic aneurysm** until proven otherwise. Perform an immediate laparotomy (90% mortality rate).
76. Conditions best viewed as **anginal equivalents:** transient ischemic attacks, claudication, and chronic mesenteric ischemia. Arterial workup and imaging are indicated.
77. **Cryptorchidism** is the main identifiable risk factor for testicular cancer and can also cause infertility. Treat with surgical retrieval and orchiopexy or orchiectomy. Treatment does not decrease the risk of cancer.
78. **Benign prostatic hyperplasia** can present as acute renal failure. Patients have a distended bladder and bilateral hydronephrosis on ultrasound (neither is present with "medical" renal disease). Drain the bladder first (catheterize), then treat with medications or perform transurethral resection of the prostate (TURP) for more advanced cases.
79. **Erectile dysfunction** may be physical (e.g., vascular, nervous system, drugs) or, less commonly, psychogenic (patients have normal nocturnal erections and a history of dysfunction only in certain settings).
80. The **overall pattern of growth** in a child is more important than any one measurement. Consider close follow-up and remeasurement of growth parameters if you do not have enough data. A stable pattern is less worrisome and less likely to be correctable than a sudden change in previously stable growth. For example, the most common cause of delayed puberty is constitutional delay, a normal variant.
81. **Findings suspicious for child abuse**, assuming that other explanations are not provided: failure to thrive, multiple injuries in different stages of healing, retinal hemorrhages plus subdural hematomas ("shaken baby" syndrome), sexually transmitted diseases, a caretaker story that does not fit the child's injury or complaint, mechanism does not fit the child's age (e.g., rolling off a table at 2 weeks old), childhood behavioral or emotional problems, and multiple personality disorder as an adult.
82. The **Apgar score** (commonly performed at 1 and 5 minutes after birth; the maximum score is 10):

CATEGORY	*Number of Points Given*		
	0	**1**	**2**
Appearance (color)	Completely cyanotic	*Acrocyanosis*: Body pink, extremities blue	Completely pink
Pulse (heart rate)	Absent	<100 beats/min	>100 beats/min
Grimace (reflex irritability)[a]	None	Excessive stimulation required	Grimace and strong cry, cough, and sneeze
Activity (muscle tone)	Flaccid limbs	Limbs are flexed but do not resist active extension	Active motion or able to partially resist active extension
Respiratory effort	Apneic	Irregular respirations or a slow, weak cry	Good, strong cry

[a]Reflex irritability usually is measured by the infant's response to stimulation of the sole of the foot or a catheter put into the nose.

83. **Diuretics** are a common cause of metabolic derangement. Thiazide diuretics cause calcium retention, hyperglycemia, hyperuricemia, hyperlipidemia, hyponatremia, hypokalemic metabolic alkalosis, and hypovolemia; because they are sulfa drugs, watch out for sulfa allergy. Loop diuretics cause hypokalemic metabolic alkalosis, hypovolemia (more potent than thiazides), ototoxicity, and calcium excretion; with the exception of ethacrynic acid, they are also sulfa drugs. Carbonic anhydrase inhibitors cause metabolic acidosis, and potassium-sparing diuretics (e.g., spironolactone) may cause hyperkalemia.

84. **Overdoses and antidotes:**

POISONING OR OVERDOSE	ANTIDOTE
Acetaminophen	N-acetylcysteine
Benzodiazepines	Flumazenil (can precipitate seizures or delirium tremens if the patient has chronic benzodiazepine dependence)
Beta-blockers	Glucagon
Carbon monoxide	Oxygen (hyperbaric if severe)
Cholinesterase inhibitors	Atropine (always first), pralidoxime
Copper or gold	D-penicillamine or trientine (zinc is an alternative)
Dabigatran	Idarucizumab
Digoxin	Replete potassium and other electrolytes; digoxin-specific antibodies
Direct factor Xa inhibitors (apixaban, rivaroxaban)	Andexanet
Heparin	Protamine sulfate
Iron	Deferoxamine
Lead	Dimercaptosuccinic acid (DMSA, succimer), dimercaprol, calcium sodium edetate (EDTA)
Methanol or ethylene glycol	Fomepizole, ethanol
Muscarinic receptor blockers	Physostigmine
Opioids	Naloxone
Quinidine or tricyclic antidepressants	Sodium bicarbonate (cardioprotective)
Salicylic acid (aspirin)	Urine alkalinization, dialysis
Warfarin	Vitamin K, fresh frozen plasma, prothrombin complex concentrate (if life-threatening bleeding)

85. **Aspirin/nonsteroidal antiinflammatory drug (NSAID) side effects:** GI bleeding, gastric ulcers, renal damage (e.g., interstitial nephritis, papillary necrosis), allergic reactions, platelet dysfunction (life of platelet for aspirin, reversible dysfunction with NSAIDs), and Reye syndrome (encephalopathy and/or liver failure in a child taking aspirin in the setting of a viral infection). Aspirin overdose can be fatal and classically leads to both metabolic acidosis and respiratory alkalosis.

86. **Osmotic demyelination syndrome** (ODS, formerly called central pontine myelinolysis), which involves brainstem damage and possibly death, may result from correcting hyponatremia too rapidly.

87. Due to cellular shifts, **alkalosis and acidosis** can cause symptoms of potassium and/or calcium derangement (e.g., alkalosis can lead to symptoms of hypokalemia or hypocalcemia). In this setting, pH correction is needed (rather than direct treatment of the calcium or potassium levels). Magnesium depletion can also make hypocalcemia and hypokalemia unresponsive to replacement therapy (until magnesium is corrected).

88. Adult patients of sound mind are allowed to **refuse any form of treatment.** Watch for depression as a cause of "incompetence." Treat depression before wishes for death are respected.

89. **If a patient is incompetent** (including younger minors who lack adequate decision-making capacity) and an emergency treatment is needed, seek a family member or court-appointed guardian to make health care decisions. If no one is available, treat as you see fit in an emergency, or contact the courts in a nonemergency setting.

90. **Respect patient wishes and living wills** (assuming that they are appropriate) even in the face of dissenting family members, but take time to listen to family members' concerns.

91. **Always be a patient advocate** and treat patients with respect and dignity, even if they refuse your proposed treatment or are noncompliant. If patients' actions puzzle you, do not be afraid to question them.

92. Break doctor-patient confidentiality only in the following situations:
    - The patient asks you to do so.

- Child abuse is suspected.
- The courts mandate you to do so.
- You must fulfill the duty to warn or protect (if a patient says that he is going to kill someone or himself, you have to tell the someone, the authorities, or both).
- The patient has a reportable disease.
- The patient is a danger to others (e.g., if a patient is blind or has seizures, let the proper authorities know so that they can revoke the patient's license to drive; if the patient is an airplane pilot and is a paranoid, hallucinating schizophrenic, then authorities need to know).

93. **Causes of "false" lab disturbances:** hemolysis (hyperkalemia), pregnancy (elevated sedimentation rate and alkaline phosphatase), hypoalbuminemia (hypocalcemia), and hyperglycemia (hyponatremia).

94. **ECG findings of myocardial infarction:** flipped or flattened T waves, ST segment elevation (depression means ischemia; elevation means injury), and/or Q waves in a segmental distribution (e.g., leads II, III, and AVF for an inferior infarct). ST depression may also be seen in "reciprocal"/opposite leads.

95. Drugs that may be useful in the setting of **acute coronary syndrome:** aspirin, morphine, nitroglycerin, beta-blocker, angiotensin-converting enzyme inhibitor, clopidogrel, HMG-CoA reductase inhibitor, glycoprotein IIb/IIIa receptor inhibitors, heparin (unfractionated or low-molecular-weight heparin), and tissue-plasminogen activator (t-PA; strict criteria for use).

96. **Cholesterol management guidelines:** the following information is from the 2019 American College of Cardiology/American Heart Association (ACC/AHA) Guidelines on the Treatment of Blood Cholesterol to Reduce Atherosclerotic Cardiovascular Risk in Adults. This new guideline differs from the previous recommendations in that it moves away from specific low-density lipoprotein (LDL) targets. Instead, overall LDL reductions are recommended.

GROUP	LDL REDUCTION GOAL	RECOMMENDED STATIN THERAPY
Anyone with an LDL level ≥190 mg/dL	Reduce by >50%	High-intensity statin
Patients with diabetes aged 40–75 yr and LDL ≥70 mg/dL	Reduce by 30%–50%	Moderate-intensity statin
Anyone with 7.5%–20% chance of developing atherosclerotic CVD in the next 10 yr, using a specific calculator*	Reduce by 30%–50%	Moderate-intensity statin
Anyone with ≥20% ASCVD	Reduce LDL by ≥50%	High-intensity statin

ASCVD, atherosclerotic cardiovascular disease; *CVD*, Cardiovascular disease; *LDL,* low-density lipoprotein

* The Pooled Cohort Equations. Available at http://my.americanheart.org/professional/StatementsGuidelines/Preventin-Guidelines_UCM_457698_SubHomePage.jsp.

97. Type 1 vs. type 2 diabetes:

	TYPE 1 (10% OF CASES)	TYPE 2 (90% OF CASES)
Age at onset	Most commonly <30 yr	Most commonly >30 yr
Associated body habitus	Thin	Obese
Development of ketoacidosis	Yes	Less likely
Development of hyperosmolar state	No	Yes
Level of endogenous insulin	Low to none	Normal to high (insulin resistance)
Twin concordance	<50%	>50%
HLA association	Yes	No
Response to oral hypoglycemics	No	Yes
Antibodies to insulin	Yes (at diagnosis)	No
Risk for diabetic complications	Yes	Yes
Islet cell pathology	Insulitis (loss of most B cells)	Normal number, but with amyloid deposits

Remember, however, that these findings may overlap.
HLA, Human leukocyte antigen.

98. "Hypertension" was redefined in the updated ACC/AHA guidelines published in 2017. There are now four blood pressure categories for adults, based on systolic blood pressure (SBP) and diastolic blood pressure (DBP):
    - **Normal**: SBP <120 mm Hg **and** DBP <80 mm Hg
    - **Elevated**: SBP between 120 and 129 mm Hg **and** DBP <80 mm Hg
    - **Hypertension stage 1**: SBP between 130 and 139 mm Hg **or** DBP between 80 and 89 mm Hg
    - **Hypertension stage 2**: SBP ≥140 mm Hg **or** DBP ≥90 mm Hg

    Note that patients with SBP and DBP in two separate categories are considered to be in the higher of the two categories.

99. Word associations (not 100%, but they can help when you have to guess):

BUZZ PHRASE OR SCENARIO	CONDITION
Friction rub	Pericarditis
Kussmaul breathing (deep, rapid breathing)	Diabetic ketoacidosis
Kayser-Fleischer ring in the eye	Wilson disease
Bitot spots	Vitamin A deficiency
Dendritic corneal ulcers on fluorescein stain of the eye	Herpes keratitis
Cherry-red spot on the macula without hepatosplenomegaly	Tay-Sachs disease
Cherry-red spot on the macula with hepatosplenomegaly	Niemann-Pick disease
Bronze skin plus diabetes	Hemochromatosis
Malar rash on the face	Systemic lupus erythematosus
Heliotrope rash (purplish rash on the eyelids)	Dermatomyositis
Clue cells	*Gardnerella vaginalis* infection
Meconium ileus	Cystic fibrosis
Rectal prolapse	Cystic fibrosis
Salty-tasting infant	Cystic fibrosis
Café au lait spots with normal IQ	Neurofibromatosis
Café au lait spots with mental retardation	McCune-Albright syndrome or tuberous sclerosis
Worst headache of the patient's life	Subarachnoid hemorrhage
Abdominal striae	Cushing syndrome or pregnancy
Honey ingestion	Infant botulism
Left lower quadrant tenderness/rebound	Diverticulitis
Children who torture animals	Conduct disorder
Currant jelly stools in children	Intussusception
Ambiguous genitalia and hypotension	21-hydroxylase deficiency in girls
Catlike cry in an infant	Cri-du-chat syndrome
Infant weighing >10 lb	Maternal diabetes
Anaphylaxis from immunoglobulin therapy	IgA deficiency
Postpartum fever unresponsive to broad-spectrum antibiotics	Septic pelvic thrombophlebitis
Increased hemoglobin A2 and anemia	Thalassemia
Heavy young woman with papilledema and negative CT/MRI of head	Pseudotumor cerebri
Low-grade fever in the first 24 hr after surgery	Atelectasis
Vietnam veteran	Posttraumatic stress disorder
Bilateral hilar adenopathy in a black patient	Sarcoidosis

BUZZ PHRASE OR SCENARIO	CONDITION
Sudden death in a young athlete	Hypertrophic obstructive cardiomyopathy
Fractures or bruises in different stages of healing in a child	Child abuse
Absent breath sounds in a trauma patient	Pneumothorax
Shopping sprees	Mania
Constant clearing of throat in a child or teenager	Tourette syndrome
Intermittent bursts of swearing	Tourette syndrome
Koilocytosis	Human papillomavirus or cytomegalovirus
Rash develops after administration of ampicillin or amoxicillin for sore throat	Epstein-Barr virus infection
Daytime sleepiness and occasional falling down (cataplexy)	Narcolepsy
Facial port wine stain and seizures	Sturge-Weber syndrome

100. Signs and syndromes:

SIGN/SYNDROME	EXPLANATION
Babinski sign	Stroking the bottom of the foot yields extension of the big toe and fanning of other toes (upper motor neuron lesion)
Beck triad	Jugular venous distention, muffled heart sounds, and hypotension (cardiac tamponade)
Brudzinski sign	Pain on neck flexion with meningeal irritation (meningitis)
Charcot triad	Fever/chills, jaundice, and right upper quadrant pain (cholangitis)
Courvoisier sign	Painless, palpable gallbladder plus jaundice (pancreatic cancer)
Chvostek sign	Tapping on the facial nerve elicits tetany (hypocalcemia)
Cullen sign	Bluish discoloration of periumbilical area (pancreatitis with retroperitoneal hemorrhage)
Cushing reflex	Hypertension, bradycardia, and irregular respirations (high intracranial pressure)
Grey Turner sign	Bluish discoloration of flank (pancreatitis with retroperitoneal hemorrhage)
Homan sign	Calf pain on forced dorsiflexion of the foot (deep venous thrombosis)
Kehr sign	Pain in the left shoulder (ruptured spleen)
Leriche syndrome	Claudication and atrophy of the buttocks with impotence (aortoiliac occlusive disease)
McBurney sign	Tenderness at McBurney point (appendicitis)
Murphy sign	Arrest of inspiration during palpation under the rib cage on the right (cholecystitis)
Ortolani sign/test	Abducting an infant's flexed hips causes a palpable/audible click (congenital hip dysplasia)
Prehn sign	Elevation of a painful testicle relieves pain (epididymitis vs testicular torsion)
Rovsing sign	Pushing on left lower quadrant then releasing your hand produces pain at McBurney point (appendicitis)
Tinel sign	Tapping on the volar surface of the wrist elicits paresthesias (carpal tunnel syndrome)
Trousseau sign	Pumping up a blood pressure cuff causes carpopedal spasm (tetany from hypocalcemia)
Virchow triad	Stasis, endothelial damage, and hypercoagulability (risk factors for deep venous thrombosis)

CHAPTER 1

ACID-BASE AND ELECTROLYTES

1. How do you analyze arterial blood gas values?
   Remember three points:
   1. The pH tells you whether the primary process is an acidemia or an alkalemia. The body will compensate as much as it can (secondary process) but will never perfectly compensate or overcompensate.
   2. CO_2. If the carbon dioxide (CO_2) is high, the patient either has respiratory acidosis (pH <7.4) or is compensating for a metabolic alkalosis (pH >7.4). If CO_2 is low, the patient either has a respiratory alkalosis (pH >7.4) or is compensating for a metabolic acidosis (pH <7.4).
   3. HCO_3. If the bicarbonate (HCO_3) is high, the patient either has a metabolic alkalosis (pH >7.4) or is compensating for a respiratory acidosis (pH <7.4). If bicarbonate is low, the patient either has a metabolic acidosis (pH <7.4) or is compensating for a respiratory alkalosis (pH >7.4).

2. True or false: The body does not compensate beyond a normal pH
   True. For example, a patient with metabolic acidosis will eliminate CO_2 (the body will increase the respiratory rate to help "blow off" CO_2) to help restore a normal pH, and a compensatory respiratory alkalosis will develop. However, the compensatory alkalosis will not correct the pH to greater than 7.4. Overcorrection does not occur.

3. List the common causes of acidosis.
   Respiratory acidosis: hypoventilation, chronic obstructive pulmonary disease, asthma, drugs (e.g., opioids, benzodiazepines, barbiturates, alcohol, other respiratory depressants), chest wall and neuromuscular problems (paralysis, pain), and sleep apnea.
   Metabolic acidosis: ethanol, diabetic ketoacidosis, uremia, lactic acidosis (e.g., sepsis, shock, bowel ischemia), methanol/ethylene glycol, aspirin/salicylate overdose, isoniazid, diarrhea, and carbonic anhydrase inhibitors.

4. What is the anion gap and why is it useful?
   The anion gap is the calculated difference between the major cations and anions in the blood. The formula used to determine it is $[Na^+] - ([HCO_3^-] + [Cl^-])$. The normal value of the anion gap is 8 to 12 mEq/L. The anion gap is a useful measure to know when evaluating a metabolic acidosis because differential diagnoses can be included based on the value.

5. What is the differential diagnosis for a high anion gap metabolic acidosis? What is the differential diagnosis for a normal anion gap metabolic acidosis?
   An anion gap >12 mEq/L is considered high and occurs in several disease states. The **MUDPILES** mnemonic can be used to remember the offending diseases: **m**ethanol toxicity, **u**remia, **d**iabetic ketoacidosis, **p**ropylene glycol toxicity, **i**ron or **i**soniazid toxicity, **l**actic acidosis, **e**thylene glycol toxicity, and **s**alicylate toxicity (late).
   The **HARDASS** mnemonic can be used to remember the disorders that cause a normal anion gap metabolic acidosis: **h**yperalimentation, **A**ddison disease, **r**enal tubal acidosis, **d**iarrhea, **a**cetazolamide, **s**pironolactone, and **s**aline infusion.

6. List the common causes of alkalosis.
   Respiratory alkalosis: anxiety/hyperventilation and aspirin/salicylate overdose
   Metabolic alkalosis: diuretics (except carbonic anhydrase inhibitors), vomiting, volume contraction, antacid abuse/milk-alkali syndrome, and hyperaldosteronism

7. What type of acid-base disturbance does aspirin overdose cause?
   Respiratory alkalosis and anion gap metabolic acidosis (two different primary disturbances). Look for coexisting tinnitus, hypoglycemia, vomiting, and a history of "swallowing several pills." Anion gap will be elevated. Alkalinization of the urine with bicarbonate speeds excretion. Consider dialysis if a patient has a pH <7.1, altered mental status, pulmonary edema, initial salicylate level >100, renal failure, or if acidosis is refractory to medical management.

8. What happens to the blood gas of patients with chronic lung conditions?
   Many people with chronic lung disease (e.g., chronic obstructive pulmonary disease) develop a chronic respiratory acidosis because of CO_2 retention. During an exacerbation of a respiratory disorder, the respiratory acidosis worsens, and a compensatory metabolic alkalosis develops. As the respiratory acidosis improves with treatment

of the exacerbation, the metabolic alkalosis is no longer a compensatory mechanism and becomes a primary disturbance. However, in certain people with chronic lung conditions (especially those with sleep apnea), pH may be alkaline during the day because breathing improves when awake. As a side note, remember that sleep apnea, like other chronic lung diseases, can cause right-sided heart failure (cor pulmonale) by causing pulmonary hypertension.

9. Should you give bicarbonate to a patient with acidosis?
For purposes of Step 2, almost never. First, give intravenous (IV) fluids, and treat the underlying disorder. If all other measures fail and the pH remains <7.0, bicarbonate may be given.

10. The blood gas of a patient with asthma has changed from alkalotic to normal, and the patient seems to be sleeping. Is the patient ready to go home?
For Step 2, this scenario means that the patient is probably crashing. Asthmatic patients are supposed to be slightly alkalotic during an asthma attack. Remember that pH is initially high in patients with an asthma exacerbation because they are breathing rapidly, eliminating CO_2, and developing a respiratory alkalosis. If the patient becomes tired and breathing slows, CO_2 will begin to rise, and pH will begin to normalize. Eventually the patient becomes acidotic and requires emergency intubation if appropriate measures are not taken. If this scenario is mentioned on boards, the appropriate response is to prepare for possible elective intubation and to continue aggressive medical treatment with beta$_2$-agonists, steroids, and oxygen. Fatigue secondary to work of breathing is an indication for intubation.

11. List the signs and symptoms of hyponatremia.
  - Lethargy
  - Seizures
  - Mental status changes or confusion
  - Cramps
  - Anorexia
  - Coma

12. How do you determine the cause of hyponatremia?
The first step in determining the cause is to assess the patient's volume status:

	Hypovolemic	*Euvolemic*	*Hypervolemic*
Think of	Dehydration, diuretics, diabetes, Addison disease/ hypoaldosteronism (high potassium)	SIADH, psychogenic polydipsia, oxytocin use, hypothyroidism	Heart failure, nephrotic syndrome, cirrhosis, toxemia, renal failure

SIADH, Syndrome of inappropriate antidiuretic hormone secretion

13. How is hyponatremia treated?
For hypovolemic hyponatremia, the Step 2 treatment is normal saline to restore the intravascular volume. Euvolemic and hypervolemic hyponatremia are treated with water/fluid restriction; diuretics may be needed for hypervolemic hyponatremia.

14. What medication is used to treat SIADH if water restriction fails?
Demeclocycline, which induces nephrogenic diabetes insipidus

15. What happens if hyponatremia is corrected too quickly?
You may cause osmotic demyelination syndrome (ODS, formerly called central pontine myelinolysis), which can result in irreversible or only partially reversible neurologic symptoms such as dysarthria, paresis, behavioral disturbances, lethargy, confusion, and coma (remember the saying "from low to high [Na$^+$], the pons will die"). Hypertonic saline is used only when a patient has seizures from severe hyponatremia (usually Na <120 mEq/L)—and even then, only briefly and cautiously. Normal saline is a better choice 99% of the time for board purposes. In chronic severe symptomatic hyponatremia, the rate of correction should not exceed 0.5 to 1 mEq/L/hr.

16. What causes spurious (false) hyponatremia?
  - Hyperglycemia (once glucose is >200 mg/dL, sodium decreases by 1.6 mEq/L for each rise of 100 mg/dL in glucose). Make sure you know how to make this correction.
  - Hyperproteinemia
  - Hyperlipidemia
  - Mannitol
  In these instances, the lab value is low, but the total body sodium is normal. Do not give the patient extra salt or saline.

17. **What causes hyponatremia in postoperative patients?**
The most common cause is the combination of pain and narcotics (causing SIADH) with overaggressive administration of IV fluids. A rare cause that you may see on the USMLE is adrenal insufficiency, particularly in a patient who is on chronic steroids and had medications stopped before surgery. In this instance, potassium is high and blood pressure is low.

18. **What is the classic cause of hyponatremia in pregnant patients about to deliver?**
Oxytocin, which has an antidiuretic hormone-like effect

19. **What are the signs and symptoms of hypernatremia?**
Basically, the same as the signs and symptoms of hyponatremia:
- Mental status changes or confusion
- Seizures
- Hyperreflexia
- Coma

20. **What causes hypernatremia?**
The most common cause is dehydration (free water loss) due to inadequate fluid intake relative to bodily needs. Watch for diuretics, diabetes insipidus, diarrhea, and renal disease as well as iatrogenic causes (administration of too much hypertonic IV fluid). Sickle cell disease, which may lead to renal damage and isosthenuria (inability to concentrate urine), is a rare cause of hypernatremia, as are hypokalemia and hypercalcemia, which also impair the kidney's concentrating ability. Cushing syndrome and primary hyperaldosteronism are potential endocrine causes of hypernatremia.

21. **How is hypernatremia treated?**
Treatment involves water replacement, but the patient is often severely dehydrated, therefore normal saline is used most frequently. Once hemodynamically stable, the patient is often switched to dextrose 5% (D5) one-half normal saline. Dextrose 5% in water (D5W) should not be used for hypernatremia since dextrose is not an effective osmole and would just worsen hypernatremia.

22. **What are the signs and symptoms of hypokalemia?**
Hypokalemia causes muscular weakness, which can lead to paralysis and ventilatory failure. When smooth muscles are also affected, patients may develop ileus and/or hypotension. Best known and most tested, however, is the effect of hypokalemia on the heart. Electrocardiogram (ECG) findings include loss of the T wave or T-wave flattening, ST depressions, the presence of U waves, premature ventricular and atrial complexes, and ventricular and atrial tachyarrhythmias.

23. **What is the effect of pH on serum potassium?**
Changes in pH cause changes in serum potassium as a result of cellular shift. Alkalosis causes hypokalemia, whereas acidosis causes hyperkalemia. For this reason, bicarbonate is given to severely hyperkalemic patients. If the pH is deranged, normalization will most likely correct the potassium derangement automatically without the need to give or restrict potassium.

24. **Describe the interaction between digoxin and potassium**
The heart is particularly sensitive to hypokalemia in patients taking digoxin because digoxin binds to the K^+ site on the Na^+/K^+ ATPase, so hypokalemia leads to increased binding. Potassium levels should be monitored carefully in all patients taking digoxin, especially if they are also taking diuretics (a common occurrence).

25. **How should potassium be replaced?**
Like all electrolyte abnormalities, hypokalemia should be corrected slowly. Oral replacement is preferred, but if the potassium must be given intravenously for severe derangement, do not give more than 20 mEq/hr. Put the patient on an ECG monitor when giving IV potassium because potentially fatal arrhythmias may develop.

26. **When hypokalemia persists even after administration of significant amounts of potassium, what should you do?**
Check the magnesium level. When magnesium is low, the body cannot retain potassium effectively. Correction of a low magnesium level allows the potassium level to return to normal.

27. **What are the signs and symptoms of hyperkalemia?**
Weakness and paralysis may occur, but the cardiac effects are the most tested. ECG changes (in order of increasing potassium value) include **tall, peaked T waves,** widening of QRS, prolongation of the PR interval, loss of P waves, and a sine wave pattern ECG (Fig. 1.1). Arrhythmias include asystole and ventricular fibrillation.

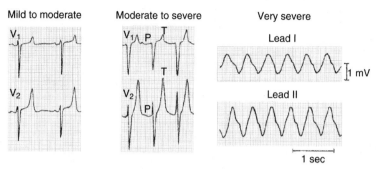

Mild to moderate   Moderate to severe   Very severe

Fig. 1.1 The earliest electrocardiogram (ECG) change with hyperkalemia is peaking of the T waves. As the serum potassium concentration increases, the QRS complexes widen, the P waves decrease in amplitude and may disappear, and finally a sine wave pattern leads to asystole unless emergency therapy is given. (From Goldberger A. *Clinical Electrocardiography: A Simplified Approach.* 7th ed. Philadelphia: Mosby; 2006 [fig. 10.6].)

28. What causes hyperkalemia?
    - Renal failure (acute or chronic)
    - Severe tissue destruction such as rhabdomyolysis or hemolysis (because potassium has a high intracellular concentration)
    - Hypoaldosteronism (watch for hyporeninemic hypoaldosteronism in diabetes)
    - Medications (stop potassium-sparing diuretics, beta-blockers, nonsteroidal antiinflammatory drugs, angiotensin-converting enzyme inhibitors, angiotensin receptor blockers, trimethoprim-sulfamethoxazole, cyclosporine, digoxin, and succinylcholine)
    - Adrenal insufficiency (also associated with low sodium and low blood pressure)
    - Insulin deficiency

29. What should you suspect if an asymptomatic patient has hyperkalemia?
    With hyperkalemia, the first consideration (especially if the patient is asymptomatic and the ECG is normal) is whether the lab specimen is hemolyzed. Hemolysis causes a false hyperkalemia due to high intracellular potassium concentrations. Repeat the test.

30. The specimen was not hemolyzed. What is the first treatment?
    Get an ECG first to look for cardiotoxicity. In general, the best therapy for hyperkalemia is decreased potassium intake and administration of a gastrointestinal cation exchange (e.g., patiromer or zirconium cyclosilicate). The oral sodium polystyrene resin, Kayexalate, is only used in rare instances due to increased risk of bowel necrosis. If the potassium level is >6.5 or cardiac toxicity is apparent (more than peaked T waves), however, immediate IV therapy is needed. First give **calcium gluconate** (which is cardioprotective, although it does not change potassium levels); then give **glucose with insulin** (insulin forces potassium inside cells, and glucose prevents hypoglycemia). Beta$_2$-agonists also drive potassium into cells and can be given if the other choices are not listed on the test. If the patient has renal failure (high creatinine) or initial treatment is ineffective, prepare to institute dialysis emergently.

31. What are the signs and symptoms of hypocalcemia?
    Hypocalcemia produces neurologic findings, the most tested of which is tetany. Tapping on the facial nerve at the angle of the jaw elicits contraction of the facial muscles (**Chvostek sign**), and inflation of a tourniquet or blood pressure cuff elicits hand and foot muscle (carpopedal) spasms (**Trousseau sign**). Other signs and symptoms are perioral tingling, hyperreflexia, depression, encephalopathy, dementia, laryngospasm, and convulsions/seizures. The classic ECG finding is QT-interval prolongation.

32. What should you do if the calcium level is low?
    Check the albumin and correct the calcium as necessary to account for hypoalbuminemia. Remember that hypoproteinemia (i.e., low albumin) of any etiology can cause hypocalcemia because the protein-bound fraction of calcium is decreased. In this instance, however, the patient is asymptomatic because the ionized (unbound, physiologically active) fraction of calcium is unchanged. Thus you should first check the albumin level and/or the ionized or free calcium level to make sure "true" hypocalcemia is present. For every 1-g/dL decrease in albumin <4 g/dL, correct the calcium by adding 0.8 mg/dL to the given calcium value.

33. What causes hypocalcemia?
    - DiGeorge syndrome (tetany 24–48 hours after birth, absent thymic shadow on x-ray, cardiofacial abnormalities)
    - Renal failure (remember the kidney's role in vitamin D metabolism)
    - Hypoparathyroidism (watch for a postthyroidectomy patient; all four parathyroids may have been accidentally removed)
    - Vitamin D deficiency

- Pseudohypoparathyroidism (short fingers, short stature, intellectual disability, and elevated parathyroid hormone [PTH] level with end-organ unresponsiveness to PTH)
- Acute pancreatitis
- Renal tubular acidosis

34. **Describe the relationship between low calcium and low magnesium**
It is difficult to correct hypocalcemia until hypomagnesemia (of any cause) is also corrected, as magnesium is needed to produce PTH.

35. **How does pH affect calcium levels?**
Alkalosis can cause symptoms similar to hypocalcemia through effects on the ionized fraction of calcium (alkalosis causes calcium to shift intracellularly or because alkalosis induces the dissociation of hydrogen ions from albumin, allowing free Ca^{2+} to bind, which lowers ionized Ca^{2+}). Clinically, this scenario is most common with hyperventilation/anxiety syndromes, in which the patient eliminates too much CO_2, becomes alkalotic, and develops perioral and extremity tingling. Treat by correcting the pH. Treat anxiety if hyperventilation is the cause.

36. **Describe the relationship between calcium and phosphorus**
Phosphorus and calcium levels usually go in opposite directions (when one goes up, the other goes down), and derangements in one can cause problems with the other. This relationship becomes clinically important in patients with chronic renal failure, in whom you must not only try to raise calcium levels (with vitamin D and calcium supplements) but also restrict/reduce phosphorus.

37. **What are the signs and symptoms of hypercalcemia?**
Hypercalcemia is often asymptomatic and discovered by routine lab tests. When symptoms are present, recall the following rhyme:

Bones (bone changes such as osteopenia, pathologic fractures, and osteitis fibrosa cystica)
Stones (kidney stones and polyuria)
Groans (abdominal pain, anorexia, constipation, ileus, nausea, vomiting)
Psychiatric overtones (depression/anxiety, psychosis, delirium/confusion)

   Abdominal pain may also be due to peptic ulcer disease and/or pancreatitis, both of which have an increased incidence with hypercalcemia. The ECG classically shows QT-interval shortening when hypercalcemia is present.

38. **What causes hypercalcemia?**
Primary hyperparathyroidism is the most common cause of hypercalcemia in outpatients. In inpatients, the most common cause is malignancy. Check the PTH level to differentiate hyperparathyroidism from other causes.
   Other causes include vitamin A or D intoxication, sarcoidosis, thiazide diuretics, familial hypocalciuric hypercalcemia (look for low urinary calcium, which is rare with hypercalcemia), and immobilization. Hyperproteinemia (e.g., high albumin) of any etiology can cause hypercalcemia because of an increase in the protein-bound fraction of calcium, but the patient is asymptomatic because the ionized (unbound) fraction is unchanged.

39. **Why is asymptomatic hypercalcemia usually treated?**
Prolonged hypercalcemia can cause nephrocalcinosis, urolithiasis, and renal failure due to calcium salt deposits in the kidney and may result in bone disease secondary to loss of calcium.

40. **How is hypercalcemia treated?**
First, give IV fluids. Then, once the patient is well hydrated, give furosemide (a loop diuretic) to cause calcium diuresis. Thiazides are contraindicated because they increase serum calcium levels. Other treatments include phosphorus administration (use oral phosphorus; IV administration can be dangerous), calcitonin, bisphosphonates (e.g., etidronate, which is often used in Paget disease), plicamycin, or prednisone (especially for malignancy-induced hypercalcemia). Correction of the underlying cause of hypercalcemia is the ultimate goal. The previous measures are all temporary until definitive treatment can be given. For hyperparathyroidism, surgery is the treatment of choice.

41. **In what clinical scenario is hypomagnesemia usually seen?**
Alcoholism. Magnesium is wasted through the kidneys.

42. **What are the signs and symptoms of hypomagnesemia?**
Signs and symptoms are similar to those of hypocalcemia (prolonged QT interval on ECG and possibly tetany).

43. **In what clinical scenario is hypermagnesemia seen?**
Hypermagnesemia is classically iatrogenic in pregnant patients who are treated for preeclampsia with magnesium sulfate. It also commonly occurs in patients with renal failure. Patients who receive magnesium sulfate should be monitored carefully because the physical findings of hypermagnesemia are progressive. The initial sign is a decrease in deep tendon reflexes; then hypotension and respiratory failure occur sequentially.

44. How is hypermagnesemia treated?

First, stop any magnesium infusion! Remember the ABCs (airway, breathing, circulation), and intubate the patient if respiratory failure is pending. If the patient is stable, start IV fluids. Furosemide can be given next, if needed, to cause a magnesium diuresis. The last resort is dialysis.

45. In what clinical scenarios is hypophosphatemia seen? What are the signs and symptoms?

Uncontrolled diabetes (especially diabetic ketoacidosis) and alcoholism. Signs and symptoms of hypophosphatemia include neuromuscular disturbances (encephalopathy, weakness), rhabdomyolysis (especially in alcoholics), anemia, and white blood cell and platelet dysfunction.

46. What is the IV fluid of choice in hypovolemic patients?

Normal saline or lactated Ringer solution (regardless of other electrolyte problems). First, fill the tank; then, correct the imbalances that the kidney cannot sort out on its own.

47. What is the maintenance fluid of choice for patients who are not eating?

One-half normal saline with D5 in adults. Typically, one-fourth normal saline with D5 in children <10 kg; one-third or one-half normal saline with D5 in children >10 kg.

48. Should anything be added to the IV fluid for patients who are not eating?

Potassium chloride, 10 or 20 mEq, is usually added to a liter of IV fluid each day to prevent hypokalemia (assuming that the baseline potassium level is normal).

CHAPTER 2

ALCOHOL

1. With which cancers is alcohol intake associated?
   Cancers of the oral cavity, larynx, pharynx, esophagus, liver, and lung. It also may be associated with gastric, colon, pancreatic, and breast cancer.

2. Describe the relationship between alcohol and accidental or intentional death (i.e., suicide and murder).
   Alcohol is involved in roughly 50% of fatal car accidents, 67% of drownings, 67% of homicides, 35% of suicides, and 70% to 80% of deaths caused by fire.

3. True or false: Alcohol can precipitate hypoglycemia.
   True. But give thiamine first and then glucose in a patient with significant alcohol use disorder.

4. What may happen if you give glucose to a person with alcohol use disorder without giving thiamine first?
   You may precipitate Wernicke encephalopathy. Always give thiamine before glucose to avoid this complication.

5. What is the difference between Wernicke and Korsakoff syndromes? What causes each?
   Wernicke syndrome is an acute encephalopathy characterized by ophthalmoplegia (paralysis of extraocular muscles), nystagmus, ataxia, and/or confusion. It can be fatal but is often reversible with thiamine.
   Korsakoff syndrome is a chronic psychosis characterized by anterograde amnesia (inability to form new memories) and confabulation (making up stories) to cover up the amnesia. Korsakoff syndrome is generally irreversible and is thought to be due to damage to the mammillary bodies and thalamic nuclei. Both conditions result from thiamine deficiency.

6. True or false: Alcohol withdrawal can be fatal.
   True. Alcohol withdrawal needs to be treated on an inpatient basis because it can result in death (mortality rate of 1%–5% with delirium tremens).

7. How is alcohol withdrawal treated?
   With benzodiazepines (or, in rare cases, barbiturates). The dose is tapered gradually over several days until symptoms have resolved.

8. What are the stages of alcohol withdrawal?
   Minor withdrawal (6–36 hours after the last drink): tremors, mild anxiety, sweating, gastrointestinal upset, headache, and normal mental status.
   Seizures (6–48 hours after the last drink): single or brief generalized tonic-clonic seizures. Status epilepticus is rare.
   Alcoholic hallucinosis (12–24 hours after last drink): visual, auditory, or tactile hallucinations without autonomic signs (stable vital signs).
   Delirium tremens (48–72 days after last drink, possibly longer): hallucinations, confusion, insomnia, and autonomic lability (sweating, increased pulse and temperature). Fatality is usually associated with this stage.

   Of course, these stages may overlap. Delirium tremens may occur several days after the last drink. The classic example is a patient who develops delirium on postoperative day 2 but was fine before the surgery. The patient could have undisclosed alcohol use disorder, assuming other causes for delirium have been ruled out.

9. What are the classic physical stigmata of liver disease in those with alcohol use disorder?
   - Abdominal wall varices (caput medusae)
   - Testicular atrophy
   - Esophageal varices
   - Encephalopathy
   - Hemorrhoids (internal)
   - Asterixis
   - Jaundice
   - Scleral icterus
   - Ascites
   - Edema
   - Palmar erythema

- Spider angiomas
- Gynecomastia
- Terry nails (white nails with a ground-glass appearance and no lunula)
- Fetor hepaticus ("breath of the dead," which is a sweet, fecal smell)
- Dupuytren contractures

10. **What are the classic laboratory findings of liver disease in those with alcohol use disorder?**
- Anemia (classically macrocytic)
- Prolonged prothrombin time
- Hyperbilirubinemia
- Hypoalbuminemia
- Thrombocytopenia
- Leukocytosis (predominantly neutrophils)

11. **What diseases and conditions may be caused by chronic alcohol intake?**
- Gastritis
- Fatty change in the liver
- Hepatitis
- Mallory-Weiss tears
- Cirrhosis
- Pancreatitis (acute or chronic)
- Peripheral neuropathy (via thiamine deficiency and a direct effect)
- Wernicke or Korsakoff syndrome
- Cerebellar degeneration (ataxia, past-pointing)
- Dilated cardiomyopathy
- Rhabdomyolysis (acute or chronic)

12. **Describe the classic derangement of aspartate aminotransferase (AST) and alanine aminotransferase (ALT) in alcoholic hepatitis.**
The ratio of AST (also known as serum glutamate oxaloacetate transaminase [SGOT]) to ALT (also known as serum glutamate pyruvate transaminase [SGPT]) is at least 2:1, although both may be modestly elevated (almost always <500 IU/L). Other causes of hepatitis are usually associated with the opposite ratio or equal elevation of both AST and ALT.

13. **What is the best treatment for alcohol use disorder?**
Alcoholics Anonymous or other peer-based support groups have had the best success rates. Disulfiram (an aldehyde dehydrogenase enzyme inhibitor that makes people sick when they drink) can be used in some patients. Be sure to warn patients that metronidazole and certain cephalosporins have a similar effect on those who drink alcohol.

14. **Describe the effects of alcohol on pregnancy.**
Alcohol is a teratogen and the most common cause of preventable mental retardation in the United States. You should be able to recognize the classic presentation of a child affected by fetal alcohol syndrome: intellectual disability, smooth philtrum, thin vermilion border, microcephaly, short palpebral fissures, and cardiac defects (Fig. 2.1). No amount of alcohol consumption can be considered safe during pregnancy. Fetal alcohol syndrome rates vary but may affect as many as 1 in 1000 births in the United States.

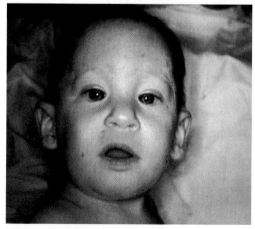

Fig. 2.1 Infant with fetal alcohol syndrome. Note short palpebral fissures, mild ptosis, smooth philtrum, and narrow vermilion of the upper lip. (From Gilbert-Barness E. *Potter's Pathology of the Fetus, Infant and Child.* 2nd ed. Philadelphia: Mosby; 2007 [fig. 4.1.12].)

15. Discuss the epidemiology of alcohol use disorder.

    Roughly 10% to 15% of the population abuses alcohol. Alcohol use disorder is more common in men. The genetic component is passed most easily from father to son.

16. What kind of pneumonia should you suspect in a homeless patient with alcohol use disorder?

    Aspiration pneumonia. Look for enteric organisms (anaerobes, *Escherichia coli*, streptococci, staphylococci) as the cause. Think of *Klebsiella* spp. if the sputum resembles currant jelly or if thick mucoid capsules are mentioned in culture reports.

17. What are the classic electrolyte and vitamin/mineral abnormalities in those with alcohol use disorder?

    Electrolytes: low magnesium, low potassium, low sodium, elevated uric acid (resulting in gout)
    Vitamins: deficiencies of folate and thiamine

    Remember that patients with severe alcohol use disorder tend to have poor nutrition and may develop just about any deficiency.

18. How are bleeding esophageal varices treated?

    First, think of the ABCs (airways, breathing, and circulation). Stabilize the patient with intravenous fluids and blood if needed. If indicated, correct clotting factor deficiencies with fresh frozen plasma, fresh blood, and vitamin K. Patients with cirrhosis and upper GI bleeding should be given prophylactic antibiotics to reduce all-cause mortality, bacterial infection, and rebleeding. Somatostatin analogues (octreotide) can be given intravenously to inhibit release of vasodilator hormones and indirectly decrease portal blood flow through splanchnic vasoconstriction. Next, upper endoscopy is performed to determine the cause of the upper gastrointestinal bleed (there are many possibilities for the bleeding). Once varices are identified on endoscopy, sclerotherapy of the veins is attempted with cauterization, banding, or vasopressin. The mortality rate is high, and rebleeding is common. If you must choose, try a transjugular intrahepatic portosystemic shunt (TIPS) over an open surgical portacaval shunt for more definitive management, if needed. The most physiologic shunt type among surgical options is the splenorenal shunt. However, open surgical shunt procedures are now rarely performed.

19. How are varices with no history of bleeding treated?

    With nonselective beta-blockers (e.g., propranolol, nadolol, timolol) to relieve portal hypertension provided that there is no contraindication to the use of beta-blockers.

CHAPTER 3

BIOSTATISTICS

1. **How is the sensitivity of a test defined? What are highly sensitive tests used for clinically?**
   Sensitivity is defined as the ability of a test to detect disease mathematically as the number of true positives divided by the number of people with the disease. Tests with high sensitivity are used for disease screening. False positives occur, but the test does not miss many people with the disease (low false-negative rate). One way to remember this is the word *snout*, written "Sn-N-out," meaning with high **sen**sitivity (Sn) a **n**egative (N) test rules **out** (out) the disease.

2. **How is the specificity of a test defined? What are highly specific tests used for clinically?**
   Specificity is defined as the ability of a test to detect health (or nondisease) mathematically as the number of true negatives divided by the number of people without the disease. Tests with high specificity are used for disease confirmation. False negatives occur, but the test does not identify anyone who is actually healthy as sick (low false-positive rate). The ideal confirmatory test must have high sensitivity and high specificity; otherwise, people with the disease may be called healthy. One way to remember this is the word *spin*, written "Sp-P-in," meaning that with high **sp**ecificity (Sp) a **p**ositive (P) test rules **in** (in) the disease.

3. **Explain the concept of a trade-off between sensitivity and specificity.**
   The trade-off between sensitivity and specificity is a classic statistics question. For example, you should understand how changing the cutoff glucose value in screening for diabetes (or changing the value of any of several screening tests) will change the number of true- and false-negative as well as true- and false-positive results. If the cutoff value is raised, fewer people will be identified as diabetic (more false negatives, fewer false positives), whereas if the cutoff glucose value is lowered, more people will be identified as diabetic (fewer false negatives, more false positives) (Fig. 3.1). As an example, if the diagnostic threshold for a fasting blood sugar for diabetes were raised from ≥125 mg/dL to ≥300 mg/dL, most people with diabetes would be missed (low sensitivity because a patient with a blood sugar of 285 mg/dL would be negative for diabetes according to this criterion). In addition, the test would be very specific for patients with blood sugar ≥300 mg/dL (a patient would certainly have diabetes if the test is positive).

4. **Define positive predictive value (PPV). On what does it depend?**
   When a test is positive for disease, the PPV measures how likely it is that the patient has the disease (probability of having a condition, given a positive test). PPV is calculated mathematically by dividing the number of true positives by the total number of people with a positive test. PPV depends on the prevalence of a disease (the higher the

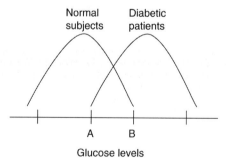

Glucose levels

Fig. 3.1 If the cutoff serum glucose value for a diagnosis of diabetes mellitus is set at point A, no cases of diabetes will be missed, but many people without diabetes will be mislabeled as diabetics (i.e., higher sensitivity, lower specificity, lower positive predictive value, higher negative predictive value). If the cutoff is set at B, the diagnosis of diabetes will not be made in healthy people, but many cases of true diabetes will go undiagnosed (i.e., lower sensitivity, higher specificity, higher positive predictive value, lower negative predictive value). The optimal diagnostic value lies somewhere between points A and B.

prevalence, the higher the PPV) and the sensitivity and specificity of the test (e.g., an overly sensitive test that gives more false positives has a lower PPV).

5. **Define negative predictive value (NPV). On what does it depend?**
When a test comes back negative for disease, the NPV measures how likely it is that the patient is healthy and does not have the disease (probability of not having a condition given a negative test). It is calculated mathematically by dividing the number of true negatives by the total number of people with a negative test. NPV also depends on the prevalence of the disease and the sensitivity and specificity of the test (the higher the prevalence, the lower the NPV). In addition, an overly sensitive test with many false positives leads to a higher NPV.

6. **Define attributable risk. How is it measured?**
Attributable risk is the number of cases of a disease attributable to one risk factor (in other words, the amount by which the incidence of a condition is expected to decrease if the risk factor in question is removed). For example, if the incidence rate of lung cancer is 1/100 in the general population and 10/100 in smokers, the attributable risk of smoking in causing lung cancer is 9/100 (assuming a properly matched control group).

7. **Develop the habit of drawing a 2 × 2 table for Step 2 statistics questions.**
Given the following 2 × 2 table, define the formulas for calculating the test values.

Disease	Test Name	Formula
Test or exposure	Sensitivity	$A/(A + C)$
	Specificity	$D/(B + D)$
	PPV	$A/(A + B)$
	NPV	$D/(C + D)$
	Odds ratio	$(A \times D)/(B \times C)$
	Relative risk	$[A/(A + B)]/[C/(C + D)]$
	Attributable risk	$[A/(A + B)] - [C/(C + D)]$

8. **Define relative risk. From what types of studies can it be calculated?**
Relative risk compares the disease risk in people exposed to a certain factor with the disease risk in people who have not been exposed to the factor in question. Relative risk can be calculated only after prospective or experimental studies; it cannot be calculated from retrospective data. If a Step 2 question asks you to calculate the relative risk from retrospective data, the answer is "cannot be calculated" or "none of the above."

9. **What is a clinically significant value for relative risk?**
Any value for relative risk other than 1 is clinically significant. For example, if the relative risk is 1.5, a person is 1.5 times more likely to develop the condition if exposed to the factor in question. If the relative risk is 0.5, the person is only half as likely to develop the condition when exposed to the factor; in other words, the factor is protective.

10. **Define odds ratio. From what types of studies is it calculated?**
Odds ratio attempts to estimate relative risk with retrospective studies (e.g., case control). An odds ratio compares two factors ([1] the incidence of disease in persons exposed to the factor and the incidence of nondisease in persons not exposed to the factor, and [2] the incidence of disease in persons unexposed to the factor and the incidence of nondisease in persons exposed to the factor) to see whether there is a difference between the two. As with relative risk, values other than 1 are significant. The odds ratio is a less than perfect way to estimate relative risk (which can be calculated only from prospective or experimental studies). You can remember that an **o**dds ratio is commonly used in **c**ase **c**ontrol studies through the mnemonic: **CC** (or **c**ritical **c**are) patients often go to the **OR** (**o**perating **r**oom).

11. **What do you need to know about standard deviation (SD) for the USMLE?**
You need to know that for a normal or bell-shaped distribution, the mean ±1 SD contains 68% of the values, the mean ±2 SD contains 95% of the values, and the mean ±3 SD contains 99.7% of the values. A classic question gives the mean and SD and asks what percentage of values will be above a given value. For example, if the mean score on a test is 80 and the SD is 5, 68% of the scores will be within 5 points of 80 (scores of 75–85), and 95% of the scores will be within 10 points of 80 (scores of 70–90). The question may ask what percentage of scores are over 90. The answer is 2.5% because 2.5% of the scores fall below 70 and 2.5% of the scores are over 90. Variations of this question are common.

12. **Define mean, median, and mode.**
The mean is the average value, the median is the middle value, and the mode is the most common value. A question may give several numbers and ask for their mean, median, and mode. For example, if the question gives the numbers 2, 2, 4, and 8:
  The mean is the average of the four numbers: $(2 + 2 + 4 + 8)/4 = 16/4 = 4$.

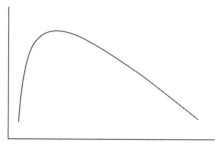

Fig. 3.2 Positive skew. An excess of higher values makes this a nonnormal distribution.

The median is the middle value. Because there are four numbers, there is no true middle value. Therefore take the average between the two middle numbers (2 and 4), so the median is 3. The mode is 2 because the number 2 appears twice (more times than any other value). Remember that in a normal distribution, mean = median = mode.

13. What is a skewed distribution? How does it affect mean, median, and mode?

A skewed distribution implies that the distribution is not normal; in other words, the data do not conform to a perfect bell-shaped curve. **Positive skew** is an asymmetric distribution with an excess of high values; in other words, the tail of the curve is on the right (mean > median > mode) (Fig. 3.2). **Negative skew** is an asymmetric distribution with an excess of low values; in other words, the tail of the curve is on the left (mean < median < mode). Because they are not normal distributions, SD and mean are less meaningful values.

14. Define test reliability. How is it related to precision? What reduces reliability?

Practically speaking, the reliability of a test is synonymous with its precision. Reliability measures the reproducibility and consistency of a test. For example, if the test has good interrater reliability, the person taking the test will get the same score even if two different people administer the same test. Random error reduces reliability and precision (e.g., limitation in significant figures).

15. Define test validity. How is it related to accuracy? What reduces validity?

Practically speaking, the validity of a test is synonymous with its accuracy. Validity measures the trueness of measurement, in other words, whether the test measures what it claims to measure. For example, if a valid IQ test is administered to a genius, the test should not indicate that the person has an intellectual disability. Systematic error reduces validity and accuracy (e.g., when the equipment is miscalibrated).

16. Define correlation coefficient. What is the range of its values?

A correlation coefficient measures to what degree two variables are related. The value of the correlation coefficient ranges from −1 to +1.

17. True or false: A correlation coefficient of −0.6 is a stronger correlation coefficient than +0.4

True. The important factor in determining the strength of the relationship between two variables is the distance of the value from zero. A correlation coefficient of 0 equates to no association whatsoever; the two variables are totally unrelated. A correlation coefficient of +1 equates to a perfect positive correlation (when one variable increases, so does the other), whereas −1 corresponds to a perfect negative correlation (when one variable increases, the other decreases). Therefore the absolute value indicates the strength of the correlation (e.g., the strength of −0.3 is the same as that of +0.3).

18. Define confidence interval. Why is it used?

When you take a set of data from a subset of the population and calculate the mean, you may want to say that it is equivalent to the mean for the whole population. In fact, however, the two means are usually not exactly equal. A confidence interval of 95% (the value used in most medical literature before data are accepted by the medical community) indicates that there is 95% certainty that the mean for the entire population is within a certain range (usually 2 SD of the experimental or derived mean, calculated from the subset of the population examined). For example, if the heart rate of 100 people is sampled and the mean is calculated as 80 beats per minute with an SD of 2, the confidence interval (also known as confidence limits) is written as 76 < X < 84 = 0.95. In other words, there is 95% certainty that the mean heart rate of the whole population (X) is between 76 and 84 (within 2 SD of the mean).

19. What five types of studies should you know for the Step 2 exam?

From highest to lowest quality and desirability: (1) experimental studies, (2) prospective studies, (3) retrospective studies, (4) case series, and (5) prevalence surveys.

20. What are experimental studies?

    Experimental studies are the gold standard. They compare two equal groups in which one variable is manipulated and its effect is measured. Experimental studies use double blinding (or at least single blinding) and well-matched controls to ensure accurate data. It is not always possible to do experimental studies because of ethical concerns.

21. What are prospective studies? Why are they important?

    Prospective studies (also known as observational, longitudinal, cohort, incidence, or follow-up studies) involve choosing a sample and dividing it into two groups based on the presence or absence of a risk factor and following the groups over time to see what diseases they develop. For example, individuals with and without asymptomatic hypercholesterolemia may be followed to determine if those with hypercholesterolemia have a higher incidence of myocardial infarction later in life. The relative risk and incidence can be calculated from this type of study. Prospective studies are time consuming and expensive but practical for common diseases.

22. What are retrospective studies? Discuss their advantages and disadvantages

    Retrospective (case control) studies choose population samples after the fact according to the presence (cases) or absence (controls) of disease. Information can be collected about risk factors. For example, you can compare individuals with lung cancer and individuals without lung cancer to determine if those with lung cancer smoked more before they developed lung cancer. In a retrospective study, an odds ratio can be calculated, but true relative risk cannot be calculated, and incidence cannot be measured. Compared with prospective studies, retrospective studies are less expensive, less time consuming, and more practical for rare diseases.

23. What is a case series study? How is it used?

    A case series study simply describes the clinical presentation of people with a certain disease. This type of study is good for extremely rare diseases (as are retrospective studies) and may suggest a need for a retrospective or prospective study.

24. What is a prevalence survey? How is it used?

    A prevalence (cross-sectional) survey looks at the prevalence of a disease and the prevalence of risk factors. When used to compare two different cultures or populations, a prevalence survey may suggest a possible cause of a disease. The hypothesis then can be tested with a prospective study. For example, researchers have found a higher prevalence of colon cancer and a diet higher in fat in the United States versus a lower prevalence of colon cancer and a diet lower in fat in Japan.

25. What is the difference between incidence and prevalence?

    Incidence is the number of new cases of a disease in a unit of time (generally 1 year, but any time frame can be used). The incidence of a disease is equal to the absolute (or total) risk of developing a condition (as distinguished from relative or attributable risk).

    Prevalence is the total number of cases of a disease (new or old) at a certain point in time.

26. If a disease can be treated only to the point that people can be kept alive longer without being cured, what happens to the incidence and prevalence of the disease?

    This is the classic question about incidence and prevalence on the Step 2 exam. Nothing happens to the incidence (the same number of people contract the disease every year), but the prevalence will increase because people with the disease live longer. For short-term diseases (e.g., influenza), the incidence may be higher than the prevalence, whereas for chronic diseases (e.g., diabetes or hypertension), the prevalence is greater than the incidence.

27. Define epidemic

    In an epidemic, the observed incidence greatly exceeds the expected incidence.

28. When are a chi-square test, *t*-test, and analysis of variance (ANOVA) test used?

    All of these tests are used to compare different sets of data.

    Chi-square test: used to compare percentages or proportions (nonnumeric or nominal data)

    ***t*-test:** used to compare two means

    ANOVA test: used to compare three or more means

29. What is the difference between nominal, ordinal, and continuous types of data?

    Nominal data have no numeric value (e.g., the day of the week). Ordinal data give a ranking but no quantification (e.g., class rank, which does not specify how far number 1 is ahead of number 2). Most numeric measurements are continuous data (e.g., weight, blood pressure, and age). This distinction is important because of question 28: Chi-square tests must be used to compare nominal or ordinal data, whereas a *t*-test or ANOVA test is used to compare continuous data.

30. Define *P*-value.

The significance of the *P*-value is high yield on the Step 2 exam. If *P* is <0.05 for a set of data, there is <5% chance (0.05 = 5%) that the data were obtained by random error or chance. If *P* is <0.01, the chance is <1%. For example, if the blood pressure in a control group is 180/100 mm Hg but falls to 120/70 mm Hg after drug X is given, a *P*-value <0.10 means that the chance that this difference was due to random error or chance is <10%. It also means, however, that the chance that the result is random and unrelated to the drug may be as high as 9.99%. A *P*-value <0.05 is generally used as the cutoff for statistical significance in the medical literature.

31. What three points about *P*-value should be remembered for the Step 2 exam?
    1. A study with a *P*-value <0.05 may still have serious flaws.
    2. A low *P*-value does not imply causation.
    3. A study that has statistical significance does not necessarily have clinical significance. For example, if drug X can lower blood pressure from 130/80 to 129/80 mm Hg with *P* <0.0001, drug X is unlikely to be used because the result is not clinically important given the minimal blood pressure reduction, the costs, and probable side effects.

32. Explain the relationship of the *P*-value to the null hypothesis.

The *P*-value is also related to the null hypothesis (the hypothesis of no difference). For example, in a study of hypertension, the null hypothesis says that the drug under investigation does not work; therefore, any difference in blood pressure is due to random error or chance. If the drug works well and lowers blood pressure by 60 points, the null hypothesis must be rejected because clearly the drug works. When *P* is <0.05, the null hypothesis can be rejected with confidence because the *P*-value indicates that there is a <5% chance that the null hypothesis is correct. If the null hypothesis is wrong, the difference in blood pressure is not due to chance, therefore it must be due to the drug.

In other words, the *P*-value represents the chance of making a type I error—that is, claiming an effect or difference when none exists or rejecting the null hypothesis when it is true. If *P* is <0.07, there is a <7% chance of a type I error if a true difference (not due to random error) in blood pressure between the control and experimental groups is claimed.

33. What is a type II error?

In a type II error, the null hypothesis is accepted when in fact it is false. In the previous example, this would mean that the antihypertensive drug works but the experimenter says that it does not.

34. What is the power of a study? How do you increase the power of a study?

Power measures the probability of rejecting the null hypothesis when it is false (a good thing). The best way to increase power is to **increase the sample size.**

35. What are confounding variables?

Confounding variables are unmeasured variables that affect both the independent (manipulated, experimental) variable and dependent (outcome) variable. For example, an experimenter measures the number of ashtrays owned and the incidence of lung cancer and finds that people with lung cancer have more ashtrays. The experimenter concludes that ashtrays cause lung cancer. Smoking tobacco is the confounding variable because it causes the increase in ashtrays and lung cancer.

36. Discuss nonrandom or nonstratified sampling

City A and city B can be compared, but they may not be equivalent. For example, if city A is a retirement community and city B is a college town, of course city A will have higher rates of mortality and heart disease if the groups are not stratified into appropriate age-specific comparisons.

37. What is nonresponse bias?

Nonresponse bias is a type of selection bias that occurs when people do not return printed surveys or answer the phone in a phone survey. If nonresponse accounts for a significant percentage of the results, the experiment will suffer. The first strategy in this situation is to visit or call the nonresponders repeatedly. If this strategy is unsuccessful, list the nonresponders as unknown in the data analysis, and determine if any results can be salvaged. *Never* make up or assume responses.

38. Explain lead-time bias.

Lead-time bias is due to time differentials. The classic example is a cancer screening test that claims to prolong survival compared with older survival data, when in fact the difference is due only to earlier detection and not to improved treatment or prolonged survival.

39. Explain admission rate bias.

The classic admission rate bias occurs when an experimenter compares the mortality rates for myocardial infarction (or some other disease) in hospitals A and B and concludes that hospital A has a higher mortality rate. But the higher rate may be due to tougher admission criteria at hospital A, which admits only the sickest patients with myocardial infarction. Hence hospital A has higher mortality rates, although their care may be superior. The same bias can apply to morbidity and mortality rates for a surgeon who takes on only difficult cases.

40. Explain recall bias.

Recall bias is a risk in all retrospective studies. When people cannot remember exactly, they may inadvertently overestimate or underestimate risk factors. For example, John died of lung cancer and his angry widow remembers him as smoking "like a chimney," whereas Mike died of causes not related to smoking and his loving wife denies that he smoked "much." In fact, both men smoked one pack per day.

41. Explain interviewer bias.

Interviewer bias occurs in the absence of blinding. The scientist receives a large amount of money to perform a study and wants to find a difference between cases and controls. Thus the scientist may inadvertently call the same patient comment or outcome "not significant" in the control group and "significant" in the treatment group.

42. What is unacceptability bias?

Unacceptability bias occurs when people do not admit to embarrassing behavior. For example, they may claim to exercise more than they do to please the interviewer, or they may claim to have taken experimental medications when they actually spat them out.

43. What is attrition bias and intention-to-treat analysis?

Attrition bias occurs in prospective studies when a substantial number of subjects are lost to follow-up. This type of bias may be minimized by conducting a study that will likely be important to participants, fostering good communication between participants and study staff and using intention-to-treat analysis. Intention-to-treat analysis dictates that all participants who are randomized are included in statistical analysis and are analyzed in the groups to which they were allocated regardless of which treatment (if any) they received. Generally, an attrition rate of <5% leads to little bias, whereas >20% likely threatens the validity of a study.

CHAPTER 4

CARDIOLOGY

1. **When USMLE Step 2 describes a patient with nontraumatic chest pain, what is your first step?**
   Make sure that the chest pain is not due to acute coronary syndrome by ordering a 12-lead electrocardiogram (ECG) and serial troponins.

2. **What elements of the history and physical exam steer you away from a diagnosis of myocardial infarction (MI)?**
   Wrong age: A patient age <40 is very unlikely to have an MI without known heart disease, strong family history, or multiple risk factors for coronary artery disease.
   Lack of risk factors: A 60-year-old marathon runner who eats well and has a high level of high-density lipoprotein (HDL) and no cardiac risk factors (other than age) is unlikely to have an MI.
   Physical characteristics of pain: If the pain is reproducible by palpation, it is from the chest wall, not the heart. If the pain worsens with inspiration, that is pleuritic chest pain, not the heart. If the pain is associated with meals or certain foods, it is likely a gastrointestinal cause such as gastroesophageal reflux disease (GERD), not the heart. The pain associated with an MI is usually not sharp or well localized.

   Many physicians still want to make sure that a heart attack has not occurred by obtaining an ECG and possibly one or more sets of cardiac enzyme levels. For your licensing exams, however, the clues mentioned earlier should steer you toward an alternative diagnosis.

3. **What findings on ECG should make you suspect an MI?**
   Inverted or flattened T waves, ST-segment elevation (depression means ischemia; elevation means injury), and/or Q waves in a segmental distribution (e.g., leads II, III, and aVF for an inferior infarct) suggest a MI has or is occurring (Fig. 4.1). A new left bundle branch block is also considered an MI equivalent.

4. **Describe the classic pattern of MI chest pain.**
   The pain is classically described as a crushing or pressure sensation; it is a poorly localized substernal pain that may radiate to the shoulder, arm, or jaw. The pain is usually not reproducible on palpation and in patients with a heart attack often does not resolve with nitroglycerin (as it often does in angina). The pain usually lasts at least half an hour.

5. **What tests are used to diagnose an MI?**
   Other than an ECG, serum levels of the troponin enzyme are typically drawn three times in 8-hour intervals for the first 24 hours after presentation before an MI is ruled out. Troponin levels stay elevated for >24 hours but take about 2 hours to reach their peak. Do not be fooled by an initial troponin measurement in the normal range if the patient's chest pain began only a few minutes ago. Chest radiographs may show cardiomegaly and/or pulmonary congestion; echocardiography may show ventricular wall motion abnormalities.

6. **Describe the classic physical exam findings in patients with MI.**
   Patients are often diaphoretic, anxious, tachycardic, tachypneic, pale, and appear anxious; they may also have nausea and vomiting. A large MI can cause heart failure; look for bilateral pulmonary rales in the absence of other pneumonia-like symptoms, distended neck veins, a new S3 or S4 heart sound, new murmurs, and/or cardiogenic shock.

7. **What historical points should steer you toward a diagnosis of MI?**
   Patients often have a history of angina or previous chest pain, murmurs, arrhythmias, risk factors for coronary artery disease, hypertension, or diabetes. They may also be taking digoxin, furosemide, cholesterol medications (e.g., statins), antihypertensives, or other cardiac medications.

8. **Describe the management of an MI.**
   These patients should be admitted to the intensive or cardiac care unit. Several basic principles should be kept in mind:
   - Early reperfusion is indicated if the time from onset of symptoms is <12 hours, and choice of reperfusion therapy is determined by patient and medical center criteria. Early reperfusion (<4–6 hours) is preferred to try to salvage myocardium ("time is myocardium"). Reperfusion may be accomplished by fibrinolysis or percutaneous coronary intervention (i.e., balloon angioplasty or stent). Coronary artery bypass grafting (CABG) may be required.

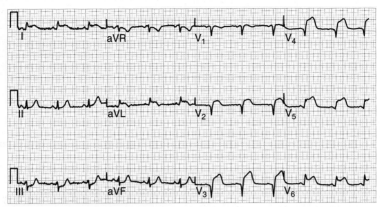

Fig. 4.1 An anterolateral acute myocardial infarction caused by a lesion in the proximal left anterior descending artery. ST-segment elevation is seen in leads I, aVL, and V2 through V6. (From Marx J, Hockberger R, Walls R. *Rosen's Emergency Medicine: Concepts and Clinical Practice.* 6th ed. Philadelphia: Mosby; 2006 [fig. 77.6].)

- ECG monitoring is essential. If ventricular tachycardia occurs, use amiodarone.
- Use the mnemonic **MONA BASH** to remember the eight medications that may be used to manage an MI:
  1. Control pain with **morphine**, which may improve pulmonary edema, if present.
  2. Give **oxygen** by nasal cannula and maintain an oxygen saturation >90%.
  3. Administer **nitroglycerin** unless there is evidence of right-sided heart failure; nitroglycerin in these patients will cause their blood pressure to bottom out.
  4. Administer **aspirin** (or clopidogrel).
  5. **Beta-blockers**, which patients without contraindications should take for life, reduce the mortality rate of MI as well as the incidence of a second MI.
  6. An **angiotensin-converting enzyme (ACE) inhibitor** or **angiotensin receptor blocker (ARB)** should be started within 24 hours.
  7. Administer an HMG-CoA reductase inhibitor (**statin**).
  8. Administer unfractionated or low-molecular-weight **heparin** (LMWH).

9. Which cardiac biomarker is the most sensitive for recurrent MI within a few days of the initial MI?
   CK-MB. Serum levels of CK-MB return to baseline after 48 to 72 hours; if serum levels of CK-MB are elevated >72 hours after hospital admission, the patient may have experienced a second MI.

10. When is heparin indicated in the setting of chest pain and MI?
    For unstable angina, a cardiac thrombus, or if severe congestive heart failure (CHF) is seen on echocardiogram. The USMLE Step 2 will not ask about other indications, which are not as clear-cut. Do not give heparin to patients with contraindications to its use (e.g., active bleeding).

11. What clues suggest the common noncardiac causes of chest pain?
    Gastroesophageal reflux/peptic ulcer disease: Look for a relation to certain foods (e.g., spicy foods, chocolate), smoking, caffeine, or lying down. Pain is relieved by antacids or acid-reducing medications. Patients with peptic ulcer disease often test positive for *Helicobacter pylori.*
    Chest wall pain (costochondritis, bruised or broken ribs): Pain is well localized and reproducible with chest wall palpation or with inspiration.
    Esophageal problems (achalasia, nutcracker esophagus, or esophageal spasm): This is often a difficult differential. The question will probably give a negative workup for MI or mention the lack of atherosclerosis risk factors. Look for abnormalities with barium swallow (achalasia) or esophageal manometry. Achalasia is treated with pneumatic dilatation or botulism toxin administration. Treat nutcracker esophagus or esophageal spasm with calcium channel blockers (e.g., diltiazem). If medical treatments are ineffective, endoscopic or surgical myotomy may be needed.
    Pericarditis: Look for a history suggesting viral upper respiratory infection prodrome within the last month. The ECG shows diffuse ST-segment elevation in all leads, the erythrocyte sedimentation rate is elevated, and a low-grade fever will likely be present. Classically, the pain is positional and is relieved by sitting forward. A triphasic pericardial rub is heard on auscultation. The most common cause is infection with coxsackievirus

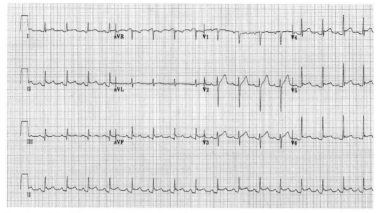

Fig. 4.2 Acute pericarditis in a 30-year-old man presenting with pleuritic chest pain. The electrocardiogram demonstrates ST-segment elevation most clearly seen in leads I, II, aVF, V3 through V6, diffuse PR-segment depression, and PR-segment elevation in lead aVR. (From Demangone D. EKG manifestations: noncoronary heart disease. *Emerg Med Clin North Am.* 2006;24(1):113 [fig. 1].)

B virus. Other causes include tuberculosis, uremia, malignancy, and lupus erythematosus or other autoimmune diseases (Fig. 4.2).

Pneumonia: Pneumonia-related chest pain is due to pleuritis. Patients may also present with cough, fever, and/or sputum production. Ask about possible sick contacts and obtain a chest radiograph.

Aortic dissection: This is associated with severe tearing or ripping pain that may radiate to the back. Look for hypertension or evidence of Marfan syndrome (tall, thin patient with hyperextensible joints). Blunt chest trauma can cause aortic laceration and pseudoaneurysm, which are different conditions that are often managed similarly (Fig. 4.3). Look for a widened mediastinum on chest radiograph.

12. **How can you recognize stable angina?**
    The chest pain of stable angina begins with exertion or stress, is reproduced predictably at the same level of exertion, and does not occur at rest or after calming down. The pain is described as a pressure or squeezing pain in the substernal area and may radiate to the shoulders, neck, and/or jaw. It is often accompanied by shortness of breath, diaphoresis, and/or nausea. The pain is usually relieved by nitroglycerin. An ECG done during an acute attack often shows ST-segment depression, but in the absence of pain the ECG is often normal. In angina, the pain should last <20 minutes or be relieved after a sublingual nitroglycerin; otherwise, suspect progression to unstable angina or MI.

13. **Define unstable angina. How is it diagnosed and treated?**
    Unstable angina is similar to the presentation of stable angina, but chest pain is present at rest. Unstable angina typically presents with normal or only minimally elevated cardiac enzymes, minor ECG changes (e.g., ST depression without evidence of ST elevation), and prolonged chest pain that may not respond to nitroglycerin. Management for unstable angina is similar to that for MI. The patient is admitted to the coronary or intensive care unit and typically receives the MONA BASH medications discussed in question 8. Consider emergent percutaneous transluminal coronary angioplasty (PTCA) if the pain does not resolve. Almost all patients have a history of stable angina with risk factors for coronary artery disease.

14. **Describe vasospastic angina (previously called Prinzmetal or variant angina).**
    This rare type of angina is characterized by pain at rest (unrelated to exertion), often occurs in the middle of the night or early morning, and presents with ST-segment elevation; cardiac enzymes are normal. Patients are usually younger, and the cause is coronary artery spasm. Vasospastic angina usually responds to nitroglycerin and is managed chronically with calcium channel blockers, which reduce arterial spasm.

15. **Define silent MI. How common is it?**
    Patients with a silent MI do not develop chest pain. They present with CHF, shock, or confusion and delirium (especially elderly patients). MIs are silent in up to 25% of cases (especially in diabetics with neuropathy). Diabetic, elderly, and female patients are more likely to experience silent or atypical MI symptoms, so have a lower threshold for checking an ECG and troponins if these patients present with vague symptoms such as abdominal discomfort, nausea, or diaphoresis.

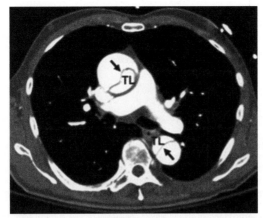

Fig. 4.3 Contrast-enhanced computed tomography scan demonstrating acute aortic dissection with enlargement of the ascending aorta and intimal flaps *(arrows)* in the ascending and descending aorta. Both the true lumen *(TL)* and the false lumen are opacified with contrast material in this example. (From Mann DL, et al. *Braunwald's Heart Disease.* 10th ed. Philadelphia: Elsevier; 2015.)

16. Describe the etiology and classic history of the various heart valve abnormalities.

Valve Problem	Etiology	History
Mitral stenosis	Rheumatic fever is most common etiology.	Dyspnea, orthopnea, and PND
Mitral regurgitation	Typically results from rheumatic fever or chordate tendineae rupture after MI.	Fatigue, dyspnea, orthopnea
Aortic stenosis	Typically seen in the elderly due to valvular calcification. Bicuspid or unicuspid valves may present with symptoms in childhood.	Usually asymptomatic for years and begins with dyspnea on exertion. Progresses to angina, syncope, and heart failure, with the mortality rate increasing through this progression.
Aortic regurgitation	**CREAM** mnemonic: **c**ongenital **r**heumatic damage, **e**ndocarditis, **a**ortic dissection/**a**ortic root dilatation, **M**arfan syndrome	Can present acutely with severe dyspnea, acute pulmonary congestion, and cardiogenic shock. Can also present chronically with DOE, orthopnea, and PND.

DOE, Dyspnea on exertion; *MI,* myocardial infarction; *PND,* paroxysmal nocturnal dyspnea.

17. What physical exam findings are associated with various heart valve abnormalities?

Valve Problem	Physical Characteristics	Other Findings
Mitral stenosis	Late diastolic blowing murmur (best heard at apex)	Opening snap, loud S1, AF, LAE, PH
Mitral regurgitation	Holosystolic murmur (radiates to axilla)	Soft S1, LAE, PH, LVH
Aortic stenosis	Harsh systolic ejection murmurs (best heard in aortic area; radiates to carotids)	Slow pulse upstroke, S3/S4, ejection click, LVH, cardiomegaly; syncope, angina, heart failure. Murmur will *increase with increased preload* (e.g., hand grip; sitting position) to distinguish AS from hypertrophic cardiomyopathy (HCM).

Valve Problem	Physical Characteristics	Other Findings
Aortic regurgitation	Early diastolic decrescendo murmur (best heard at apex); patient may be described in a vignette as "bobbing" the head.	Widened pulse pressure, LVH, LV dilatation, S3, Waterhammer pulse
Mitral prolapse	Midsystolic click, late systolic murmur	Panic disorder

AF, Atrial fibrillation; *LAE*, left atrial enlargement; *LV*, left ventricle; *LVH*, left ventricular hypertrophy; *PH*, pulmonary hypertension.

18. Describe the treatment of each of the aforementioned valvular disorders.
    Mitral stenosis is a mechanical problem that requires balloon valvotomy or surgery if it becomes severe. Medical management (diuretics, digoxin, beta-blockers) are only adjunctive to either percutaneous or surgical intervention. **Mitral regurgitation** is treated with corrective surgery if certain indications such as flail leaflet or severe regurgitation are present. Vasodilators (e.g., nitroprusside, hydralazine) may be used in symptomatic patients. Atrial fibrillation is common due to the resulting left atrial enlargement, which should be managed medically, if present. Patients with **aortic stenosis** should almost universally receive surgical aortic valve replacement. Aortic valve replacement or repair is also indicated in symptomatic patients with chronic **aortic regurgitation.** Aortic valve replacement or repair may be indicated for asymptomatic patients under certain circumstances, such as progressive left ventricular enlargement (along with specific echocardiographic findings that are beyond the scope of the USMLE). Vasodilators may be used to reduce the hemodynamic burden and possibly delay the need for surgery in asymptomatic patients.

19. True or false: An understanding of the pathophysiology behind the various changes associated with long-standing valvular heart disease is high yield for the Step 2 exam.
    True. This is not memorization, but rather the ability to fundamentally understand which physiologic or anatomic changes are associated with each type of valvular dysfunction. For example, it is advisable to understand why right-heart failure may occur with long-standing mitral stenosis.

20. Who should receive endocarditis prophylaxis?
    The American Heart Association and American College of Cardiology (AHA/ACC) recommendations from 2017 conclude that a minimal number of cases of infective endocarditis might be prevented by antibiotic prophylaxis for dental procedures. Antibiotic prophylaxis should only be considered if one of the following cardiac conditions is present prior to the dental procedure:
    - Prosthetic cardiac valve or prosthetic material used in valve repair
    - History of previous endocarditis
    - Cardiac transplantation recipients with cardiac valvular disease
    - Congenital heart disease only in the following categories:
      - Unrepaired cyanotic congenital heart disease, including those with palliative shunts and conduits
      - Completely repaired congenital heart disease with prosthetic material or device, whether placed by surgery or catheter intervention, during the first 6 months after the procedure
      - Repaired congenital heart disease with residual defects at the site or adjacent to the site of a prosthetic patch or prosthetic device (which inhibit endothelialization)
        Based on these AHA/ACC recommendations, there is no evidence to support antibiotic prophylaxis prior to genitourinary or gastrointestinal procedures.

21. Describe the protocols for endocarditis prophylaxis, if indicated.
    An antibiotic for prophylaxis should be administered in a single dose before the procedure. Amoxicillin is the preferred choice for oral therapy; cephalexin, clindamycin, azithromycin, or clarithromycin may be used in patients with penicillin allergy. Ampicillin, cefazolin, ceftriaxone, or clindamycin may be used for patients who cannot tolerate oral medication.

22. What is the Virchow triad?
    The Virchow triad describes three key predisposing factors that may lead to deep venous thrombosis (DVT): endothelial damage, venous stasis, and hypercoagulability. These three broad categories should help you remember when to think about the possibility of DVT.

23. List the common clinical scenarios leading to the development of DVT.
    - Surgery (especially orthopedic, pelvic, abdominal, or neurosurgery)
    - Malignancy
    - Trauma
    - Immobilization (e.g., hospitalization)
    - Pregnancy

- Use of birth control pills
- Disseminated intravascular coagulation
- Hypercoagulable states such as factor V (Leiden), antithrombin III deficiency, protein C deficiency, protein S deficiency, prothrombin *G20210A* gene mutation, hyperhomocysteinemia, or antiphospholipid syndrome

24. **Describe the physical signs and symptoms of DVT. How is it definitively diagnosed?**
Signs and symptoms of DVT include unilateral leg swelling, unilateral calf pain or tenderness, and/or **Homan sign** (calf tenderness with passive ankle dorsiflexion; present in 30% of cases). Superficial palpable cords imply superficial thrombophlebitis as a more likely diagnosis. DVT is best diagnosed by Doppler compression ultrasonography or by impedance plethysmography of the veins of the affected extremity. The gold standard is venography, but this invasive test is reserved for situations in which the diagnosis is not clear.

25. **True or false: Superficial thrombophlebitis is a risk factor for pulmonary embolus (PE).**
False. As the name implies, superficial thrombophlebitis (erythema, tenderness, edema, and palpable clot in a superficial vein) affects superficial veins, which pose no risk of progression to pulmonary emboli. It is considered a benign condition, although recurrent superficial thrombophlebitis can be a marker for underlying malignancy (e.g., Trousseau syndrome, or migratory thrombophlebitis, is a classic marker for pancreatic cancer). Treat affected patients with nonsteroidal antiinflammatory drugs (NSAIDs) and warm compresses.

26. **How is DVT managed? For how long?**
Systemic anticoagulation is necessary to manage DVT. Use intravenous heparin or subcutaneous LMWH initially, followed by crossover to oral warfarin. Fondaparinux and factor Xa inhibitors (rivaroxaban, apixaban) may also be used. Patients should be maintained on anticoagulation for at least 3 months and possibly for life if more than one episode of clotting occurs or other risk factors are present.

27. **What is the best way to prevent DVT in patients undergoing surgery?**
Prophylactic measures for patients undergoing surgery depend on the risk for developing deep venous thrombosis or pulmonary embolism. Early ambulation is recommended for low-risk patients. LMWH, low-dose unfractionated heparin, or fondaparinux is recommended for patients at moderate risk. High-risk patients should be given LMWH, fondaparinux, or an oral vitamin K antagonist. If the patient is at a high risk of bleeding, pneumatic compression stockings should be used instead.

28. **In what clinical settings might pulmonary embolus occur?**
PE commonly follows DVT, obstetric delivery (amniotic fluid embolus), or long-bone fractures (fat emboli). The classic patient in an exam vignette recently went on a long car ride, took a long airplane flight, or has been immobilized. Symptoms include sudden-onset tachypnea, dyspnea, chest pain, hemoptysis (if a lung infarct has occurred), hypotension, syncope, or death in severe cases. In rare instances, the chest radiograph or computed tomography (CT) scan shows a wedge-shaped defect due to pulmonary infarct, and the ECG shows evidence of right-heart strain such as the classic S1Q3T3 of a prominent S wave in lead 1 and both a Q wave and inverted T wave in lead 3.

29. **True or false: DVT typically leads to a stroke.**
False, with one rare exception. Embolization of left-sided heart clots (due to atrial fibrillation, ventricular wall aneurysm, severe CHF, or endocarditis) may cause arterial infarcts (e.g., cerebral, renal, gastrointestinal, or extremity infarcts). DVT, on the other hand, may embolize to cause pulmonary emboli—**not** arterial emboli. The one rare exception occurs in patients with a right-to-left shunt (e.g., patent foramen ovale, atrial or ventricular septal defect, or pulmonary arteriovenous fistula). In such patients, a DVT may embolize, cross through the anatomic defect, and advance into the arterial circulation, causing an arterial infarct.

30. **How is pulmonary embolism diagnosed?**
Use a CT pulmonary angiogram (Fig. 4.4) or ventilation/perfusion (V/Q) scan to evaluate for PE. If either test is positive, PE is diagnosed and treatment started. If the test is indeterminate, a conventional pulmonary angiogram is used to clinch the diagnosis. Conventional pulmonary angiography is the gold standard, but it is invasive and carries substantial risks. If a CT angiogram or V/Q scan is negative, it is highly unlikely that the patient has a significant PE, thus no treatment is needed. In the setting of a low-probability V/Q scan and high clinical suspicion, a CT angiogram or conventional pulmonary angiogram is needed.

31. **How is pulmonary embolism managed?**
Oxygenation is essential to PE management. Anticoagulants (e.g., LMWH or intravenous unfractionated heparin) are also critical in PE management to prevent further clots and emboli. The patient should be gradually switched to oral warfarin, which must be continued for at least 3 to 6 months. In patients with recurrent clots while on anticoagulation or with contraindications to anticoagulation, an inferior vena cava filter (e.g., Greenfield filter) should be placed. In patients with massive PE, embolectomy (surgical or catheter embolectomy) or pharmacologic thrombolysis (e.g., giving tissue plasminogen activator [t-PA]) may be attempted.

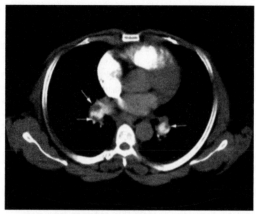

Fig. 4.4 Computed tomography pulmonary angiography showing multiple filling defects *(arrows)* consistent with pulmonary emboli within the bilateral lobar and segmental branches. (Courtesy Dr. Justin Shafa; from Ferri F. *Ferri's Clinical Advisor 2020*. Philadelphia: Elsevier; 2020:1469.e2-1469.e4.)

32. **What is the most important adverse effect of heparin to be aware of?**
Heparin can cause two types of thrombocytopenia. The first is a nonimmune form that is of no clinical consequence and is characterized by a slight reduction in platelet count during the first 2 days. This does not require intervention, as the platelet count generally returns to normal with continued heparin administration. The second form is much less common but much more serious: heparin-induced thrombocytopenia (HIT). In this immune-mediated disorder, antibodies are formed against the heparin-platelet factor 4 complex. In immune-mediated HIT, platelet count falls by >50%, typically 5 to 10 days after heparin therapy is initiated and may lead to both arterial and venous thrombosis. The diagnosis of HIT is made on clinical grounds but can be confirmed with a functional assay. If HIT is suspected, heparin (and LMWH) should be discontinued immediately. Be sure to repeatedly measure complete blood counts (CBCs) in patients receiving heparin treatment to monitor platelet counts for the possibility of HIT.

33. **How are the effects of heparin, warfarin, and aspirin monitored?**
Heparin is monitored with the **partial thromboplastin time (PTT)**, a measure of the intrinsic coagulation pathway. Warfarin is monitored with the **prothrombin time (PT)**, a measure of the extrinsic coagulation pathway. Aspirin prolongs the **bleeding time**, a measure of platelet function. Clinically, the effect of aspirin is not monitored with lab testing, but be aware that it prolongs the bleeding time test.

34. **How are the effects of LMWH monitored?**
LMWH does not significantly affect PT, PTT, or bleeding time but may be monitored using an antifactor Xa assay.

35. **In an emergency, how can you reverse the effects of heparin, warfarin, and aspirin?**
Heparin (and to some degree LMWH) can be reversed with **protamine**. Warfarin can be revered with fresh frozen plasma (FFP) and/or vitamin K. FFP contains clotting factors and has an immediate effect, while vitamin K takes a few days to work. The antiplatelet effects of aspirin may be reversed with platelet transfusions.

36. **How do the conditions listed in the table affect coagulation studies?**

Condition	Prolongs	Aids to Diagnosis
Hemophilia A	PTT	Low levels of factor VIII (think "factor ate"); normal PT and bleeding time; X linked
Hemophilia B	PTT	Low levels of factor IX; normal PT and bleeding time; X linked
vWF deficiency	Bleeding time (and PTT if severe)	Normal or low levels of factor VIII; normal PT; autosomal dominant
Disseminated intravascular coagulation (DIC)	PT, PTT, bleeding time	Positive d-dimer or FDPs; postpartum, infection, malignancy; schistocytes and fragmented cells on peripheral smear

Condition	Prolongs	Aids to Diagnosis
Liver disease	PT	PTT normal or prolonged; all factors but VIII are low; stigmata of liver disease; no correction with vitamin K
Vitamin K deficiency	PT, PTT (slight)	Normal bleeding time; low levels of factors II, VII, IX, and X, as well as proteins C and S; look for a neonate who did not receive prophylactic vitamin K; malabsorption, alcoholism, or prolonged antibiotic use (which kills vitamin K-producing bowel flora)

FDPs, Fibrin degradation products; *PT,* prothrombin time; *PTT,* partial thromboplastin time; *vWF,* von Willebrand factor. Remember that uremia causes a qualitative platelet defect and that vitamin C deficiency and chronic corticosteroid therapy can cause bleeding tendency with normal coagulation tests.

37. What are the typical signs and symptoms of congestive heart failure?
    Typical signs and symptoms of CHF include:
    - Fatigue
    - Ventricular hypertrophy on ECG
    - Dyspnea
    - S3 or S4 heart sounds
    - Cardiomegaly on chest radiograph
    - Specific left- and right-sided findings (discussed in question 38)

38. What signs and symptoms help to determine whether CHF is due to left or right ventricular failure?
    Left ventricular failure (heart failure with reduced ejection fraction [HFrEF]): orthopnea (shortness of breath when lying down; the patient sleeps on more than one pillow or even sitting up); paroxysmal nocturnal dyspnea (patients may sleep with either multiple pillows or in a reclining chair to keep themselves propped up); pulmonary congestion (bilateral basilar rales on auscultation); Kerley B lines on chest radiograph; pulmonary vascular congestion and edema; bilateral pleural effusions
    Right ventricular failure (heart failure with preserved ejection fraction [HFpEF]: peripheral edema, jugular venous distention, hepatomegaly, ascites, underlying lung disease (cor pulmonale; see question 42)

    Note: Both ventricles are commonly affected in CHF, so a mixed pattern is commonly seen. Remember that the most common cause of right-sided heart failure is left-sided heart failure.

39. How is chronic congestive heart failure treated?
    Chronic CHF is treated on an outpatient basis, with dietary modifications (e.g., sodium restriction) and medical management as the mainstay of therapy. ACE inhibitors (first-line agents proven to reduce mortality rate by preventing cardiac myocyte remodeling), beta-blockers (somewhat counterintuitive but proven to effectively manage left-sided CHF), diuretics (e.g., furosemide, spironolactone, metolazone), digoxin (not used in diastolic dysfunction; usually reserved for moderate to severe CHF with low ejection fraction or systolic dysfunction), and vasodilators (arterial and venous) may all be used.

40. How is acute congestive heart failure treated?
    Acute CHF is treated on an inpatient basis with oxygen, diuretics, and positive inotropes as the mainstay of therapy. Digoxin may be used if the patient is stable. Intravenous sympathomimetics (dobutamine, dopamine, amrinone) may be considered for severe CHF.

41. What factors precipitate CHF exacerbations in previously stable patients?
    The most common precipitator of CHF exacerbation is dietary or mediation nonadherence, but watch for **MI**, severe hypertension, arrhythmias, infections and fever, pulmonary embolus, anemia, thyrotoxicosis, and myocarditis.

42. Define cor pulmonale. With what clinical scenarios is it associated?
    Cor pulmonale is right ventricular enlargement, hypertrophy, and right-sided heart failure due to primary lung disease. Chronic lung disease leads to right heart strain, which eventually becomes right-sided heart failure. Common causes are chronic obstructive pulmonary disease (COPD) and PE, which lead to pulmonary hypertension and then cor pulmonale. Sleep apnea and obesity hyperventilation syndrome may also lead to cor pulmonale; look for an obese snorer who reports feeling sleepy during the day. Patients with cor pulmonale may have tachypnea, cyanosis, digital clubbing, parasternal heave, loud P2, and a right-sided S4 in addition to the signs and symptoms of pulmonary disease. Cor pulmonale can be managed with prostacyclins (e.g., parenteral epoprostenol), antiendothelins (e.g., bosentan), phosphodiesterase 5 inhibitors (e.g., sildenafil), and calcium channel blockers (e.g., diltiazem) while awaiting heart-lung transplantation.

43. What causes restrictive cardiomyopathy? How is it different from constrictive pericarditis?
Restrictive cardiomyopathy involves a problem with the ventricle musculature (e.g., myocardium) itself and is typically due to pathologic deposition/infiltrative disease such as amyloidosis, sarcoidosis, hemochromatosis, or myocardial fibroelastosis. A ventricular biopsy will be abnormal in all of these conditions. Cardiac magnetic resonance imaging may also be useful. **Constrictive pericarditis** occurs in a setting of completely normal myocardium, but an irritated pericardium is preventing proper ventricular filling. Constrictive pericarditis can be fixed simply by removing an abnormal pericardium; look for a pericardial knock on exam, with calcification of the pericardium, and a normal ventricular biopsy. Watch for an S4 heart sound (which indicates stiff ventricles) and signs of right-sided heart failure (e.g., jugular venous distention and peripheral edema) in both conditions. These two disorders are mentioned together because both can cause a "restrictive"-type cardiac physiology, but the etiologies and management strategies are quite different.

44. What is the most common type of cardiomyopathy? What causes it?
Dilated cardiomyopathy is the most common type of cardiomyopathy. It is most commonly caused by chronic coronary artery disease or ischemia, though by strict definition this is not a true cardiomyopathy. On the USMLE Step 2, watch for Chagas disease, alcohol abuse, myocarditis, or chronic doxorubicin use as the cause of dilated cardiomyopathy.

45. Which type of cardiomyopathy most likely causes a young person to pass out or die while exercising or playing sports? How is this condition managed?
Hypertrophic cardiomyopathy (CM), which may be autosomal dominant. This idiopathic condition causes an asymmetric ventricular hypertrophy that partially obstructs left ventricular outflow, reducing cardiac output and causing diastolic dysfunction. Look for a systolic ejection murmur along the left sternal border (similar to aortic stenosis) that decreases with increased preload (e.g., squatting, hand grip) and increases with decreased preload (e.g., standing, Valsalva maneuver). Note that this is the opposite of how aortic stenosis murmurs change with the same maneuvers. Manage HCM with beta-blockers or disopyramide (to allow the ventricle more time to fill). Competitive sports should be avoided. Surgical correction may be considered. Positive inotropes (e.g., digoxin), diuretics, and vasodilators are contraindicated because they worsen the condition.

46. What ECG abnormalities do I need to know about for USMLE Step 2? How are they treated?
Figs. 4.5 through 4.17 demonstrate the same ECG strips of the arrhythmias described in the following table. Always check for electrolyte disturbances (e.g., potassium, calcium) as a cause for any arrhythmia.

Arrhythmia	Treatment and Warnings
Atrial fibrillation	In symptomatic patients, first control the ventricular rate with a beta-blocker, nondihydropyridine calcium channel blocker, or digoxin: • If **acute** (onset <24 hr), cardiovert with amiodarone, procainamide, or DC cardioversion. • If **chronic**, first anticoagulate, then cardiovert; if this approach fails or atrial fibrillation recurs, leave the patient on rate control medications (beta-blocker, calcium channel blocker, or digoxin) and anticoagulation.
Atrial flutter	Treat like atrial fibrillation. You may try to stop the arrhythmia with vagal maneuvers (e.g., carotid massage, Valsalva maneuver).
Heart block First degree	No treatment; avoid beta-blockers and calcium channel blockers, both of which slow conduction and may worsen a first-degree block.
Second degree	For Mobitz type I (Wenckebach), use pacemaker or atropine only in symptomatic patients; remember the characteristic PR interval changes with "longer, longer, longer, drop; now you've got a Wenckebach." Use pacemaker in all patients with Mobitz type II.
Third degree	Use pacemaker.
WPW syndrome	Use **procainamide** or quinidine; avoid digoxin and verapamil.
Ventricular tachycardia	If pulseless, treat with immediate defibrillation followed by epinephrine, vasopressin, amiodarone, or lidocaine as you initiate CPR. If a pulse is present, treat with amiodarone and synchronized cardioversion.
Ventricular fibrillation	Immediate defibrillation followed by epinephrine, vasopressin, amiodarone, or lidocaine as you initiate CPR.

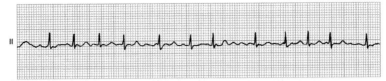

Fig. 4.5 Atrial fibrillation. There are no true P waves, and the ventricular rate is irregular. (From Goldberger AL. *Clinical Electrocardiography: A Simplified Approach.* 7th ed. Philadelphia: Mosby; 2006 [fig. 15.4].)

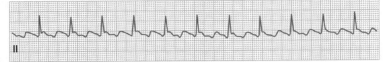

Fig. 4.6 An example of atrial flutter. In contrast to atrial fibrillation, atrial flutter is regular. The baseline has a sawtooth shape. (From Walsh D. *Palliative Medicine.* Philadelphia: Saunders; 2008 [fig. 80.2].)

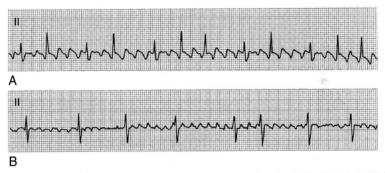

Fig. 4.7 Atrial flutter with variable block (A) and coarse atrial fibrillation (B) may be easily confused. Notice that with atrial fibrillation the ventricular rate is erratic, and the atrial waves are not identical from segment to segment, while these atrial waves are identical with atrial flutter. (From Goldberger A. *Clinical Electrocardiography: A Simplified Approach.* 7th ed. Philadelphia: Mosby; 2006 [fig. 23.3].)

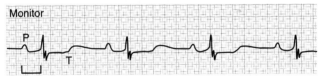

Fig. 4.8 First-degree atrioventricular block with a PR interval of 0.32 second (normal is 0.12–0.20 second). (From Goldberger E. *Treatment of Cardiac Emergencies.* 5th ed. St. Louis: Mosby; 1990.)

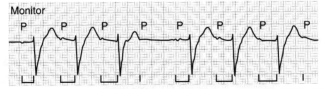

Fig. 4.9 Mobitz type I second-degree atrioventricular block (Wenckebach; a second-degree AV block in which the PR interval becomes progressively longer from cycle to cycle until the AV node no longer conducts a stimulus from above). Notice the progression of the PR interval before the impulse is completely blocked. (From Goldberger E. *Treatment of Cardiac Emergencies.* 5th ed. St. Louis: Mosby; 1990.)

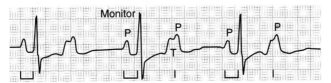

Fig. 4.10 Mobitz type II second-degree atrioventricular block (an intermittent dropped QRS). Notice that every alternate P wave is blocked (2:1 block in this case). (From Goldberger E. *Treatment of Cardiac Emergencies.* 5th ed. St. Louis: Mosby; 1990.)

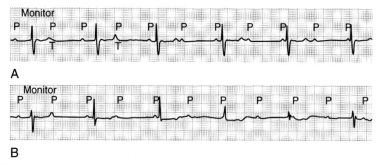

Fig. 4.11 Third-degree atrioventricular block (none of the atrial depolarizations conduct to the ventricles). Strips A and B were taken several hours apart. Strip A demonstrates an atrial rate of 75 bpm, but the ventricles are beating independently at a slow rate of approximately 40 bpm. Strip B, taken a few hours later in the same patient, demonstrates variations in the shape of QRS complex from beat to beat. (From Goldberger E. *Treatment of Cardiac Emergencies.* 5th ed. St. Louis: Mosby; 1990.)

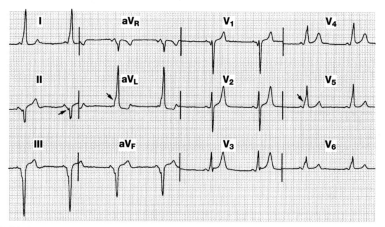

Fig. 4.12 Wolff-Parkinson-White syndrome. Triad of a wide QRS complex, a short PR interval, and delta waves *(arrows).* (From Goldberger AL. *Clinical Electrocardiography: A Simplified Approach.* 7th ed. Philadelphia: Mosby; 2006 [fig. 12.3].)

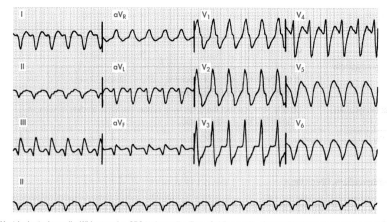

Fig. 4.13 Ventricular tachycardia. Wide complex QRS tachycardia. (From Goldberger AL. *Clinical Electrocardiography: A Simplified Approach.* 7th ed. Philadelphia: Mosby; 2006 [part 4, case 3].)

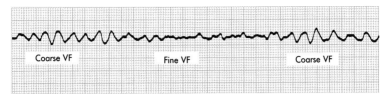

Fig. 4.14 Ventricular fibrillation. Fibrillatory waves in an irregular pattern. (From Goldberger AL. *Clinical Electrocardiography: A Simplified Approach.* 7th ed. Philadelphia: Mosby; 2006 [fig. 16.13].)

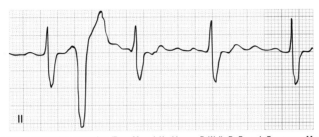

Fig. 4.15 A single premature ventricular contraction. (From Marx J, Hockberger R, Walls R. *Rosen's Emergency Medicine.* 7th ed. Mosby; 2009 [fig. 77.22].)

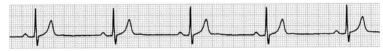

Fig. 4.16 Sinus bradycardia at a rate of about 40 beats per minute. (From Goldberger AL. *Clinical Electrocardiography: A Simplified Approach.* 8th ed. Philadelphia: Mosby; 2006 [fig. 20.1].)

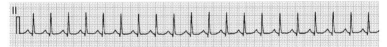

Fig. 4.17 Sinus tachycardia at a rate of about 150 beats per minute. (From Goldberger AL. *Clinical Electrocardiography: A Simplified Approach.* 8th ed. Philadelphia: Mosby; 2006 [fig. 13.2].)

Arrhythmia	*Treatment and Warnings*
PVCs	Usually not treated; if severe and symptomatic, consider beta-blockers or amiodarone.
Sinus bradycardia	Usually not treated; use atropine or pacing if severe and symptomatic (e.g., after MI). Avoid beta-blockers, calcium channel blockers, and other conduction-slowing medications.
Sinus tachycardia	Usually none; correct the underlying cause. Use beta-blocker or calcium channel blocker if symptomatic.

CPR, Cardiopulmonary resuscitation; *DC,* direct current; *PVCs,* premature ventricular complexes; *WPW,* Wolff-Parkinson-White.

47. What endocrine disease is suggested when a patient presents with sinus tachycardia or atrial fibrillation?
Hyperthyroidism. Check the level of thyroid-stimulating hormone (TSH) as a screening test.

48. Which patients with atrial fibrillation should receive anticoagulation? What medications are recommended for this purpose?
The **CHADS$_2$-VASc** score is used to estimate the risk of stroke in patients with nonrheumatic atrial fibrillation. The score is used to determine whether the patient should be managed with anticoagulation.

The points in the following table are added to determine the CHADS$_2$-VASc score.
- A **score of 0** is low risk for stroke; no anticoagulant therapy is recommended in most cases.
- A **score of 1** is moderate risk; oral anticoagulation therapy or aspirin should be considered.
- A **score of ≥2** is high risk; oral anticoagulant therapy is recommended unless contraindicated (e.g., significant fall risk; bleeding risk; use HASBLED score).

When indicated for a CHADS$_2$-VASc score of ≥2, anticoagulation by medical management has transitioned toward preferring **n**onvitamin K antagonist **o**ral **antic**oagulants (NOACs; e.g., apixaban, rivaroxaban, dabigatran) over warfarin.

	Condition	Points
C	**C**ongestive heart failure	1
H	Current **h**ypertension or taking antihypertensive medication	1
A	**A**ge >75 yr	2
D	**D**iabetes mellitus	1
S$_2$	Prior **s**troke or transient ischemic attack	2
V	**V**ascular disease	1
A	**A**ge 65–74 yr	1
Sc	Female **s**ex confers higher risk	1

49. **How does Wolff-Parkinson-White (WPW) syndrome classically present?**
A child becomes dizzy, dyspneic, or passes out after playing and then recovers and has no other symptoms. The cause is a transient reentrant tachyarrhythmia via an accessory pathway (bundle of Kent). ECG shows the pathognomonic sloping delta wave with shorted PR interval. The treatment of choice for these patients is radiofrequency catheter ablation of the pathway, but look for mentions of **procainamide** for medical management on your licensing exams.

50. **What do you need to know about the common congenital heart defects?**

Defect	Symptoms, Treatment, and Other Information
Patent ductus arteriosus (PDA)	Constant, **machine-like** murmur in upper left sternal border; dyspnea and possible CHF. Close with indomethacin or surgery (if indomethacin fails). Keep the ductus open with prostaglandin E1. Associated with congenital rubella and high altitudes. *Preserve the PDA with prostaglandins; end the PDA with indomethacin.*
Ventricular septal defect (VSD)	*Most common congenital heart defect.* Characterized by a holosystolic murmur next to sternum. Most cases resolve on their own. Watch for fetal alcohol, TORCH, or Down syndrome.
Atrial septal defect (ASD)	Often asymptomatic until adulthood. Characterized by fixed, split S2 and palpitations. Most defects do not require correction (unless very large).
Tetralogy of Fallot	*Most common cyanotic congenital heart defect.* Characterized by four anomalies: pulmonary stenosis, RVH, overriding aorta, and VSD (mnemonic: PROVe the tetralogy). Look for "tet" spells (children whose oxygenation improves with squatting).
Coarctation of aorta	Upper extremity hypertension only; radiofemoral delay; systolic murmur heard over mid-upper back; possibly cyanotic lower extremities; rib notching on radiograph; associated with Turner syndrome.

CHF, Congestive heart failure; *RVH*, right ventricular hypertrophy; *TORCH*, toxoplasma, other, rubella, cytomegalovirus, and herpes simplex.

51. Name the noncyanotic congenital heart defects
Noncyanotic heart diseases result in left-to-right shunts in which oxygenated blood from the lungs is shunted back into the pulmonary circulation, resulting in a "pink baby." These noncyanotic heart conditions can be remembered by the three Ds: VS**D**, AS**D**, and P**DA**. These risk conversion to cyanotic right-to-left shunts (Eisenmenger syndrome) if the right ventricle hypertrophies to the point that it becomes stronger than the left ventricle.

52. Name the cyanotic congenital heart defects
Cyanotic heart disease causes right-to-left shunts in which deoxygenated blood is shunted into the systemic circulation, resulting in a "blue baby." These cyanotic heart conditions can be remembered by the mnemonic **1-2-3-4-5**:
1. Truncus arteriosus: there is just **one** common vessel leaving both ventricles.
2. Transposition of the great vessels: the **two** great vessels (aorta and pulmonary artery) are transposed.
3. Tricuspid atresia: **three** for **tri**cuspid.
4. Tetralogy of Fallot: **four** for **tetra**logy.
5. Total anomalous pulmonary venous return (TAPVR): there are **five** words in TAPVR.

53. What is important to remember about tachycardia in children?
Heart rates >100 beats per minute are often normal in a child until they reach adolescence (age 12–13). Respiratory rates >20 respirations per minute are also typically normal findings unless additional clinical findings raise your suspicion for disease.

54. In the fetal circulation, where is the highest and lowest oxygen content?
The **highest** oxygen content in fetal circulation is in the **umbilical vein** (the blood coming from the mother), and the **lowest** is in the **umbilical arteries** (blood leaving fetus/placenta). Also remember that oxygen content is higher in blood going to the upper extremities than in blood going to the lower extremities.

55. What circulatory changes occur in the circulation as an infant goes from intrauterine to extrauterine life?
An infant's first breaths inflate the lungs, causing decreased pulmonary vascular resistance, which increases blood flow to the pulmonary arteries. This, along with the clamping of the umbilical cord, increases left-sided heart pressures and induces the functional closure of the foramen ovale. Increased oxygen concentration shuts off prostaglandin production in the ductus arteriosus, leading to gradual closure.

CHAPTER 5

CHOLESTEROL

1. **When is cholesterol screening done in adults? Children?**
   Although no protocol is universally accepted, measurement of total cholesterol and high-density lipoprotein (HDL) cholesterol every 5 years once a person turns 35 years old for men and 45 years old for women is considered reasonable by most authorities. Start sooner and screen more frequently for obese patients and patients with a family history of hypercholesterolemia.

   Children without risk factors for cardiovascular disease should be screened once between the ages of 9 and 11 and a second time between the ages of 17 and 21. Children with risk factors should be screened when the risk factor is first identified.

2. **Why is cholesterol so important?**
   Cholesterol is one of the main known modifiable risk factors for atherosclerosis. Atherosclerosis is involved in about one-half of all deaths in the United States and one-third of deaths between the ages of 35 and 65 years. Atherosclerosis is the most important cause of permanent disability and accounts for more hospital days than any other illness. (*Translation: Atherosclerosis and high cholesterol are high-yield USMLE topics.*)

3. **What physical findings will Step 2 test use as clues to hypercholesterolemia?**
   Xanthelasma (Fig. 5.1), tendon xanthomas (cholesterol deposits in the skin, classically over tendons in the lower extremities), corneal arcus in younger patients, "milky"-appearing serum, and obesity are possible markers for familial hypercholesterolemia. Family members should be tested if a case of familial hypercholesterolemia is found. Pancreatitis in the absence of obvious risk factors may be a marker for familial hypertriglyceridemia.

4. **What are the current recommendations for management of cholesterol levels?**
   The following information is from the 2019 American College of Cardiology/American Heart Association (ACC/AHA) Guidelines on the Treatment of Blood Cholesterol to Reduce Atherosclerotic Cardiovascular Risk in Adults. This new guideline differs from the previous recommendations in that it moves away from specific low-density lipoprotein (LDL) targets. Instead, overall LDL reductions are recommended.

Group	LDL Reduction Goal	Recommended Statin Therapy
Anyone with an LDL level ≥190 mg/dL	Reduce by >50%	High-intensity statin
Patients with diabetes aged 40–75 yr and LDL ≥70 mg/dL	Reduce by 30%–50%	Moderate-intensity statin
Anyone with 7.5%–20% chance of developing atherosclerotic CVD in the next 10 yr, using a specific calculator*	Reduce by 30%–50%	Moderate-intensity statin
Anyone with ≥20% ASCVD	Reduce LDL by ≥50%	High-intensity statin

ASCVD, Atherosclerotic cardiovascular disease; *CVD*, cardiovascular disease; *LDL*, low-density lipoprotein; *MI*, myocardial infarction; *PAD*, peripheral arterial disease.
*The Pooled Cohort Equations. Available at http://my.americanheart.org/professional/StatementsGuidelines/Preventin-Guidelines_ UCM_457698_SubHomePage.jsp.

5. **What is meant by high-intensity and moderate-intensity statins?**
   High-dose statin means a statin at a sufficient dose to reduce LDL by at least 50%. This includes atorvastatin 40 to 80 mg and rosuvastatin 20 to 40 mg. Moderate-dose statin means a statin at a sufficient dose to reduce LDL by 30% to 50%. This includes atorvastatin 10 to 20 mg, simvastatin 20 to 40 mg, rosuvastatin 5 to 10 mg, pravastatin 40 to 80 mg, and lovastatin 40 mg.

6. **List the major risk factors for coronary heart disease (CHD).**
   Although elevated levels of LDL and total cholesterol are risk factors for CHD, do not count them as risk factors when deciding to treat or not to treat high cholesterol. The following factors should be counted:
   - **Age** (men aged ≥45 years; women aged ≥55 years or with premature menopause and no estrogen replacement therapy)
   - **Family history of premature heart attacks** (defined as definite myocardial infarction or sudden death in father or first-degree male relative <55 years old or mother or first-degree female relative <65 years old)
   - **Cigarette smoking**
   - **Hypertension** (≥140/90 mm Hg or prescription for antihypertensive medications)

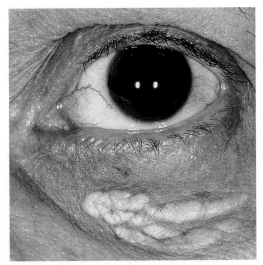

Fig. 5.1 Xanthelasma. Multiple soft yellow plaques involving the lower eyelid. Xanthelasma is usually a normal finding with no significance but is classically seen on the USMLE because of its association with hypercholesterolemia. Screen affected patients with a fasting lipid profile. (From Yanoff M, Duker JS. *Ophthalmology.* 3rd ed. Philadelphia: Mosby; 2008 [fig. 12.9.18].)

- **Diabetes mellitus**
- **Low HDL** (<40 mg/dL)
  Note: An HDL level of ≥60 mg/dL is considered protective and negates one risk factor.

7. Discuss other possible risk factors for heart disease.
   The 2019 ACC/AHA cholesterol guidelines address other factors that may indicate an elevated risk for atherosclerotic cardiovascular disease (ASCVD). In selected individuals who are in one of the four statin benefit groups and for whom a decision to initiate statin therapy is otherwise unclear, additional factors may be considered to inform treatment decision making. These factors include:
   - Primary LDL ≥160 mg/dL
   - Family history of premature ASCVD with onset age <55 years in a first-degree male relative or <65 years in a first-degree female relative
   - Comorbid conditions such as chronic kidney disease, metabolic syndrome, inflammatory diseases (e.g., rheumatoid arthritis, psoriasis, human immunodeficiency virus)
   - Ethnicity (i.e. South Asian ancestry)
   - Triglycerides ≥175 mg/dL
   - Lipoprotein(a) >50 mg/dL or 125 nmol/L
   - Apolipoprotein B (apoB) ≥130 mg/dL
   - High-sensitivity C-reactive protein ≥2 mg/L
   - Coronary artery calcium (CAC) score ≥100 Agatston units or ≥75th percentile for age, sex, and ethnicity
   - Ankle-brachial index >0.9
   - Elevated lifetime risk of ASCVD (yes, this is vague)

8. How is LDL calculated?
   Lipoprotein analysis involves measuring total cholesterol, HDL, and triglycerides. LDL can then be calculated from the following formula:

   $$LDL = total\ cholesterol - HDL - (triglycerides/5)$$

9. How is HDL affected by alcohol? Estrogens? Exercise? Smoking? Progesterone?
   High HDL is protective against atherosclerosis and is increased by moderate alcohol consumption (one to two drinks/day) but not by high alcohol intake, exercise, and estrogens. HDL is decreased by smoking, androgens, progesterone, and hypertriglyceridemia.

10. What causes hypercholesterolemia?
    Genetics certainly plays a role, but most cases are thought to be multifactorial. The most common secondary causes of increased cholesterol are uncontrolled diabetes and excessive alcohol intake. Other secondary causes include hypothyroidism, uremia, nephrotic syndrome, obstructive liver disease, excessive alcohol intake (which increases triglycerides), and medications (e.g., birth control pills, glucocorticoids, thiazides, beta-blockers).

11. What are some other medications that affect cholesterol metabolism?

Medication Class	Examples	Mechanism of Action	Lipid Effect	Side Effects
Fibrates	Gemfibrozil, fenofibrate	Lipoprotein lipase activator	↓TGs, ↑HDL	Myositis (↑ risk with concomitant statin use), hepatitis, GI upset, cholelithiasis
Cholesterol absorption inhibitors	Ezetimibe	Inhibits absorption of cholesterol in small intestine	↓LDL	Diarrhea, abdominal pain
Bile acid resins	Cholestyramine, colestipol, colesevelam	Binds bile in the gastrointestinal tract to prevent reabsorption	↓LDL	GI side effects
Niacin	Niacin, Niaspan (extended release)		↓TGs, ↓LDL, ↑HDL	Facial flushing (can be prevented with aspirin)
PCSK9 inhibitors	Evolocumab, alirocumab	Inhibit PCSK9, which is a protein responsible for degrading LDL-Rs	↓↓LDL	Injection site swelling, rash, myalgias

GI, Gastrointestinal; *HDL,* high-density lipoprotein; *LDL,* low-density lipoprotein; *LDL-Rs,* low-density lipoprotein receptors; *PCSK9,* proprotein convertase subtilisin/kexin type 9 serine protease; *TGs,* triglycerides.

CHAPTER 6

DERMATOLOGY

1. Cover the two right-hand columns and define the following common terms used in dermatology to describe skin findings:

Term	Definition	Examples
Macule	Flat spot <1 cm (nonpalpable, just visible)	Freckles, tattoos
Patch	Same as macule but >1 cm	Port-wine birthmarks
Papule	Solid, elevated lesion <1 cm (palpable)	Wart, acne, lichen planus
Plaque	Same as papule but >1 cm and flat topped	Psoriasis
Nodule	Palpable, solid lesion >1 cm and not flat topped	Small lipoma, erythema nodosum
Vesicle	Elevated, circumscribed lesion <5 mm containing clear fluid (small blister)	Chickenpox, genital herpes
Bulla	Same as vesicle but >5 mm (large blister)	Contact dermatitis, pemphigus
Wheal	Itchy, evanescent, transiently edematous area	Allergic reaction

2. Define vitiligo. With what diseases is it associated? What is the treatment?
Vitiligo is characterized by well-demarcated macules or patches of skin depigmentation due to autoimmune destruction of melanocytes of unknown etiology (Fig. 6.1). It is an acquired condition associated with autoimmune diseases such as pernicious anemia, hypothyroidism, Addison disease, and type I diabetes. Patients often have antibodies to melanin, parietal cells, thyroid, or other factors. Vitiligo can be treated with topical corticosteroids, topical calcineurin inhibitors (e.g., tacrolimus, pimecrolimus), and phototherapy.

3. Name several conditions to think about on the Step 2 exam in patients with pruritus
Think of serious conditions first, such as obstructive biliary disease, uremia, and polycythemia rubra vera (classically seen after a warm shower or bath due to mast cell degranulation). Pruritus may also be caused by contact or atopic dermatitis, scabies, and lichen planus.

4. Define contact dermatitis. How do you recognize it? What are the classic culprits?
Contact dermatitis is usually due to a type IV hypersensitivity reaction, although it may also be due to an irritating or toxic substance. Look for a new exposure to a classic offending agent, such as poison ivy, nickel earrings, or deodorant. Allergic contact dermatitis requires a previous sensitizing event as opposed to irritant contact dermatitis, which does not. The rash is well circumscribed and occurs only in the area of exposure. The skin is red and itchy and often has vesicles or bullae (Fig. 6.2). Avoidance of the agent is required. Patch testing can be done, if needed, to determine the antigen.

5. Define atopic dermatitis. What history points to this diagnosis? What is the treatment?
Atopic dermatitis, also known as eczema, is a chronic allergic-type condition that begins in the first year of life with red, itchy, weeping skin on the head, upper extremities on extensor surfaces, and sometimes around the diaper area. In children and adults, it usually develops on the flexor surfaces. The clue to diagnosis is a family and/ or personal history of allergies (e.g., hay fever) and asthma. The biggest problem is scratching of affected skin, which leads to skin breaks and possible bacterial infection. Treatment involves avoidance of drying soaps and use of antihistamines, moisturizing creams, topical steroids, and immune modulating agents (topical pimecrolimus or tacrolimus).

6. Define seborrheic dermatitis. What part of the body does it involve? How is it treated?
Seborrheic dermatitis causes the common conditions known as cradle cap and dandruff as well as blepharitis (eyelid inflammation). Look for scaling skin with or without erythema on the hairy areas of the head (scalp, eyebrows, eyelashes, mustache, beard) as well as on the forehead, nasolabial folds, external ear canals, and postauricular creases (Fig. 6.3). Treat with dandruff shampoo (e.g., selenium sulfide or tar shampoo), topical corticosteroids, and/or ketoconazole cream.

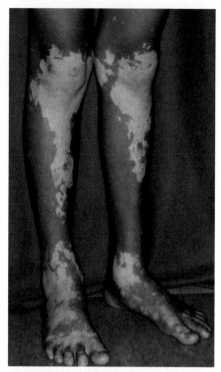

Fig 6.1 Vitiligo. Symmetric depigmentation of the knees and lower extremities. (From Paller AS, Mancini AJ. *Hurwitz Clinical Pediatric Dermatology, A Textbook of Skin Disorders of Childhood and Adolescence.* 5th ed. Philadelphia: Elsevier; 2016.)

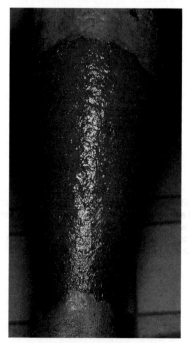

Fig. 6.2 Allergic contact dermatitis of the leg caused by an elastic wrap. Notice the well-marginated distribution that differentiates it from cellulitis. (From Auerbach PS. *Wilderness Medicine.* 6th ed. Philadelphia: Mosby; 2011.)

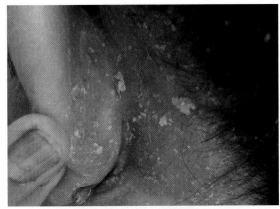

Fig. 6.3 Adult seborrheic dermatitis. Fairly sharply demarcated pink plaque with white and greasy scale. Note the fissure in the retroauricular fold. (From Bolognia J, Schaffer J. *Dermatology Essentials*. Philadelphia: Saunders; 2014:103-108. Photo courtesy of Norbert Reider, MD, and Peter O Fritcsch, MD.)

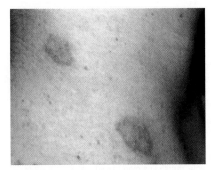

Fig. 6.4 Tinea corporis. Red ring-shaped lesions with scaling and some central clearing. (From Kliegman RM. *Nelson Textbook of Pediatrics*. 19th ed. Philadelphia: Saunders; 2011.)

7. Name the various dermatologic fungal infections

Known as dermatophytosis, tinea, and ringworm. Fungal infections include the following:

Tinea corporis (body/trunk): look for red ring-shaped lesions with raised borders that tend to clear centrally while they expand peripherally (Fig. 6.4).

Tinea pedis (athlete's foot): look for macerated, scaling web spaces between the toes that often itch and may be associated with thickened, distorted toenails (onychomycosis). It may be acquired from using locker rooms or swimming pools. Treatment includes good foot hygiene and disposal of old footwear (or treatment with antifungal powder).

Tinea unguium (onychomycosis): thickened, distorted, and discolored nails with debris under the nail edges.

Tinea capitis (scalp): mainly affects children (highly contagious), who have scaly patches of hair loss with residual "black dots" in the affected area and may have an inflamed, boggy granuloma of the scalp (known as a kerion) that usually resolves on its own.

Tinea cruris (jock itch): more common in obese males; is usually found in the crural folds of the upper, inner thighs. Increased prevalence in patients with diabetes or other immunodeficiency.

8. What organisms cause fungal infections?

Most fungal infections are due to *Trichophyton* species. In tinea capitis, if the hair fluoresces green under the Wood lamp, *Microsporum* species is the cause; if not, it is probably *Trichophyton*.

9. How are fungal infections diagnosed and treated?

Formal diagnosis of any fungal infection can be made by scraping the lesion and doing a potassium hydroxide (KOH) preparation to visualize the fungus via a microscope or by doing a culture. Because they are so common clinically, empiric treatment without a formal diagnosis is common, but for the United States Medical Licensing

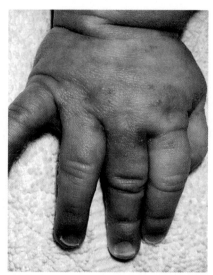

Fig. 6.5 Scabies. Itchy papules and pustules on the web spaces of the hand. (From Paige D, Wakelin S. *Kumar and Clark's Clinical Medicine*. Philadelphia: Elsevier; 2017:1337–1386.)

Examination (USMLE), get a formal diagnosis before treating. Oral antifungals (e.g., griseofulvin) must be used to treat tinea capitis and onychomycosis; the others can be treated with topical antifungals (imidazoles such as miconazole, clotrimazole, and ketoconazole or allylamines such as terbinafine) or oral griseofulvin, which is better for severe or persistent infections.

10. True or false: Candidiasis is often a normal finding in some women and children
    True. Oral thrush (creamy white patches on the tongue or buccal mucosa that can be scraped off) is seen in normal children, and *Candida* vulvovaginitis is seen in normal women, especially during pregnancy or after taking antibiotics. However, at other time periods and in different patients, candidal infections may be a sign of diabetes or immunodeficiency; for example, thrush in a man should make you think about the possibility of AIDS, and recurrent vulvovaginal candidiasis should prompt screening for diabetes.

11. How is candidiasis diagnosed and treated?
    Diagnose with KOH prep and look for pseudohyphae. Treat with local/topical nystatin or imidazoles (e.g., miconazole, clotrimazole). Oral therapy (nystatin or ketoconazole) is used for extensive or resistant disease.

12. What causes scabies? How do you recognize it?
    Scabies is caused by the mite *Sarcoptes scabiei*, which tunnels into the skin and leaves visible burrows on the skin, classically in the finger web spaces and flexor surface of the wrists (Fig. 6.5). You should know what these burrows look like. Facial involvement is sometimes seen in infants. Patients also have severe pruritus, and scratching can lead to secondary bacterial infection. Crusted or Norwegian scabies typically occurs in patients who are immunocompromised, elderly, or living in institutions. In this form of scabies, there are hundreds to thousands of mites in the skin (as opposed to 15–20 with regular scabies), leading to a scaly rash or plaque, which may resemble psoriasis.

13. How do you diagnose and treat scabies?
    Diagnosis is made by scraping a mite out of a burrow and viewing it under a microscope, though it is often a clinical diagnosis. Treat scabies with 5% permethrin cream applied to the whole body. Remember to treat all contacts (e.g., the whole family). Do *not* use lindane unless permethrin is not an option. Lindane used to be the treatment of choice but can cause neurotoxicity, especially in young children. Oral ivermectin can also be used. Close contacts may also require treatment. The patient's clothing, bedding, and towels must be cleaned or placed in a plastic bag for >3 days (mites can only live for 2–3 days away from human skin) to prevent reinfection.

14. How do you recognize and treat tinea versicolor?
    Tinea versicolor (also known as pityriasis versicolor) is usually caused by the *Malassezia globosa* fungus, presenting most commonly with multiple patches of various size and color (brown, tan, and white) on the torso of young adults (Fig. 6.6). It often becomes noticeable in the summer because the affected areas fail to tan and look white. Diagnose from lesion scrapings (KOH preparation yields septated hyphae and yeast in a "spaghetti and meatball" pattern). Treat with selenium sulfide shampoo or topical imidazoles.

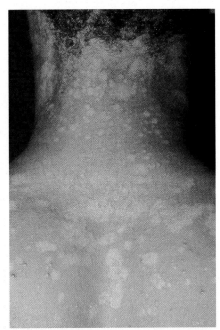

Fig. 6.6 Tinea versicolor. Hypopigmented macules and patches of seborrheic areas of the trunk. (From Paller AS, Mancini AJ. *Hurwitz Clinical Pediatric Dermatology, A Textbook of Skin Disorders of Childhood and Adolescence.* 5th ed. Philadelphia: Elsevier; 2016.)

15. **What causes lice? How is lice treated?**
    Lice (pediculosis) can involve the hair of the head (caused by *Pediculus capitis;* common in school-aged children), body (caused by *Pediculus corporis;* unusual in people with good hygiene), or pubic area (crabs, caused by *Phthirus pubis* and transmitted sexually). Infected areas tend to itch. Diagnosis is made by seeing the lice (live mites or nits) on hair shafts. Treat with permethrin cream (preferred over lindane because of lindane's neurotoxicity) and decontaminate sources of reinfection (wash or sterilize combs, hats, bed sheets, clothing).

16. **What causes warts? How are they treated?**
    Warts are caused by the human papillomavirus (HPV). They are infectious and are most commonly seen in older children, classically on the hands. They are spread by skin-to-skin contact. The most common serotypes are 6 and 11. Multiple treatments are available, including salicylic acid, liquid nitrogen, curettage, cytostatic treatment (5-fluorouracil, trichloroacetic acid), and immune response modifiers (imiquimod and interferon-α). Genital warts are also caused by HPV. Approximately 15 of the HPV serotypes are considered to be high-risk types for the development of cervical cancer; serotypes 16 and 18 are associated with the majority of cases of cervical cancer.

17. **Define molluscum contagiosum. How do you recognize it? How is it treated?**
    Molluscum contagiosum is a poxvirus infection that is common in children but may also be sexually transmitted. Diagnosis is made by the characteristic appearance of the lesions (skin-colored, smooth, waxy, dome-shaped papules with a central depression [umbilicated] that are roughly 0.5 cm) or by looking at contents of the lesion, which include cells with characteristic inclusion bodies (Fig. 6.7). The usual treatment is freezing or curettage. Consider immunodeficiency if the lesions are giant or very diffuse.

18. **True or false: A child with genital molluscum is probably a victim of sexual abuse**
    False. A child who has genital molluscum may or may not have contracted the disease from sexual contact. The more common mechanism is autoinoculation, in which the child has a lesion on the hand that spreads to the genital area from scratching. Do *not* automatically assume child abuse, although it must be ruled out.

19. **How is acne described in medical terms? What bacteria may be partially involved in its pathogenesis?**
    Acne vulgaris can be broken down into various subtypes, including comedonal, inflammatory, and nodular (cystic) acne. Comedonal acne presents with closed (whitehead) or open (blackhead) comedones primarily on the forehead, nose, and chin. Inflammatory acne presents with small (<5 mm), erythematous papules and pustules. Nodular (cystic) acne presents with large (>5 mm) nodules that may merge to form sinus tracts and subsequent scarring. *Propionibacterium acnes* is thought to be partially involved in pathogenesis, as is blockage of pilosebaceous glands.

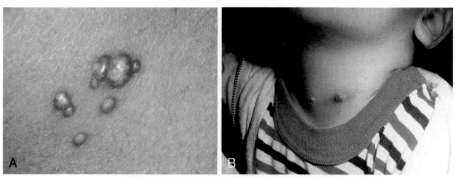

Fig. 6.7 Molluscum contagiosum. (A) Multiple papules of molluscum contagiosum demonstrating a characteristic central keratotic core. (B) Inflammatory molluscum contagiosum in a young child demonstrating both small, waxy, umbilicated papules and an inflammatory lesion simulating a furuncle. (From Nguyn N, Reed B. *Dermatology Secrets Plus*. Philadelphia: Elsevier; 2016:229-234. A, Courtesy James E. Fitzpatrick MD; B, courtesy Fitzsimons Army Medical Center teaching files.)

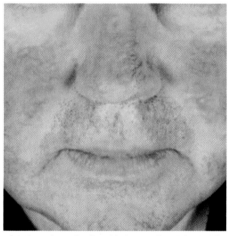

Fig. 6.8 Rosacea. Telangiectasias and erythema due to chronic actinic damage. (From Bolognia J, Schaffer J. *Dermatology Essentials*. Phildelphia: Saunders; 2014:261-267.)

20. True or false: Acne is not related to food, exercise, or sex
    True. Acne has *not* been proven to be related to food, exercise, or sex (including masturbation). However, if the patient relates acne to a food, you can try discontinuing it. Cosmetics may aggravate acne.

21. What are the treatment options for acne?
    Treatment options are multiple. Start with topical retinoids and salicylic or azelaic acids; then try topical benzoyl peroxide, topical clindamycin or erythromycin, either with or without an oral antibiotic (typically a tetracycline or erythromycin for *Propionibacterium acnes* eradication). Oral isotretinoin is the *last resort*. Although highly effective, isotretinoin is teratogenic; pregnancy testing in women before and during therapy as well as contraceptive use is mandatory. Women of childbearing age must be on two forms of contraception. In addition, it may cause dry skin and mucosae, muscle and joint pain, and liver function test abnormalities.

22. Define rosacea. In what age group is it seen? How do you treat it?
    Rosacea often looks like acne but begins in middle age. There are several different subtypes (papulopustular, erythematotelangiectasia, ocular) of rosacea. The most common is the papulopustular subtype. Typically, patients present with facial erythema and flushing (Fig. 6.8). There are numerous triggers for rosacea, including sun exposure, emotional stress, alcohol consumption, spicy foods, and hot weather. Also look for **rhinophyma** (bulbous red nose) and coexisting blepharitis. Treat the papulopustular subtype with topical metronidazole or oral tetracycline. Treat the erythematotelangiectasia subtype with topical brimonidine. The pathogenesis is incompletely understood.

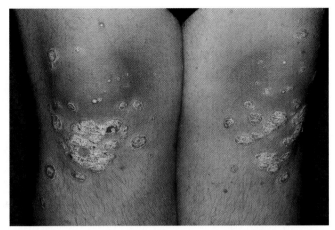

Fig. 6.9 Typical plaques of psoriasis with thick scale overlying erythema. (From Paller AS, Mancini AJ. *Hurwitz Clinical Pediatric Dermatology, A Textbook of Skin Disorders of Childhood and Adolescence.* 5th ed. Philadelphia: Elsevier; 2016.)

23. **What should you think about if hirsutism is described on the Step 2 exam?**
    Hirsutism is most commonly idiopathic, but other signs of virilization (e.g., deepening voice, clitoromegaly, frontal balding) suggest an androgen-secreting ovarian tumor (check serum androgen levels). The most common cause of hirsutism in a female is polycystic ovary syndrome. Also consider Cushing syndrome and drugs (minoxidil, corticosteroids, and phenytoin).

24. **What are the common pathologic causes of baldness?**
    Watch out for trichotillomania (a psychiatric disorder in which patients pull out their hair; baldness is patchy and irregular), alopecia areata (idiopathic but associated with antimicrosomal and other autoantibodies), and telogen effluvium (caused by stress). Baldness may also be seen in patients with lupus erythematosus or syphilis and after cancer chemotherapy.

25. **What causes ordinary male pattern baldness?**
    Although the exact pathophysiology is still not clear, male pattern baldness is considered a genetic disorder that requires androgens for expression.

26. **Describe the classic psoriatic lesion**
    Psoriatic lesions are classically described as dry, well-circumscribed, erythematous, silvery, scaling papules and plaques that are *not* pruritic (Fig. 6.9). Classic lesions are found on the scalp, lumbosacral region, intergluteal clefts, and extensor surfaces of the elbows and knees. Look for Auspitz sign, which is a small amount of bleeding when a psoriatic scale is scraped away. It is caused by abnormal proliferation of keratinocytes.

27. **What other historical points and physical findings may be seen with psoriasis? How is it diagnosed and treated?**
    A family history of psoriasis is often present, and the disease mostly occurs in Whites with onset in early adulthood. Affected patients may have pitting of the nails and an arthritis that resembles rheumatoid arthritis but is rheumatoid factor negative. Diagnosis of psoriasis can often be made by appearance alone, but a biopsy can be used in doubtful cases. Certain types of psoriasis are associated with infectious causes. For example, diffuse, sudden-onset psoriasis is associated with human immunodeficiency virus (HIV) infection. Guttate psoriasis (scaly, droplike plaques/papules) typically occurs after a streptococcal infection. Treatment is complex but involves exposure to ultraviolet light, lubricants, topical corticosteroids, calcipotriene, and keratolytics (e.g., coal tar, salicylic acid, anthralin). Oral therapies may include immunosuppressive and immunomodulating drugs such as methotrexate, cyclosporine, and biologic agents.

28. **Give the classic description and natural course of pityriasis rosea**
    Pityriasis rosea is typically seen in young adults. Look for a herald patch (slightly erythematous, scaly, ring-shaped or oval patch classically seen on the trunk), followed 1 week later by many similar lesions that tend to itch (Fig. 6.10). Look for lesions on the back with a long axis that parallels the Langerhans skin cleavage lines, typically in a Christmas tree pattern. The condition usually remits spontaneously in about 1 month. The etiology is unknown, but some think it is related to human herpesvirus 6 (HHV-6) and HHV-7. Think about syphilis (which presents with a maculopapular rash in the secondary form) in the differential diagnosis. Treat with reassurance.

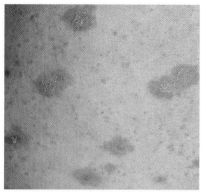

Fig. 6.10 Pityriasis rosea. Both small, oval plaques and multiple, small papules are present. (From Habif TP. *Clinical Dermatology.* 5th ed. St. Louis: Mosby; 2009.)

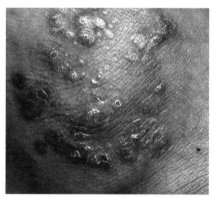

Fig. 6.11 Lichen planus. Flat-topped, purple polygonal papules of lichen planus. (From Kliegman RM. *Nelson Textbook of Pediatrics.* 19th ed. Philadelphia: Saunders; 2011.)

29. What are the four Ps that clinch a diagnosis of lichen planus?
    Pruritic, **p**urple, **p**olygonal **p**apules (or plaques) classically on the wrists, lower legs, or genitalia, usually of adults (Fig. 6.11). Oral mucosal lesions with a whitish, lacelike pattern (Wickham striae) may also be present. These oral lesions must be monitored as they may increase the risk for oral cancer. It is associated with hepatitis C virus (HCV) infection.

30. List the classic drugs that cause photosensitivity of the skin
    Tetracyclines, phenothiazines, and birth control pills. Other drugs include furosemide, hydrochlorothiazide, antipsychotics (chlorpromazine, prochlorperazine), fluoroquinolones, amiodarone, and promethazine.

31. Describe the classic lesion of erythema multiforme. What drugs classically cause it?
    Look for the classic target (iris) lesions (Fig. 6.12). The classic cause is sulfa drugs or penicillins, but herpes infections may also cause erythema multiforme, and some cases are idiopathic. Erythema multiforme exists on a spectrum. As it becomes more severe and widespread, it is known as **Stevens-Johnson syndrome (SJS)**, which is often fatal. SJS encompasses <10% of skin. Patients with SJS are treated supportively with therapy similar to what a burn victim would receive (wound care, fluid and electrolyte management, pain control, nutritional support, and monitoring for and treatment of superinfections). If >30% of skin is involved, it is classified as toxic epidermal necrolysis.

32. Describe the classic lesion of erythema nodosum. With what diseases is it commonly associated? What should the workup include?
    Erythema nodosum (Fig. 6.13) is an inflammation of the subcutaneous tissue and skin, classically over the shins (pretibial). Look for tender, red, elevated nodules. Sarcoidosis, coccidioidomycosis, or ulcerative colitis classically accompany this condition on the USMLE, though multiple other infections (e.g., streptococcal, tuberculosis [TB]) and drugs (e.g., sulfonamides) can also result in this finding. The most common vasculitis associated

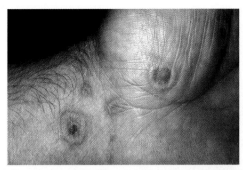

Fig. 6.12 Erythema multiforme. Bull's-eye annular lesions with central vesicles and bullae. (From Goldman L. *Goldman's Cecil Medicine.* 24th ed. Philadelphia: Saunders; 2011.)

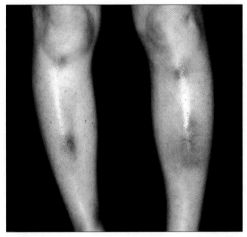

Fig. 6.13 Erythema nodosum on the legs of a young woman. (From Hochberg MC. *Rheumatology.* 5th ed. Philadelphia: Mosby; 2010.)

with it is Behcet disease. Treat the underlying disease and provide symptomatic therapies such as nonsteroidal antiinflammatory drugs (NSAIDs), leg elevation, and compressive bandages. The workup should include basic laboratory testing, TB skin testing, antistreptolysin-O antibodies, and a chest x-ray to look for sarcoidosis and TB.

33. Define and describe pemphigus vulgaris. How is it different from bullous pemphigoid?
    Pemphigus vulgaris is a potentially life-threatening autoimmune disease of middle-aged and elderly patients. It presents with multiple flaccid bullae, starting in the oral mucosa and spreading to the skin of the rest of the body. These bullae rupture easily. Look for Nikolsky sign, which is sloughing and ulcerations that occur when minor pressure is applied to the skin. Biopsy can be stained for antibody (an IgG antibody to desmoglein III, which is associated with desmosomes) and shows a lacelike or fishnet immunofluorescence pattern. Tombstone cells are seen on histology. Treat with oral corticosteroids.

    Bullous pemphigoid is a similar but milder condition that often presents as multiple tense bullae all over the body. Biopsy reveals a linear immunofluorescence pattern (different antibody), and this condition is also treated with oral corticosteroids (Fig. 6.14). Nikolsky sign is not present with bullous pemphigoid. Bullous pemphigoid is due to antibodies directed against the hemidesmosome. It is associated with certain neurologic diseases (Parkinson disease, multiple sclerosis) and malignancy. Treat with topical corticosteroids.

34. What skin disease is associated with celiac disease (gluten intolerance or sensitivity)? How is it treated?
    Dermatitis herpetiformis is associated with celiac disease. Patients have intensely pruritic vesicles, papules, and wheals on the extensor aspects of the elbows and knees and possibly on the face or neck (Fig. 6.15). Look for diarrhea and weight loss (due to gluten sensitivity). On biopsy, the skin has IgA deposits even in unaffected areas. Test for celiac disease, and treat both conditions with a gluten-free diet. Additionally, dapsone can be used for acute treatment.

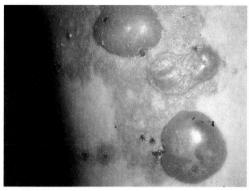

Fig. 6.14 Bullous pemphigoid. Tense subepidermal bullae on an erythematous base. (From Goldman L. *Goldman's Cecil Medicine*. 24th ed. Philadelphia: Saunders; 2011.)

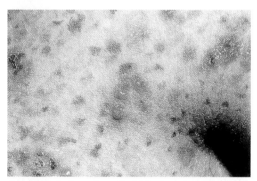

Fig. 6.15 Dermatitis herpetiformis is characterized by pruritus, urticarial papules, and small vesicles. (From Feldman M. *Sleisenger and Fordtran's Gastrointestinal and Liver Disease*. 9th ed. Philadelphia: Saunders; 2010. Courtesy of Dr. Timothy Berger, San Francisco, CA.)

35. What are decubitus ulcers? What is the best method of prevention?
    Decubitus ulcers (bedsores or pressure sores) are skin ulcers caused by prolonged pressure against the skin. The best treatment is prophylaxis. Periodic turning of paralyzed, bedridden, or debilitated patients (the populations in which they are most common) and use of special air mattresses prevents bedsores. Cleanliness and dryness also help to prevent decubitus ulcers. Periodic skin inspection ensures that the problem is recognized early. When missed, the lesions can ulcerate down to the bone and become infected, possibly leading to sepsis and death. Treat major skin breaks with aggressive surgical debridement; if signs of infection are present, administer antibiotics.

36. How are decubitus ulcers staged?
    Stage 1 is intact skin with nonblanchable redness of a localized area. Stage 2 is partial-thickness loss of the dermis presenting as a shallow open ulcer. These may also present as an intact or ruptured blister. Stage 3 is full-thickness tissue loss. Subcutaneous fat may be visible, but bone, tendon, or muscle is not exposed. Stage 4 is full-thickness skin loss with exposed bone, tendon, or muscle. An unstageable ulcer has full-thickness loss in which the base of the ulcer is covered with slough or eschar. The true depth of the ulcer cannot be determined until the slough or eschar is removed.

37. What conditions should excessive perspiration suggest on the USMLE?
    We all know people who sweat too much for no apparent reason. On the Step 2 exam, however, look for a serious cause, such as a myocardial infarction, tuberculosis or infection, hyperthyroidism, or pheochromocytoma.

38. True or false: Most melanomas start out as simple moles
    True. Moles are common and benign, but malignant transformation is possible (Fig. 6.16). **ABCDE characteristics of a mole** that should make you suspicious of malignant transformation: **a**symmetry, **b**orders (irregular), **c**olor (change in color or multiple colors), **d**iameter (the bigger the lesion, the more likely that it is malignant), and **e**volution over time. Excise any mole (or do a biopsy if the lesion is very large) if it enlarges suddenly, develops irregular borders, darkens or becomes inflamed, changes color (even if only one small area of the mole changes color), begins to bleed, begins to itch, or becomes painful.

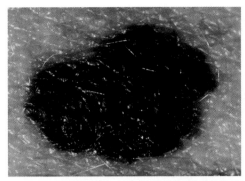

Fig. 6.16 Melanoma (superficial spreading type). (From Goldman L, Schafer AL. *Goldman's Cecil Medicine*. 24th ed. Philadelphia: Saunders; 2011.)

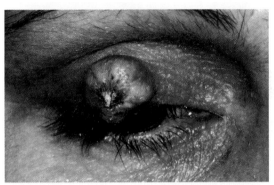

Fig. 6.17 Keratoacanthoma on the right upper lid. Lesions are solitary, smooth, dome-shaped red papules or nodules with a central keratin plug. (From Albert DM. Albert & Jakobiec's Principles and Practice of Ophthalmology. 3rd ed. Philadelphia: Saunders; 2008.)

39. **Define dysplastic nevi syndrome. How is it managed?**
Dysplastic nevus syndrome is a genetic condition with multiple dysplastic-appearing nevi (usually >100 moles). Also look for a family history of melanoma. Treat with careful and regular follow-up, excision or biopsy of any suspicious lesions, avoidance of sun exposure, and sunscreen use.

40. **Why is keratoacanthoma of note?**
Keratoacanthoma can mimic skin cancer (especially squamous cell cancer). Look for a flesh-colored lesion with a central crater that contains keratinous material, classically on the face (Fig. 6.17). Keratoacanthoma has a very rapid onset and grows to its full size in 1–2 months (which almost never happens with squamous cell cancer). The lesion involutes spontaneously in a few months and requires no treatment. If unsure, the best step is a biopsy, but choose observation as the answer in patients with a classic history of keratoacanthoma.

41. **When and where are keloids seen?**
Keloids are overgrowths of scar tissue after an injury and extend beyond the margins of the original wound. They are seen most frequently in Blacks. They are usually slightly pink and classically appear on the upper back, chest, and deltoid area. Also look for keloids to develop after ear piercing (Fig. 6.18). Do not excise these lesions because it may worsen scarring.

42. **Describe the classic lesion of basal cell cancer. What should you do if you suspect it?**
Basal cell cancer classically begins as a shiny papule on a skin-exposed area (the head is classic) and slowly enlarges and develops an umbilicated center with pearly borders (and later may ulcerate and bleed easily) with peripheral telangiectasias (Fig. 6.19). Like all skin cancers, sunlight exposure increases the risk. It is more common in elderly, light-skinned people. Treat with excision. Biopsy any suspicious skin lesions in the elderly. It is the most common type of skin cancer.

43. **True or false: Basal cell skin cancer almost never develops metastases**
True. However, it may be locally invasive and destructive.

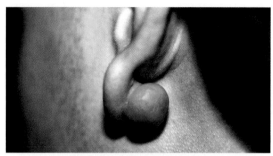

Fig. 6.18 Keloid of the ear lobe after piercing. (From Kliegman RM, Stanton BF, St. Geme JW, et al. *Nelson Textbook of Pediatrics*. 19th ed. Philadelphia: Saunders; 2011.)

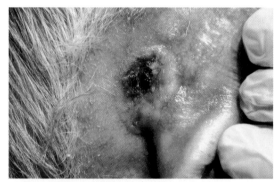

Fig. 6.19 An ulcerated basal cell carcinoma with rolled borders on the posterior ear. (From Abeloff DA, Armitage JO, Nienderhuber JE. *Abeloff's Clinical Oncology*. 4th ed. Philadelphia: Churchill Livingstone; 2008.)

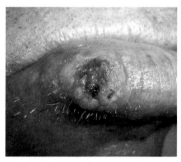

Fig. 6.20 Squamous cell carcinoma on the lower lip. (From Rakel RE. *Textbook of Family Medicine*. 8th ed. Philadelphia: Saunders; 2011. © Richard P. Usatine.)

44. **From what lesion does squamous cell cancer classically develop? What is Bowen disease?**
    Squamous cell cancer (Fig. 6.20) often develops in areas with preexisting actinic keratoses (hard, sharp, red, often scaly lesions in sun-exposed areas; Fig. 6.21) or burn scars. The lesions become nodular, warty, or ulcerated; do a biopsy if such transformation occurs. Squamous cell cancer in situ is known as Bowen disease, and lesions are typically well demarcated. Although metastases are rare in squamous cell cancer, they occur more frequently than in basal cell cancer. They can also cause numbness/paresthesias due to early perineural invasion.

45. **To what parameter is the prognosis of a malignant melanoma most closely related?**
    The Breslow thickness (or depth) of the tumor. The 10-year survival rate decreases as the thickness of the tumor increases. Tumors <1.0 mm thick have the best prognosis.

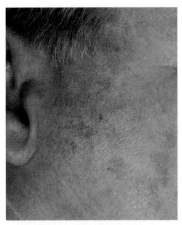

Fig. 6.21 Multiple actinic keratoses visible as thin, red, scaly lesions. (From Goldberg DJ. *Procedures in Cosmetic Dermatology: Lasers and Lights* [vol. 1]. 2nd ed. Philadelphia: Saunders; 2008.)

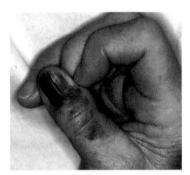

Fig. 6.22 Nailbed melanoma. (From Goldman L, Schafer AL. *Goldman's Cecil Medicine*. 24th ed. Philadelphia: Saunders; 2011.)

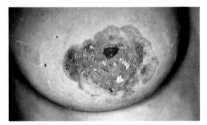

Fig. 6.23 Paget disease of the breast. Note the erythematous plaques around the nipple. (From Lentz GM, Lobo RA, Gershenson DM, et al. *Comprehensive Gynecology*. 6th ed. Philadelphia: Mosby; 2011. Originally from Callen JP. Dermatologic signs of systemic sisease. In: Bolognia JL, Jorizzo JL, Rapini RP, eds. *Dermatology*. Edinburgh: Mosby; 2003:714.)

46. What type of melanoma do Black patients tend to develop? How do you recognize it?
    Although uncommon in Blacks, melanoma tends to be of the acrolentiginous type. Look for black dots on the palms or soles or under the fingernail (Fig. 6.22) that start to change in appearance or cause symptoms.

47. Describe Paget disease of the breast. What is its significance?
    Paget disease of the breast presents as a unilateral, red, oozing or crusting nipple in an adult woman that fails to respond to typical dermatology treatments (Fig. 6.23). Though rare (roughly 1%–2% of breast cancers), it signifies an underlying breast cancer (usually invasive ductal carcinoma or ductal carcinoma in situ) with extension to the skin.

48. Define stomatitis. What does it suggest?

    Stomatitis is an inflammation of the mucous membranes of the mouth. The classic finding is fissuring of the corners of the mouth (angular stomatitis). Watch for deficiencies of B-complex vitamins (riboflavin, niacin, pyridoxine) or vitamin C. Additional causes include drugs such as methotrexate and sulfasalazine.

49. What should you think of in an elderly patient with painful and pruritic lesions that resolve only to recur at another site a month later?

    Necrolytic migratory erythema is a feature of glucagonoma along with weight loss, hyperglycemia, and diarrhea. Diagnosis is made with measurement of glucagon level (>500 pg/mL confirms the diagnosis) and abdominal imaging (magnetic resonance imaging [MRI] or computed tomography [CT] scan).

50. What dermatologic findings are classically associated with nutritional deficiencies?

    Koilonychia and diffuse hair loss: iron deficiency
    Alopecia and pustular rash of extremities and perioral region: zinc deficiency
    Brittle hair and skin depigmentation: copper deficiency
    Bitot spots: vitamin A deficiency

CHAPTER 7

DIABETES MELLITUS

1. Outline the current recommendations for diabetes mellitus screening.
   Universal screening is not generally recommended. Screening is more accepted, but not universal, in patients who are obese, people age >45 years, people with a family history of diabetes, and members of certain minority groups (Blacks, Hispanics, Pima Indians). Screening in pregnancy is mandatory!

2. Define diabetes.
   Diabetes is defined as (1) a glucose level ≥126 mg/dL after an overnight (or 8-hour) fast on two separate occasions, or (2) a random glucose level >200 mg/dL, or (3) a hemoglobin A1c (HbA$_{1c}$) level ≥6.5% on two separate occasions. If the patient has classic symptoms of diabetes (see later), one test is sufficient to make the diagnosis. In an asymptomatic patient, it is best to repeat the test. An oral glucose tolerance test is common in pregnancy; otherwise, it is rarely used because of poor reproducibility and patient compliance. With a glucose tolerance test, diabetes is diagnosed when glucose levels in the blood reach or exceed 200 mg/dL within 2 hours of receiving a 75-g oral dose of glucose.

3. What are the classic differences between type 1 and type 2 diabetes?

	Type 1 (10% of Cases)	Type 2 (90% of Cases)
Age at onset	Most commonly <30 yr	Most commonly >30 yr
Associated body habitus	Thin	Obese
Development of ketoacidosis	Yes	No
Development of hyperosmolar state	No	Yes
Level of endogenous insulin	Low to none	Normal to high (insulin resistance)
Twin concordance	<50%	>50%
HLA association	Yes	No
Response to oral hypoglycemic	No	Yes
Antibodies to insulin	Yes (at diagnosis)	No
Risk for diabetic complications	Yes	Yes
Islet-cell pathology	Insulitis (loss of most B cells)	Normal number, but with amyloid deposits

Remember, however, that these findings may overlap. *HLA*, human leukocyte antigen

4. What is the most important risk factor for developing type 2 diabetes?
   Genetic predisposition is the **most important** risk factor for developing type 2 diabetes (think high rate of twin concordance). Other risk factors include age, obesity, and physical activity. There is also increased prevalence among minority populations due to a combination of genetic and environmental factors.

5. What are the goals of treatment in terms of glucose levels?
   The goals are to keep postprandial glucose levels <180 mg/dL and fasting glucose levels 70 to 130 mg/dL. Attempts at stricter control may result in hypoglycemia; watch for symptoms of sympathetic nervous system activation and mental status changes.

6. What is a good measure of long-term diabetes control?
   HbA$_{1c}$ measures the "average" control of blood glucose level over the prior 2 to 3 months. The current recommendation is to keep the hemoglobin A$_{1c}$ level <7 in most patients. Less stringent A$_{1c}$ goals (such as <8%) may be appropriate for patients with a history of severe hypoglycemia, limited life expectancy, advanced microvascular or macrovascular complications, and extensive comorbid conditions.
   The HbA$_{1c}$ is a good way to catch patients with nocturnal hyperglycemia or less than honest patients who falsely record low glucose test readings. A rough rule of thumb is that HbA$_{1c}$ times 20 equals the average blood glucose level.

7. **When a nondiabetic patient presents with hypoglycemia, how can you distinguish between factitious disorder (exogenous insulin) and an insulinoma (endogenous insulin)?**
Measure the **C-peptide level.** C-peptide is produced whenever the body makes insulin, but it is absent in prescription insulin preparations. Therefore C-peptide is high with an insulinoma and low with factitious disorder. This is a classic USMLE question.

8. **What should you remember before giving intravenous (IV) iodinated contrast material to a diabetic patient or a patient with renal insufficiency?**
Diabetic patients and patients with renal insufficiency are prone to acute renal failure from the intravenously administered iodinated contrast agents used for intravenous pyelography (IVP), conventional angiography, and computed tomography (CT). You need to carefully weigh the risk-to-benefit ratio of using IV contrast agents. If you choose to give contrast, first hydrate the patient well with IV fluids to avoid renal shutdown. Acetylcysteine and bicarbonate may decrease the risk of contrast nephropathy in patients at high risk. The concerns about IV iodinated contrast do not apply to oral contrast agents (e.g., barium).
   Patients on metformin are at risk for development of lactic acidosis if acute renal failure were to occur after administration of IV contrast. Patients with advanced chronic kidney disease, those with acute kidney injury, or those who are undergoing a procedure that may result in emboli to the kidney, and those who require studies with IV contrast should have their metformin held before the procedure and for 48 hours afterwards. Metformin should be restarted only after kidney function has been reevaluated and no injury is identified.

9. **What is diabetic ketoacidosis (DKA)? How is it treated?**
All type I diabetics will die without insulin. DKA is what happens before they die. Clinically, look for Kussmaul breathing (deep, rapid respirations), dehydration, hyperglycemia, acidosis (due to excessive ketone formation), and increased ketones in the serum (often associated with a fruity odor of the breath) and urine.
   Treatment involves IV fluids, insulin, and replacement of electrolytes (especially potassium and phosphate). For the boards, do not use bicarbonate to correct acidosis. Remember to search for the cause of DKA, which most commonly is noncompliance with insulin therapy. The second most common cause is an infection. The mortality rate of DKA with current treatment efforts is <10%.

10. **What is nonketotic hyperglycemic hyperosmolar state? How is it treated?**
Nonketotic hyperglycemic hyperosmolar state is what happens to type II diabetics who go without adequate treatment before they die. Hyperglycemia and increased serum osmolarity are present in the absence of ketones and acidosis. Most patients are severely dehydrated; the first three treatments are thus "fluids, fluids, and fluids" (i.e., IV hydration with normal saline). Insulin and electrolyte replacement is also required. The mortality rate can approach 50% if mental status changes are present at the time of diagnosis.

11. **What are the classic presenting symptoms of new-onset diabetes?**
Polyuria, polydipsia, and polyphagia (pee a lot, drink a lot, and eat a lot). You also should be suspicious if patients present with candidal infections (e.g., thrush or vaginal yeast infection), weight loss (as a result of excessive urination), or blurry vision. Prolonged hyperglycemia causes the lenses in the eyes to swell, and the patient may become myopic. Older patients may even claim that they no longer need their reading glasses (i.e., presbyopia is temporarily corrected by lens swelling).

12. **What are the common long-term complications of diabetes mellitus?**
   - Atherosclerosis, coronary artery disease, myocardial infarction. Diabetics often have "silent" heart attacks (no chest pain because of autonomic neuropathy).
   - Retinopathy. Diabetes is the leading cause of blindness in the United States for persons age <50 years.
   - Nephropathy. Diabetes is the number-one cause of end-stage renal disease requiring hemodialysis (roughly 30% of cases; hypertension is a close second).
   - Peripheral vascular disease. Diabetes is a leading cause of limb amputation and may lead to claudication, strokes, and impotence.
   - Peripheral neuropathy. This complication causes "silent" heart attacks, numbness in the feet, and other findings (see question 13).
   - Increased risk of infection. White blood cells do not function as well in a hyperglycemic environment. Couple this dysfunction with an inability to sense pain and clogged arteries that cannot deliver white cells to the site of an early infection, and you have a recipe for disaster.
   - All of these complications can be delayed or even prevented by good glucose control.

13. **What problems may result from diabetic peripheral neuropathy?**
   - **Gastroparesis.** Because the stomach does not empty well, patients experience early satiety and vomiting. Treat with motility enhancers, such as metoclopramide.
   - **Charcot joints.** Joints in the foot and ankle are deformed secondary to lack of sensation. Patients may break a bone and not feel it.
   - **Impotence.** The causes are neuropathy and atherosclerosis.

- **Cranial nerve palsies** (especially of cranial nerves III, IV, and VI). Patients present with diplopia and extraocular muscle paralysis, which should resolve within 8 weeks without treatment.
- **Orthostatic hypotension.** This problem occurs even when the patient is well hydrated because the arteries do not "clamp down" when the patient stands up, and the heart rate fails to increase appropriately.
- **Pressure ulcers in the feet.** As with Charcot joints, lack of sensation leads to overuse or failure to rest an injured or tired foot because it is numb and the patient is unaware. All diabetics with foot numbness should wear socks and comfortably fitting shoes and inspect their feet regularly. Most cases of foot gangrene in diabetics begin as a simple callus or blister.

14. Describe the treatment for diabetic retinopathy.

If the retinopathy is proliferative (neovascularization or new, irregular vessel formation), the treatment is **panretinal laser photocoagulation.** A laser beam is used to burn tiny spots around the periphery of the retina, sparing the central retina, to prevent progression to blindness. Focal (limited) laser photocoagulation is generally done for nonproliferative retinopathy only if symptoms are present (from macular edema). All diabetics should be seen annually by an ophthalmologist to monitor retinal changes.

15. Describe the onset, peak, and duration of action of each of the insulin preparations.

Insulin Preparation	Onset (HR)	Peak (HR)	Duration (HR)
Ultrarapid Acting			
Insulin aspart	<0.25	1–3	3–5
Insulin lispro	0.25–0.5	0.5–2.5	3–5
Insulin glulisine	0.2–0.5	1.5–2.5	3–4
Rapid Acting			
Regular insulin	0.5–1	2–4	5–8
Intermediate to Long Acting			
NPH insulin	2–3	4–12	12–20
Long Acting			
Insulin glargine	1.5–4	None	24+
Insulin detemir	3–4	3–9	Dose dependent; 6–23 hr

NPH, Neutral protamine Hagedorn.

16. How do you adjust the dosage of neutral protamine Hagedorn (NPH) or regular insulin for high glucose levels?

Regular insulin starts to work in 45 minutes; its action peaks around 3 to 4 hours after injection, and the duration of action is 6 to 8 hours. NPH insulin takes 1 to 1.5 hours until onset of action; its action peaks at 6 to 8 hours, and the total duration of action is about 12 to 20 hours. For insulin adjustments, therefore the following guidelines apply:

- If the patient has high (low) glucose at 7 AM, increase (decrease) NPH insulin at dinner the night before.
- If the patient has high (low) noon glucose, increase (decrease) the morning dose of regular insulin.
- If the patient has high (low) glucose at 5 PM, increase (decrease) the morning dose of NPH insulin.
- If the patient has high (low) glucose at 9 PM, increase (decrease) the dinnertime dose of regular insulin.

17. Define the Somogyi effect and the dawn phenomenon.

The **Somogyi effect** is the body's reaction to hypoglycemia. If too much NPH insulin is given at dinnertime, the glucose level at 3 AM on the next morning will be low (hypoglycemia). The body reacts to hypoglycemia by releasing stress hormones, which cause a high glucose level at 7 AM. The treatment is to decrease evening (NPH) insulin. The **dawn phenomenon** is hyperglycemia caused by normal secretion of growth hormone early in the morning. The glucose level is high at 7 AM and normal or high at 3 AM (no hypoglycemia). The treatment is to increase evening (NPH) insulin.

18. How do you manage diabetic patients who are not allowed to eat because they are scheduled for surgery?

Generally, one-third to one-half of the normal dose of insulin is given. Glucose is monitored closely intra- and postoperatively by the anesthesiologist. Regular IV insulin can be given to control glucose levels based on blood glucose measurements.

19. **What is the deal with beta-blockers, hypoglycemia, and diabetics?**

    If you give a beta-blocker to a diabetic patient, you may mask the classic symptoms of hypoglycemia (tachycardia, diaphoresis), which are caused by catecholamine release. You must weigh the risk-to-benefit ratio of using beta-blockers in diabetics (as in all patients). If a diabetic patient is having or has had a previous myocardial infarction, the benefits outweigh the risks of treatment.

20. **What are the best oral agents to use in type 1 diabetes?**

    None. Patients with type 1 diabetes require insulin. Currently available oral agents do not work for type 1 diabetics.

21. **What is the first treatment for type 2 diabetes?**

    Weight loss, because it may reduce glucose levels by reducing insulin resistance. However, medications are usually needed, and oral agents are tried first, typically beginning with metformin. Other agents include insulin secretagogues (glipizide, glimepiride, nateglinide, glyburide, repaglinide), thiazolidinediones (rosiglitazone, pioglitazone), alpha-glucosidase inhibitors (acarbose, miglitol), GLP-1 agonists (exenatide, liraglutide), DPP-IV inhibitors (saxagliptin, sitagliptin, linagliptin), and amylin analogues (pramlintide). The thiazolidinediones are falling out of favor because of the risk of fluid retention and congestive heart failure exacerbation (rosiglitazone and pioglitazone), the risk of myocardial infarction (rosiglitazone), and the risk of bladder cancer (pioglitazone).

    Many type 2 diabetics eventually require insulin, and insulin may be required early if the blood glucose or HbA_{1c} levels are significantly elevated. In fact, current guidelines suggest using a basal insulin early in therapy (generally after one or two oral agents have been started) to get the blood glucose and HbA_{1c} under control as early as possible.

CHAPTER 8

EAR, NOSE, AND THROAT SURGERY

1. **What is the most common cause of lower motor neuron facial nerve paralysis? How does it present?**

   The most common cause is Bell palsy (Fig. 8.1). Look for sudden-onset unilateral total facial paralysis (vs. upper motor paralysis, which spares the forehead due to bilateral innervation of the forehead), usually occurring after an upper respiratory infection. The cause is thought to be a reactivation of latent herpes simplex I infection in most cases. Patients may have hyperacusis, in which everything sounds loud because the stapedius muscle in the ear is paralyzed. In severe cases, patients may be unable to close the affected eye; if so, use drops to protect the eye. Most cases resolve spontaneously in about 1 month, although some have permanent sequelae. Oral prednisone and antiviral treatment for herpes (e.g., valacyclovir, acyclovir) may improve outcomes and lessen duration of symptoms.

2. **What are the other causes of lower motor neuron facial nerve paralysis?**
   - Herpes infection (Ramsay Hunt syndrome), which commonly involves the eighth nerve. Look for vesicles on the pinna and inside the ear; encephalitis or meningitis may be present.
   - Lyme disease (one of the most common causes of bilateral facial nerve palsy)
   - Middle ear or mastoid infections
   - Meningitis
   - Temporal bone fracture (look for Battle sign and/or bleeding from the ear)
   - Tumor, classically an acoustic schwannoma (i.e., neuroma) of the cerebellopontine angle (Fig. 8.2)

   Order a computed tomography (CT) scan or magnetic resonance imaging (MRI) of the head if the cause is not apparent or if the history or physical exam raises suspicion, especially in the presence of additional neurologic signs.

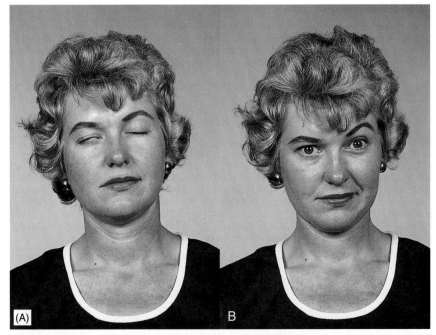

Fig. 8.1 Bell palsy. (A) When trying to shut the eyes, the right eye (on the affected side) fails to close completely but the eyeball rolls up normally. (B) When trying to smile, the mouth fails to move on the affected side, having lost all natural skin folds. The difference is made more striking by covering each side of the picture in turn. (From Odell EW. *Cawson's Essentials of Oral Pathology and Oral Medicine.* FRCPath; 2017.)

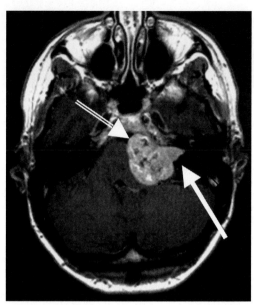

Fig. 8.2 Acoustic neuroma. On this T1-weighted magnetic resonance image, a large acoustic neuroma widens the left internal auditory canal *(solid arrow)* and compresses the brain stem *(hollow arrow)*. (From Goldman L, Ausiello D. *Cecil Medicine.* 23rd ed. Philadelphia: Saunders; 2008 [fig. 419-9].)

3. **What are the common causes of hearing loss?**
   The most common cause is **aging** (presbycusis); prescribe a hearing aid, if needed. The history may suggest other causes:
   - Prolonged or intense exposure to loud noise (e.g., work related)
   - Congenital TORCH (**t**oxoplasmosis, **o**thers, **r**ubella, **c**ytomegalovirus [CMV], **h**erpesvirus) infection
   - Ménière disease (accompanied by severe vertigo, tinnitus, sensation of ear fullness, nausea, and vomiting; treat acute episodes with benzodiazepines, anticholinergics [scopolamine] and antihistamines [meclizine or dimenhydrinate]; diuretics and salt restriction are often used for ongoing treatment; surgery may be used for refractory cases)
   - Drugs (e.g., aminoglycosides, aspirin, quinine, loop diuretics, cisplatin)
   - Tumor (classically acoustic neuroma)
   - Labyrinthitis (may be viral or follow or extend from meningitis or otitis media)
   - Miscellaneous causes (diabetes, hypothyroidism, multiple sclerosis, sarcoidosis, pseudotumor cerebri)

4. **What is the usual cause of sudden deafness?**
   Sudden sensorineural hearing loss (SSNHL) involves acute unexplained hearing loss that is usually unilateral and occurs over hours (usually <72 hours). More than 90% of patients with SSNHL report tinnitus. Most cases are idiopathic but have been postulated to be due to viral causes, microvascular events, or autoimmune causes. Physical examination is unremarkable. MRI is indicated to rule out etiologies such as acoustic neuroma, multiple sclerosis, or vascular insufficiency. Glucocorticoids (administered orally or by intratympanic injection) are considered first-line therapy; antiviral agents are sometimes used, though there is not much evidence to support their use. Two-thirds of patients will experience recovery, though the resolution is often not complete. Among those who recover, hearing usually returns within 2 weeks.

5. **What is the most common cause of acquired hearing loss in children? What is the most common cause of congenital hearing loss in children?**
   Bacterial meningitis. All children should receive formal hearing testing after a bout of meningitis. Congenital CMV infection is the most common cause of congenital hearing loss in children.

6. **What are the common causes of vertigo?**
   Vertigo can result from the same eighth cranial nerve lesions that cause hearing loss (Ménière disease, tumor, infection, multiple sclerosis). Another common cause is benign positional (paroxysmal) vertigo, which is induced by certain head positions, may be accompanied by horizontal nystagmus (never vertical nor rotatory), and is not associated with hearing loss. This condition often resolves spontaneously; no treatment is required. Epley maneuver, or modified Epley maneuvers, may help with resolution of symptoms.

7. How is a deviated nasal septum treated in patients with recurrent sinusitis?
   Surgical correction

8. What are the three common causes of rhinitis?
   Viral, allergic, and bacterial

9. How do you recognize and treat viral rhinitis?
   Viral rhinitis (the common cold) may be due to rhinovirus (the most common cause), influenza, parainfluenza, coxsackievirus, adenovirus, respiratory syncytial virus, coronavirus, or echovirus. Treatment is symptomatic. Vasoconstrictors such as phenylephrine can be used for short-term symptomatic relief, but they may cause rebound congestion when discontinued.

10. How do you recognize and treat allergic rhinitis?
    Allergic rhinitis (hay fever) is associated with seasonal flare-ups, boggy and bluish turbinates, onset before 20 years of age, nasal polyps, sneezing, pruritus, conjunctivitis, wheezing or asthma, eczema, positive family history, eosinophils in nasal mucus, and elevated serum immunoglobulin E. Skin tests may identify an allergen. Treat with avoidance of known antigens (e.g., pollen). Antihistamines, nasal steroids, and/or cromolyn may be used for more severe symptoms. Desensitization is also an option.

11. What causes bacterial rhinitis? How is it treated?
    Group A streptococci, pneumococci, or staphylococci are the most common culprits. Bacterial rhinitis is not usually due to infection of the nasal mucosa alone but is more commonly due to infection of an adjacent compartment complicated by inflammation of the nasal mucosa, hence the term *bacterial rhinosinusitis*. Look for coexisting sore throat, lymphadenopathy, fever, and tonsillar exudate. Do streptococcal throat cultures, and treat with antibiotics if appropriate.

12. What causes nosebleeds?
    The most common cause of nosebleed is trauma (e.g., nose-picking is a common cause in children). Environmental changes also commonly cause nosebleeds. Watch out for the following causes:
    - Local tumor (nasopharyngeal angiofibroma; seen in adolescent boys with no history of trauma or blood dyscrasia; signs include recurrent nosebleeds and/or obstruction)
    - Leukemia (from pancytopenia; typically in children with associated fever and anemia)
    - Other causes of thrombocytopenia (e.g., idiopathic thrombocytopenic purpura, hemolytic uremic syndrome)

13. True or false: A neck mass is more likely to be benign in a child than in an adult.
    True. Roughly 75% of neck masses are benign in children, whereas 75% are malignant in patients over age 40 years.

14. What are the common causes of a neck mass?
    In **children**, watch for thyroglossal duct cysts, which have a midline location and elevate with tongue protrusion; branchial cleft cysts, which are lateral in location and often become infected; cystic hygroma, a benign tumor also known as lymphangioma that is associated with Turner syndrome and treated with surgical resection; and cervical lymphadenitis. Cervical lymphadenitis is usually due to streptococcal pharyngitis, Epstein-Barr virus (common in the second and third decades), cat-scratch disease, or mycobacterial infection (scrofula). In terms of malignancy in children, leukemia or lymphoma may present with cervical lymphadenopathy.
    In **adults**, suspect malignancy (particularly if the mass is firm, nonmobile, and >2 cm), either lymphadenopathy from a primary tumor (lymphoma) or metastatic neoplasm (usually squamous cell carcinoma). The mass may also represent the tumor itself (especially with thyroid cancer).

15. Describe the workup for an unknown cancer in the neck.
    The workup includes random biopsy of the nasopharynx, palatine tonsils, and base of the tongue as well as laryngoscopy, bronchoscopy, and esophagoscopy (with biopsies of any suspicious lesions). This approach is known as "triple endoscopy with triple biopsy."

16. What is the scientific name for swimmer's ear? What causes it?
    Otitis externa (inflammation of the outer ear), which most often is due to infection with *Pseudomonas aeruginosa*. Patients have pain with manipulation of the auricle and erythematous, swollen skin in the auditory canal. Foul-smelling discharge and conductive hearing loss may also be present. Treat with topical antibiotics (e.g., ofloxacin, neomycin, polymyxin B) and possibly topical steroids to reduce swelling.

17. What causes otitis media? How do you recognize it?
    Otitis media (inflammation of the middle ear) is an extremely common pediatric infection, most often due to infection with *Streptococcus pneumoniae, Haemophilus influenzae,* or *Moraxella catarrhalis*. Patients have no pain with manipulation of the auricle; positive symptoms include earache, fever, erythematous and bulging tympanic membranes (the light reflex and landmarks are difficult to see with otoscopy), and nausea and vomiting.

18. **What are the complications of otitis media? How are they avoided?**
    Complications include tympanic membrane perforation (bloody or purulent discharge), mastoiditis (fluctuance and inflammation over the mastoid process, often with anterior displacement of the affected ear, roughly 2 weeks after the onset of otitis media), labyrinthitis, hearing loss (conductive hearing loss is more common than sensorineural hearing loss but both may occur), palsies of cranial nerves VII and VIII, meningitis, cerebral abscess, dural sinus thrombosis, and chronic otitis media (due to permanent perforation of the tympanic membrane). Patients with chronic otitis media may develop cholesteatomas with marginal perforations that require surgical excision.
    Otitis media is generally treated with antibiotics to avoid these complications (e.g., amoxicillin, second-generation cephalosporin such as cefuroxime, or a macrolide).

19. **What is the problem with recurrent otitis media? How is it treated?**
    Recurrent otitis media is a common pediatric problem (along with prolonged secretory otitis, a result of incompletely resolved otitis media) and can cause hearing loss with resultant developmental problems (speech, cognitive functions). Treat with prophylactic antibiotics or tympanostomy tubes. Adenoidectomy is controversial but may help in some cases; it is thought to help prevent blockage of the eustachian tubes.

20. **What causes infectious myringitis? How do you recognize and treat it?**
    Infectious myringitis, also known as bullous myringitis, is an inflammation of the tympanic membranes that can be diagnosed when otoscopy reveals vesicles on the tympanic membrane. Infectious myringitis is classically caused by *Mycoplasma* species, but *Streptococcus pneumoniae* or viruses may also be the culprit. Treat with erythromycin or clarithromycin to cover *Mycoplasma* species and *S. pneumoniae*.

21. **What are the common bacterial causes of sinusitis? How is this condition recognized clinically?**
    Bacterial sinusitis is often due to *S. pneumoniae, H. influenzae, M. catarrhalis,* or other streptococcal or staphylococcal species. Look for tenderness over the affected sinuses (and pain that is worse when bending forward), headache, and purulent nasal discharge (yellow or green) lasting 10 or more days without evidence of clinical improvement. Associated symptoms are headache and/or toothache (maxillary sinusitis), cough, anosmia, and ear fullness. Radiographs or CT are used to confirm the diagnosis and show opacification of the sinus, classically with an air-fluid level in acute sinusitis; CT scans are preferred to evaluate chronic sinusitis or suspected extension of infection outside the sinus (watch for high fever and chills). Treat with symptomatic care and observation in uncomplicated cases, as many patients improve without antibiotic therapy. For patients who fail to improve or have worsening symptoms after 1 week, treat with antibiotics (amoxicillin, trimethoprim-sulfamethoxazole, a second- or third-generation cephalosporin, a macrolide, or amoxicillin clavulanate for 10–14 days or for up to 6 weeks in chronic cases). Culture is usually not necessary unless the patient fails to respond to antibiotics. Operative intervention (drainage procedure, sinus obliteration) may be required for resistant cases.

22. **By what age are the frontal sinuses well developed in children?**
    The frontal sinuses may not be well developed until the age of 10 years.

23. **Define otosclerosis. How is it treated?**
    In otosclerosis, the otic bones become fixed together and impede hearing. The cause is unclear. Otosclerosis is the most common cause of progressive conductive hearing loss in adults, whereas presbycusis is the most common cause of sensorineural hearing loss in adults. Treat with a hearing aid or surgery.

24. **What causes parotid gland swelling?**
    The classic cause of multifocal parotid gland swelling is mumps. The best treatment for mumps and the complication of infertility is prevention through immunization. Multifocal parotid gland swelling may also be due to Sjögren syndrome, sarcoidosis, and bulimia. Alcoholism can cause parotid gland hypertrophy as well. Unifocal parotid gland swelling may be due to bacterial infection, sialolithiasis (a stone in the parotid duct), or neoplasm (of which pleomorphic adenoma is the most common type). Remember, too, that the parotid gland contains lymph nodes within its parenchyma (unique in this regard), which can become enlarged in a number of conditions, as with lymph nodes elsewhere.

25. **How do you recognize a nasal fracture? What complication may result?**
    A nasal fracture can be seen on radiographs or CT scan. Watch for a septal hematoma, which must be surgically removed to prevent pressure-induced septal necrosis.

26. **What is the Weber test used to evaluate? How is it performed and interpreted?**
    The Weber test compares bone conduction in the two ears. A vibrating tuning fork is placed on the center of the forehead, and the patient is asked where the vibrating sound is heard best. The normal response is to hear the vibration in the middle (or equally in both ears). In patients with conductive hearing loss, the sound is heard best in the affected ear, whereas in patients with sensorineural hearing loss, the sound is heard best in the unaffected ear.

27. **What is the Rinne test used to evaluate? How is it performed and interpreted?**

    The Rinne test compares air conduction with bone conduction. A vibrating tuning fork is placed on the tip of the mastoid process. When the patient can no longer hear the sound, the tuning fork is removed from the mastoid and placed next to the auditory meatus of the external ear, and the patient is asked if the sound can be heard.

    Because air conduction is normally greater than bone conduction, patients can hear the tuning fork when it is placed next to the auditory meatus (air conduction) even after they can no longer hear it vibrating on the mastoid (bone conduction). In patients with conductive hearing loss, bone conduction is greater than air conduction; thus they cannot hear the tuning fork when it is placed next to the external auditory meatus. In patients with sensorineural hearing loss, both air and bone conduction are impaired, but the normal ratio (air conduction > bone conduction) is maintained; thus they still hear the tuning fork next to the ear after they can no longer hear it on the mastoid.

CHAPTER 9

EMERGENCY MEDICINE

1. **What is a FAST exam? Explain what you are looking for when performing a FAST exam.**
   FAST is an acronym for focused assessment with sonography for trauma. It is a bedside ultrasound exam used to search for free fluid where fluid should not be—namely, pathologic pericardial, intrathoracic, and/or intraperitoneal free fluid. If detected, these fluids will appear darker than the surrounding tissue (hypoechoic or anechoic). The extended FAST exam (E-FAST) includes additional views to investigate for pneumothorax.

2. **What are the three types of burns? How should all burns be managed initially? What is the Parkland formula?**
   The three types of burns are thermal, chemical, and electrical. Initial management of all burns should begin with management of the ABCs—airway, breathing, and circulation—with a low threshold for intubation. Remove all clothing and other smoldering/exposed items on the body to ensure you can see the full breadth of the patient's injuries. For fire-related thermal burns, give 100% oxygen until carbon monoxide poisoning from smoke inhalation can be ruled out. Remember that burn patients are at an increased risk of dehydration, so administer plenty of intravenous fluids (lactated Ringer solution is first line, with normal saline as second line) and follow the **Parkland formula** (Fig. 9.1) to administer the appropriate amount of fluids over the first 24 hours: **4 cc × body weight (kg) × body surface area** (**BSA**), with half administered over the first 8 hours and the remaining half administered over the ensuing 16 hours. BSA is estimated using the rule of 9s—remember that only superficial partial-thickness burns or worse are included when using the rule of 9s.

3. **How is burn severity classified? Describe the management of each class.**
   Burn depth terminology no longer includes the use of first-, second-, and third-degree burn classifications. Burn severity is now organized into four categories: (1) superficial, (2) superficial partial-thickness, (3) deep partial-thickness, and (4) full-thickness burns.

   Superficial burns are erythematous without blister formation. They involve only the epidermis and are locally painful.
   Superficial partial-thickness burns are painful, warm, and moist with blister formation. They penetrate through the epidermis and superficial papillary dermis.
   Deep partial-thickness burns are painless and present with mottled, waxy, or whitened skin. Blisters may be present. Pressure sensation is intact.
   Full-thickness burns involve both the epidermis and dermis; have a white to gray, leathery, charred, or translucent appearance; and do not blanch with pressure. Pinprick sensation is absent.

4. **What are the important sequelae of electrical burns?**
   Because most of the tissue destruction due to electrical burns is internal, sequelae include muscle necrosis, rhabdomyolysis, compartment syndrome, dislocations (e.g., posterior shoulder dislocation), acidosis, and renal failure. Use large amounts of intravenous hydration to prevent renal shutdown. The immediate life-threatening concern with an electrical burn is a cardiac arrhythmia, so order an electrocardiogram (ECG) and monitor for seizures.

5. **How are chemical burns managed? Which is worse, acid or alkali burns?**
   All chemical burns should be treated with copious irrigation from the nearest source (e.g., tap water) because the sooner you dilute the chemical, the less damage will be done. Do not delay irrigation while searching for sterile saline for irrigation. Alkali burns are considered worse than acidic burns as they cause liquefactive necrosis. Compare this to the coagulative necrosis caused by acidic burns—the eschar that forms due to the coagulative necrosis will prevent the deeper substance penetration that occurs due to liquefactive necrosis in alkali burns.

6. **Besides dehydration, what additional complication is burned skin prone to develop?**
   Burned skin is much more prone to infection, usually by *Staphylococcus aureus* or *Pseudomonas aeruginosa*. With pseudomonal infection, look for a fruity odor and/or blue-green appearance. If given, prophylactic antibiotics should only be administered topically. Irrigation and debridement are vitally important to infection prevention. Consider a tetanus booster shot if the patient has received fewer than three lifetime doses of the tetanus vaccine or if the patient's most recent booster shot was received more than 10 years ago.

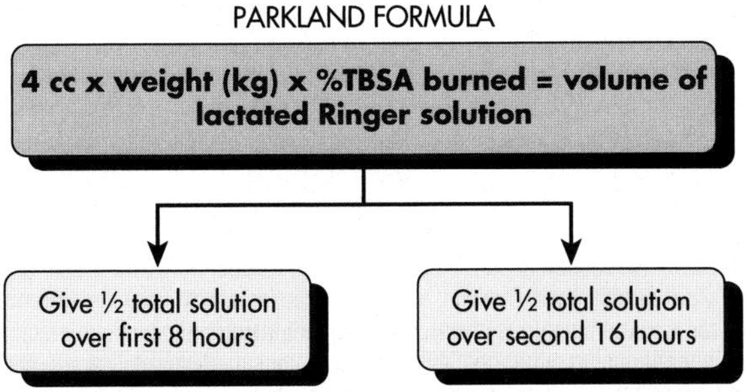

PARKLAND FORMULA

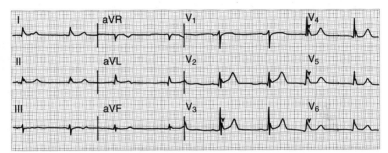

4 cc x weight (kg) x %TBSA burned = volume of lactated Ringer solution

Give ½ total solution over first 8 hours

Give ½ total solution over second 16 hours

Fig. 9.1 Parkland formula. (From Cameron JL, Cameron AM. *Current Surgical Therapy.* 12th ed. Philadelphia: Elsevier; 2017.)

Fig. 9.2 Systemic hypothermia resulting in prominent sinus bradycardia. The ars $(V_3$ through $V_6)$ point to the characteristic convex J waves, termed Osborn waves. (From Libby P, et al. *Braunwald's Heart Disease: A Textbook of Cardiovascular Medicine.* 8th ed. Philadelphia: Saunders; 2008 [fig. 12.53].)

7. **Define hypothermia. How is it managed? What are the complications?**
Hypothermia is defined as a body temperature less than 95°F (35°C), usually accompanied by mental status changes and generalized neurologic deficits. If the patient is conscious, rewarm the patient slowly with items such as blankets, radiant heat, or a Bair Hugger. If the patient is unconscious, consider gastric and bladder lavage with warm water as well as warm intravenous fluids. Additionally, be sure to monitor for cardiac arrhythmias, which are common in hypothermic patients. The most common arrhythmia is sinus bradycardia, which may deteriorate into atrial fibrillation, ventricular fibrillation, or asystole. You may (rarely) see the classic **J wave** in the ECG of hypothermic patients, which appears as a small, positive deflection following the QRS complex (Fig. 9.2). Also be sure to monitor electrolytes, renal function, and acid-base status, and consider checking thyroid function to rule out myxedema coma.

8. **Distinguish between frostnip and frostbite. How are they managed?**
Frostnip, a mild form of cold injury, occurs when there is partial skin freezing resulting in cold and painful skin. In **frostbite**, a more severe form of cold injury, the skin is cold and numb. Treat both with analgesia and slow warming of the affected areas using lukewarm or tepid water (not scalding hot, as this will cause greater tissue damage) combined with local wound care and generalized warming (e.g., blankets).

9. **True or false: You should not give up resuscitation efforts until the patient is fully warmed in the setting of hypothermic cardiac arrest**
True. An old saying in emergency medicine claims that a hypothermic patient is not considered dead "until warm and dead." Hypothermia conditions may preserve vital body functions despite what appears to be an unsuccessful resuscitation attempt. In fact, there are case reports of hypothermic patients regaining consciousness as they warmed up hours after initial resuscitation efforts in the field had stopped.

10. **Define hyperthermia. What causes it? How is it managed?**
Hyperthermia is defined as a body temperature greater than 104°F. The three primary causes are infections, medications, and heat stroke. If heat stroke is suspected, look for a history of exertion or exercise under prolonged heat exposure without clues to other underlying health problems. Treat with immediate cooling (e.g., wet blankets, ice, cold water) to a goal temperature of about 102°F to avoid overshooting and causing hypothermia. The immediate life-threatening complications are convulsions and cardiovascular collapse. Treat convulsions with benzodiazepines (e.g., diazepam) if they occur. When working up hyperthermia, always rule out infection, endocrine abnormalities, and medications—especially medications with anticholinergic activity such as antihistamines, antipsychotics, and antidepressants—as the cause.

11. **What are the two classic examples of medication-induced hyperthermia? How is each condition managed?**

Two classic examples of medication-induced hyperthermia are malignant hyperthermia and neuroleptic malignant syndrome.

Malignant hyperthermia is an idiosyncratic, life-threatening reaction to general anesthesia (e.g., succinylcholine or halothane) due to a genetic defect in the skeletal muscle ryanodine receptor (RyR), leading to extreme muscular contraction with risk of rhabdomyolysis. Reverse the effects with the RyR antagonist dantrolene.

Neuroleptic malignant syndrome is thought to be related to malignant hyperthermia and is an idiosyncratic, life-threatening reaction to an antipsychotic (e.g., haloperidol). The classic tetrad includes altered mental status, "lead pipe" rigidity, hyperthermia, and autonomic instability. Look for extremely high levels of creatine phosphokinase and mental status changes in a patient taking antipsychotic medication.

The first step when managing either condition is to stop the causative medication. The second step is supportive treatment with plenty of intravenous fluids to prevent renal shutdown secondary to rhabdomyolysis. If this is unsuccessful, proceed to treatment with dantrolene.

Drug fevers are idiosyncratic reactions to a medication that was typically started within the past week. They rarely cause fever above 104°F.

12. **How are patients managed after a near-drowning episode?**

Some, but not all, physicians believe that drowning in fresh water is worse than saltwater because aspirating fresh water may cause hypervolemia, electrolyte disturbances, and hemolysis. After a near-drowning episode, unconscious patients should be intubated whereas conscious patients should have their arterial blood gases monitored. Death due to a near-drowning episode is typically due to hypoxia and/or cardiac arrest. Remember to look for head or neck trauma and consider potential reasons why the near-drowning episode occurred (e.g., intoxication, seizure, syncope, suicide attempt).

13. **What are toxidromes? Describe the toxidromes associated with cholinergic crisis, anticholinergic crisis, sympathomimetic toxicity, and opiate toxicity.**

Toxidromes are clinical syndromes characterized by a particular constellation of classic presenting symptoms caused by exposure to toxic levels of well-documented causative substances.

- Cholinergic crisis (e.g., organophosphates or insecticides) classically presents with SLUDGE (excessive **s**alivation, **l**acrimation, **u**rination, **d**iaphoresis, **g**astrointestinal upset, and **e**mesis). Also look for pinpoint pupils and decreased heart rate.
- Anticholinergic crisis (e.g., tricyclic antidepressant overdose) presents as a patient who is blind as a bat (mydriasis), hot as a hare (temperature dysregulation), mad as a hatter (central nervous system disturbances), dry as a bone (dry mucous membranes), full as a flask (urinary retention), and red as a beet (flushing). Also look for decreased bowel sounds and increased heart rate. Note that in a question stem it may be easy to confuse the mydriasis, temperature dysregulation, and mental status change for sympathomimetic toxicity—look for dry skin to distinguish anticholinergic crisis from the diaphoretic patient with sympathomimetic toxicity.
- Sympathomimetic toxicity (e.g., cocaine or amphetamine use) can cause hypertension, tachycardia, increased activity, anxiety, dilated pupils, diaphoresis, and possibly altered mental status.
- Opiate toxicity (e.g., heroin overdose) can cause pinpoint pupils and respiratory depression. Also look for decreased bowel sounds, bradycardia, and hypotension.

14. **Cover the right-hand column of the table and name the antidote for each of the poisonings or overdoses listed.**

Poisoning or Overdose	Antidote
Acetaminophen	N-acetylcysteine
Benzodiazepines	Flumazenil (can precipitate seizures or delirium tremens if the patient has chronic benzodiazepine dependence)
Beta-blockers	Glucagon
Carbon monoxide	Oxygen (hyperbaric if severe)
Cholinesterase inhibitors	Atropine (always first), pralidoxime
Copper or gold	D-penicillamine or trientine (zinc is an alternative)
Dabigatran	Idarucizumab
Digoxin	Replete potassium and other electrolytes; digoxin-specific antibodies

Poisoning or Overdose	Antidote
Direct factor Xa inhibitors (apixaban, rivaroxaban)	Andexanet
Heparin	Protamine sulfate
Iron	Deferoxamine
Lead	Dimercaptosuccinic acid (DMSA, succimer), dimercaprol, calcium sodium edetate (EDTA)
Methanol or ethylene glycol	Fomepizole, ethanol
Muscarinic receptor blockers	Physostigmine
Opioids	Naloxone
Quinidine or tricyclic antidepressants	Sodium bicarbonate (cardioprotective)
Salicylic acid (aspirin)	Urine alkalinization, dialysis
Warfarin	Vitamin K, fresh frozen plasma, prothrombin complex concentrate (if life-threatening bleeding)

15. **How do you manage suspected acetaminophen overdose or toxicity?**
    The first step is to secure the ABCs (airway, breathing, circulation). If it has been 4 hours or less since time of ingestion, administer activated charcoal for gastric decontamination. However, usually the timing of ingestion is unknown. In that case, the first step is to obtain a serum acetaminophen (APAP) level and liver function tests. Administer N-acetylcysteine if there is any evidence of liver injury, serum APAP levels are above the "treatment line" on the Rumack-Matthew nomogram, or APAP levels are above 10 μg/mL with unknown ingestion time.

16. **What are the clinical signs of aspirin toxicity? How do you treat it?**
    Signs of aspirin toxicity include tinnitus, hyperventilation (stimulation of medullary respiratory center), nausea/vomiting, altered mental status, and sometimes pulmonary edema. Overdose initially causes a primary respiratory alkalosis that develops into a mixed respiratory alkalosis-anion gap metabolic acidosis. Treatment is via alkalinization of the urine with sodium bicarbonate. Dialysis is indicated in emergent scenarios (e.g., pulmonary edema, renal failure, severely elevated salicylate levels).

17. **What complications should you monitor for in caustic ingestion (e.g., acid or alkali)? How should these patients be managed?**
    Complications of caustic ingestion include perforation, ulcers, strictures, and carcinoma. Stricture formation is the most common complication and typically develops over several weeks. In terms of management, the first step, as always, is to secure the ABCs. All sources of chemical contamination (e.g., clothing) should be removed. Obtain a chest x-ray if the patient has or develops any respiratory symptoms to rule out perforation. All patients should receive an esophagogastroduodenoscopy within 24 hours to evaluate damage and guide management.

18. **What substances can cause methemoglobinemia? How is methemoglobinemia treated?**
    Methemoglobinemia is acquired via exposure to oxidizing substances, most commonly topical anesthetic agents (e.g., lidocaine, benzocaine), dapsone, nitrites (including nitroglycerin), and aniline dyes. Treatment includes oxygen supplementation and administration of methylene blue and vitamin C.

19. **What are the clinical signs of arsenic toxicity? What are the most common sources of exposure? How do you treat it?**
    Acute arsenic toxicity can present with abdominal pain, nausea, vomiting, diarrhea, garlic odor breath, and QTc prolongation. The most common sources include pesticides, contaminated well water, and pressure-treated wood. Treat with dimercaprol or dimercaptosuccinic acid (DMSA, succimer).

20. **What are the clinical signs associated with cyanide toxicity? When should you be suspicious for such exposure?**
    Cyanide toxicity is associated with headache, abdominal pain, flushed cherry-red skin, altered mental status, seizures, and coma. Watch for signs if a patient recently had significant smoke exposure (e.g., fire) or is on a nitroprusside drip for blood pressure control.

CHAPTER 10

ENDOCRINOLOGY

1. **What are the common signs and symptoms of hyperthyroidism?**

   Signs: enlarged thyroid gland, warm skin, thyroid stare/lid lag, exophthalmos, proptosis, ophthalmoplegia (Graves disease), pretibial myxedema (Graves disease), tremor, tachycardia, and atrial fibrillation. Check thyroid-stimulating hormone (TSH) when patients present with new-onset atrial fibrillation.

   Symptoms: nervousness, anxiety, irritability, insomnia, heat intolerance, sweating, palpitations, tremors, weight loss with increased appetite, fatigue, weakness, hair loss, emotional lability, amenorrhea, and diarrhea.

2. **What are the most common causes of hyperthyroidism?**

   The most common cause is **Graves disease**, which is characterized by a diffusely enlarged thyroid gland, the presence of thyrotropin receptor antibodies (TRAb), exophthalmos, proptosis, ophthalmoplegia, and pretibial myxedema. In elderly patients, look for toxic multinodular goiter (individual lumps instead of diffuse enlargement of the gland and "hot" nodules on thyroid nuclear scan). Other causes include adenoma (single lump that is hot on nuclear scan), multinodular goiter (multiple lumps that are hot on nuclear scan), subacute thyroiditis (viral infection with **tender**, **painful** thyroid gland), painless thyroiditis, and factitious hyperthyroidism (in which the patient takes thyroid hormone). Rare, exotic causes include amiodarone (which can cause hypo- or hyperthyroidism), TSH-producing pituitary tumor, thyroid carcinoma, and struma ovarii (an ovarian teratoma that secretes thyroid hormone).

3. **Describe the classic laboratory pattern of hyperthyroidism.**

   The TSH level is low (unless the patient has a TSH-secreting tumor), whereas triiodothyronine (T3) and thyroxine (T4) are increased.

4. **How is hyperthyroidism treated?**

   Short-term (stabilizing) treatment: Propylthiouracil (PTU) and methimazole/carbimazole can be used as suppressive agents (in pregnancy, PTU is recommended in the first trimester with transition to methimazole at the start of the second trimester). Beta-blockers are used in the setting of thyroid storm (severe hyperthyroid state—an emergency) for control of adrenergic symptoms. Iodine can also suppress the thyroid gland through negative feedback but can only be given after administering antithyroid medication and steroids (to reduce conversion of T4 to T3) during thyroid storm.

   Definitive (curative) treatment: Radioactive iodine ablation of the thyroid gland is typically used. In patients with Graves ophthalmoplegia, glucocorticoids can be used to prevent the worsening of the ophthalmopathy when radioactive iodine is administered. Surgery is preferred in pregnant patients. Hypothyroidism may result from either treatment; if so, it is treated with thyroid hormone replacement (for life).

5. **What are the signs and symptoms of hypothyroidism?**

   Signs: bradycardia; dry, coarse, cold, and pale skin; periorbital and peripheral edema; coarse, thin hair; thick tongue; slow speech; decreased and delayed reflexes; hypertension; carpal tunnel syndrome and paresthesias; vitiligo, pernicious anemia, and diabetes (remember the autoimmune association between these three conditions and Hashimoto disease); and coma (severe disease).

   Symptoms: weakness, lethargy, fatigue, cold intolerance, weight gain with anorexia, constipation, loss of hair, hoarseness, menstrual irregularity (menorrhagia is classic), myalgias and arthralgias, memory impairment, and dementia. Always rule out hypothyroidism as a cause of dementia.

   In children, congenital hypothyroidism may occur (mental, motor, and growth retardation).

6. **What are the common causes of hypothyroidism?**

   The most common known cause is Hashimoto thyroiditis (chronic autoimmune thyroiditis). Women of reproductive age outnumber men by 8:1. Histology reveals lymphocytes in the thyroid gland as well as antithyroid peroxidase, antithyroglobulin, and antimicrosomal antibodies. Other autoimmune diseases may coexist. The associated goiter is nontender. The second most common cause is iatrogenic after treatment of hyperthyroidism. Other, less common causes include iodine deficiency, amiodarone, lithium, and secondary hypothyroidism due to pituitary or hypothalamic failure (look for decreased TSH), such as with Sheehan syndrome (hypopituitarism caused by pituitary necrosis from blood loss and hypovolemic shock during and after childbirth).

7. Describe the laboratory findings in hypothyroidism.
   Elevated TSH (unless due to secondary causes), decreased T3 and T4, antithyroid and antimicrosomal antibodies (if due to Hashimoto thyroiditis), hypercholesterolemia, and anemia (which may be due to chronic disease or coexisting pernicious anemia).

8. Why is free T4 (or free T4 index) better than total T4 for measuring thyroid hormone activity?
   Free T4 (free T4 index) measures the active form of thyroid hormone. Many conditions cause a change in the amount of thyroid-binding globulin (TBG), thus changing total T4 levels in the absence of hypo- or hyperthyroidism. Common examples include pregnancy, estrogen therapy, and oral contraceptive pills, all of which increase TBG. Nephrotic syndrome, cirrhosis, and corticosteroid treatment all decrease TBG. T3 resin uptake is an older test that is not worth the effort to learn for Step 2, but if you are asked, it should rise or fall in the same way as free T4. Although an oversimplification, this principle should serve you well on the exam.

9. How is hypothyroidism treated?
   With T4 or thyroxine. T3 should not be used. In elderly patients it is important to "start low and go slow" because overtreatment can be dangerous.

10. What is nonthyroidal illness (formerly euthyroid sick syndrome)?
    Any patient with any illness may have temporary derangements in thyroid function tests that resemble hypothyroidism. Thyroid function should not be assessed in seriously ill patients unless there is a strong suspicion of thyroid dysfunction. TSH ranges from normal to mildly elevated, and serum T4 ranges from normal to mildly decreased, and T3 levels are low. Clinical circumstances and physical findings are the best guides to whether the patient has true hypothyroidism. In patients with nonthyroidal illness, simply treat the underlying illness. If the diagnosis is in doubt, either remeasure thyroid tests after the patient recovers (preferred) or try an empiric dose of levothyroxine (if the patient does not respond to treatment of the underlying illness).

11. What are the signs and symptoms of Cushing syndrome (hypercortisolism)?
    Signs: buffalo hump, truncal and central obesity with wasting of extremities, round plethoric facies ("moon facies"), purplish skin striae, acne, hirsutism, weakness (especially of the proximal muscles), hypertension, depression, psychosis, peripheral edema, poor wound healing, glucose intolerance or diabetes, osteoporosis, and hypokalemic metabolic alkalosis (due to mineralocorticoid effects of certain corticosteroids). Growth may be stunted in children.
    Symptoms: weight gain, changes in appearance, easy bruising, acne, hirsutism, emotional lability, depression, psychosis, weakness, menstrual changes, sexual dysfunction, insomnia, and memory loss.

12. What causes Cushing syndrome?
    The most common cause is iatrogenic because steroids are frequently prescribed. The second most common cause is Cushing disease (a pituitary adenoma that secretes adrenocorticotropic hormone [ACTH]), which causes roughly 60% of noniatrogenic cases. Women of reproductive age outnumber men by 5:1. Other causes include ectopic ACTH production (classically by small cell lung cancer, which is more common in men) and adrenal adenomas or carcinomas (more common in children).

13. How is Cushing syndrome diagnosed?
    Initial testing is with two of the following first-line tests: a 24-hour measurement of free cortisol in urine (free cortisol levels are abnormally elevated), late-night salivary cortisol, or an overnight low-dose (1 mg) dexamethasone suppression test (cortisol levels are not appropriately suppressed after administration of dexamethasone). Random cortisol level is an inappropriate test because of wide inter- and intrapatient as well as circadian variations. **Remember that ACTH is elevated in Cushing disease but decreased with an adrenal adenoma.** If ACTH is increased, a high-dose (8 mg) dexamethasone test should be ordered. A high-dose dexamethasone suppression test is not used to make a diagnosis of Cushing syndrome but is used to distinguish Cushing disease (suppresses) from ectopic ACTH production such as adrenal adenoma (does not suppress). Alternatively, a corticotropin-releasing hormone (CRH) test can be used. A positive response indicates Cushing disease, whereas no response indicates an ectopic source of ACTH. If Cushing disease is suspected, magnetic resonance imaging (MRI) of the brain should be obtained to look for a pituitary adenoma. Primary cancer is usually obvious when ectopic ACTH is the cause (e.g., weight loss, hemoptysis with lung mass on chest radiograph in patients with small cell lung cancer). If ACTH is decreased and the patient has no history of taking steroids, an abdominal computed tomography (CT) scan or MRI should be obtained to look for an adrenal tumor. Primary cancer is usually obvious when ectopic ACTH is the cause (e.g., weight loss, hemoptysis with lung mass on chest radiograph in patients with small cell lung cancer). Treatment is based on the cause and usually involves surgery.

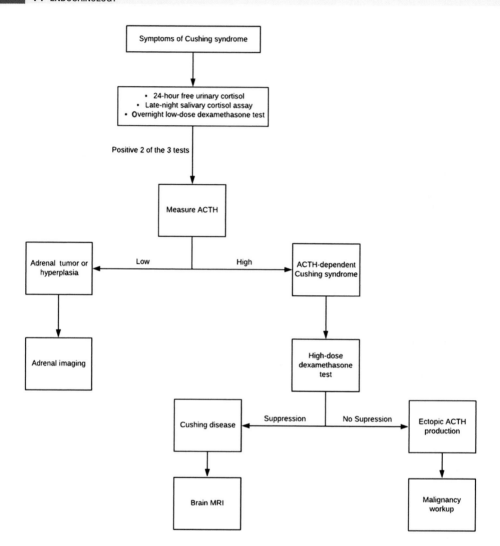

14. What are the signs and symptoms of hypoadrenalism?
    Signs: hypotension, hyperkalemia, hyponatremia, hyperpigmentation (only if the pituitary is functioning because of melanocyte-stimulating hormone), nausea and vomiting, diarrhea, abdominal pain, mild fever, hypoglycemia, acidosis, eosinophilia, orthostatic hypotension, and shock.
    Symptoms: anorexia, weight loss, weakness, dizziness, apathy.

15. What is the most common type of adrenal insufficiency (hypoadrenalism)?
    Tertiary (iatrogenic) adrenal insufficiency due to steroid treatment in which exogenous steroids inhibit the secretion of CRH by the hypothalamus. People who are removed abruptly from long-term steroid therapy may be unable to secrete an appropriate amount of corticosteroids in response to stress for up to 1 year. Watch out for the classic postoperative patient who crashes (with hypotension, shock, and hyperkalemia) shortly after surgery and has a history of a disease requiring steroid therapy within the past year. You may assess ACTH (inappropriately low) and cortisol levels (inappropriately low) to help make the diagnosis, but do not wait for the results to give steroids. The patient may die. Give prophylactic stress doses of corticosteroids in the setting of an illness, operation, or other stressor to prevent an adrenal crisis.

16. **What are the other causes of adrenal insufficiency?**
    The most common primary (noniatrogenic) cause is autoimmune (idiopathic) disease in the developed world, whereas tuberculosis is the most common cause in the developing world. Patients may have other autoimmune diseases, such as hypothyroidism, pernicious anemia, vitiligo, diabetes, or hypoparathyroidism. Secondary adrenal insufficiency can be caused by a pituitary adenoma, which decreases ACTH production, or Sheehan syndrome. Other causes include metastatic cancer (especially lung cancer), infection (tuberculosis, fungal infections, opportunistic infections in AIDS, and other immunosuppressed states), ketoconazole, and pituitary/hypothalamic failure.

17. **How is adrenal insufficiency diagnosed?**
    Measurement of morning cortisol soon after wakening can suggest the diagnosis of adrenal insufficiency. A high-dose ACTH stimulation (cosyntropin) test is the most accurate way to establish the diagnosis. Plasma cortisol is measured, ACTH is administered intravenously (IV) or intramuscularly (IM), and cortisol is measured again at either 30 minutes or 30 and 60 minutes postinjection. If adrenal function is normal, the cortisol level should rise appropriately (18–20 µg/dL for IV cosyntropin or 16 µg/dL for IM cosyntropin) and indicates a secondary or tertiary adrenal insufficiency. An inappropriate response to ACTH indicates primary adrenal insufficiency. Do not withhold treatment to make a diagnosis if the patient is crashing.

18. **Define hirsutism. What causes it?**
    Hirsutism is a male pattern hair growth in women or prepubescent children. The most common cause is familial, genetic, or idiopathic hirsutism, but on the boards watch for **polycystic ovary syndrome** (Stein-Leventhal syndrome), Cushing syndrome, and drugs (minoxidil, phenytoin, cyclosporine). These disorders do not produce virilization. If virilization (clitoral enlargement, deepening of the voice, temporal balding) accompanies the hirsutism, an androgen-secreting ovarian tumor (e.g., Sertoli-Leydig cell tumor or arrhenoblastoma) or adrenal source (congenital adrenal hyperplasia, Cushing syndrome, or adrenal tumor) is likely.

19. **What causes virilization in children?**
    In female neonates, congenital adrenal hyperplasia is a likely cause of virilization. The classic example is a female infant born with ambiguous genitalia. However, the patient may also be a male child with precocious puberty. At least 90% of cases are due to **21-hydroxylase deficiency.** Because 21-hydroxylase is involved in the production of both aldosterone and cortisol, children develop signs of hypoadrenalism, with salt wasting, hypotension, hyperkalemia, hyponatremia, hypoglycemia, acidosis, and nausea and vomiting. Abnormally high levels of serum 17-hydroxyprogesterone or urinary 17-ketosteroids (dehydroepiandrosterone [DHEA], DHEA sulfate, and androsterone), along with decreased free cortisol in the serum, clinch the diagnosis. Give corticosteroids to prevent death. In older children with virilization, worry about a testosterone-secreting gonadal neoplasm such as a Sertoli-Leydig tumor. Additionally, children with a 5-alpha reductase deficiency can present with virilization during puberty. These patients are phenotypically female, as dihydrotestosterone, which is converted from testosterone by 5-alpha reductase, is needed for external male genitalia development. Increased testosterone levels at puberty will cause clitoromegaly, voice deepening, and increased muscle mass in these patients.

20. **What are the signs and symptoms of hyperparathyroidism?**
    Since parathyroid hormone (PTH) serves to increase serum calcium, the symptoms of hyperparathyroidism are the same as those for hypercalcemia ("bones, stones, groans, thrones, and psychiatric overtones"; see question 24). In primary cases, serum calcium is high, phosphorus is normal to low, and PTH is increased. In secondary cases, calcium is low.

21. **What causes hyperparathyroidism?**
    Ninety percent of primary cases are due to a parathyroid adenoma, which can usually be confirmed with a nuclear medicine scan (Fig. 10.1). Other causes include parathyroid hyperplasia and (rarely) parathyroid carcinoma. Secondary cases include low calcium levels (e.g., from renal failure), to which an increase in PTH is a normal physiologic response. Tertiary hyperparathyroidism occurs when PTH has been elevated for too long (secondary to long-standing hypocalcemia) and continues to be oversecreted via parathyroid hyperplasia even when calcium is normalized with treatment. Translation: Put all patients with renal failure on calcium supplements to prevent this complication.

22. **What are the signs and symptoms of hypoparathyroidism?**
    The same as those for hypocalcemia (tetany, prolonged QT interval on electrocardiogram [ECG]; see question 26). Calcium is low, phosphorus is high, and PTH is low.

23. **What causes hypoparathyroidism?**
    The most common cause is accidental removal or damage during thyroid surgery. Watch for tetany after thyroid surgery. Rare causes are genetic. Watch for **DiGeorge syndrome** (22q11.2 deletion syndrome) in children with congenital absence of parathyroid glands, tetany in the first 48 hours of life, absent thymus gland, immunodeficiency, cardiac anomalies, and midline facial defects.

24. **What are the signs and symptoms of hypercalcemia?**

Signs: shortened QT interval on ECG, weakness, polyuria, bone changes and kidney stones on radiograph, and renal failure.

Symptoms: "bones, stones, groans, thrones, and psychiatric overtones." In other words: bone resorption with osteomalacia and osteitis fibrosa cystica (a condition where calcified portions of bone are replaced by fibrosis and cystlike brown tumors, which are masses of fibrosis, form); kidney stones; abdominal pain secondary to nausea and vomiting, ileus, nephrolithiasis, peptic ulcer disease, constipation, or pancreatitis (all increased with hypercalcemia); increased urination; and emotional lability, delirium, depression, and/or psychosis.

25. **What causes hypercalcemia?**

In outpatients, the most common cause is hyperparathyroidism. In hospitalized patients, the most common cause is malignancy. The first test to order is the PTH, which helps differentiate hyperparathyroidism (high PTH) from other causes of hypercalcemia such as malignancy, vitamin D intoxication, or thiazide diuretic use (low PTH). Multiple types of cancers can cause hypercalcemia, but the classic board question involves either multiple myeloma or paraneoplastic secretion of PTH-related hormone (PTHrP) by a squamous cell carcinoma, especially in the lung. Familial hypocalciuric hypercalcemia is characterized by hypercalcemia with low calcium levels in the urine (opposite of other hypercalcemias). Other causes include vitamin A or D intoxication, sarcoidosis or other granulomatous diseases, and excessive calcium intake (milk-alkali syndrome).

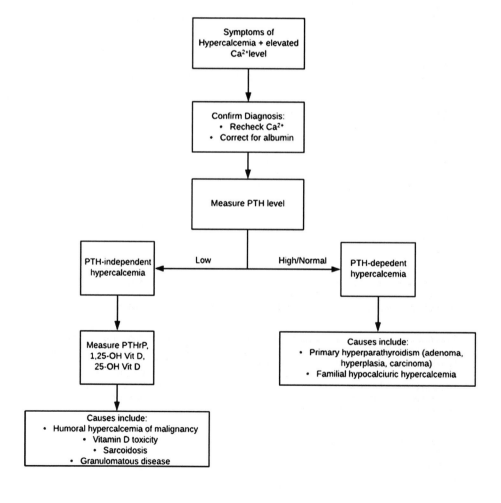

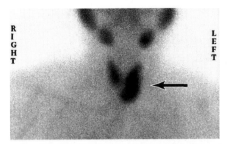

Fig. 10.1 Parathyroid adenomas are almost always solitary lesions. This technetium-99m-sestamibi radionuclide scan demonstrates an area of increased uptake corresponding to the left inferior parathyroid gland *(arrow).* This patient had a parathyroid adenoma. (From Kumar V, Abbas A, Fausto N. *Robbins and Cotran: Pathologic Basis of Disease.* 7th ed. Philadelphia: Saunders; 2005 [fig. 24.24].)

26. What are the signs and symptoms of hypocalcemia?

Signs: prolonged QT interval on ECG, tetany, **Chvostek sign** (tetany elicited by tapping on the facial nerve to cause facial muscle contraction), **Trousseau sign** (carpopedal spasm caused by inflation of a blood pressure cuff or application of a tourniquet), dementia, depression, psychosis, seizures, and papilledema.

Symptoms: paresthesias (the classic pattern is perioral or distal extremities), muscle aches, dementia, depression, and psychosis.

27. What causes hypocalcemia?

- Hypoparathyroidism (usually after thyroid gland surgery)
- Pseudohypoparathyroidism (genetic end-organ unresponsiveness to PTH with normal PTH levels, shortened metacarpal bones, short stature, and intellectual disability)
- DiGeorge syndrome (22q11.2 deletion syndrome)
- Vitamin D deficiency (osteomalacia, rickets)
- Renal failure of any cause and certain renal tubular problems
- Acute pancreatitis (one of the Ranson criteria)
- Secondary to hypomagnesemia

    Hypoproteinemia of any cause may lead to low levels of total serum calcium, but levels of ionized calcium (the active form) are normal. In any patient with low serum calcium, the first step is to determine whether the serum albumin level is decreased. If it is, no treatment is required, and no symptoms will develop.

28. What specific problems are caused by obesity?

Obesity causes an increase in overall mortality (at any age) and increases the risk for insulin resistance and type 2 diabetes, hypertension, hypertriglyceridemia, coronary artery disease, gallstones, sleep apnea and hypoventilation, osteoarthritis, thromboembolism, varicose veins, and cancer (especially endometrial cancer due to aromatase action in adipose tissue).

29. Define precocious puberty and pseudoprecocious puberty.

True precocious puberty is defined as activation of the hypothalamic-pituitary axis with sexual maturation before the age of 8 years in females and before the age of 9 years in males. In **pseudoprecocious puberty**, secondary sex characteristics develop prematurely because of high circulating levels of androgen or estrogen.

30. How is precocious puberty different from pseudoprecocious puberty?

True precocious puberty is usually idiopathic but can be caused by central nervous system (CNS) lesions. A general rule of thumb is that true precocious puberty causes testicular or ovarian enlargement, which does not occur with pseudoprecocious puberty (ovarian cysts are not considered true ovarian enlargement). All patients with suspected precocious puberty should have a gonadotropin-releasing hormone (GnRH) stimulation test. If a dose of GnRH produces the typical pubertal response of increased follicle-stimulating hormone (FSH) and luteinizing hormone (LH), true precocious puberty is diagnosed. An MRI of the brain should be obtained to rule out CNS disease (e.g., hamartomas, tumors, cysts, trauma) as the cause.

31. What causes pseudoprecocious puberty?

Pseudoprecocious puberty may be caused by exogenous hormones, adrenal tumors, congenital adrenal hyperplasia (e.g., 21-hydroxylase deficiency), hormone-secreting tumors, or **McCune-Albright syndrome** in females (ovarian cysts, pseudoprecocious puberty, polyostotic fibrous dysplasia of bone, and café au lait spots) (Fig. 10.2).

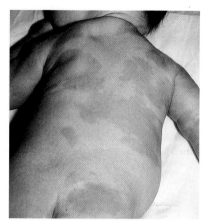

Fig. 10.2 Multiple patterned café au lait spots in a child with McCune-Albright syndrome. (From Eichenfield LF. *Neonatal Dermatology*. 2nd ed. Philadelphia: Saunders; 2008 [fig. 22.3].)

32. How is precocious puberty treated?

Because premature puberty causes premature fusion of growth plates in the bone and can cause serious social problems for affected children, treatment is indicated. Treatment of any underlying disorders is indicated for pseudoprecocious puberty. For true idiopathic precocious puberty, treatment with long-acting GnRH agonists is indicated to suppress the pituitary-hypothalamic axis and to delay the onset of puberty until an appropriate age.

33. What is the difference between a primary and a secondary endocrine disorder?

In **primary disorders**, the problem is in the gland; the hypothalamic-pituitary axis is functioning appropriately. In primary hypothyroidism, for example, the thyroid gland does not function properly for whatever reason, but the pituitary and hypothalamus respond appropriately. Therefore thyroid hormone is low (as in all cases of hypothyroidism), but TSH and thyroid-releasing hormone (TRH) are high (the appropriate response from the pituitary and hypothalamus to low levels of thyroid hormone).

In **secondary disorders**, the true dysfunction is outside the gland itself. For example, in secondary hypothyroidism, thyroid hormone is low, but TSH and/or TRH is also low (inappropriate in the setting of low thyroid hormone). If the pituitary is destroyed or surgically removed, secondary hypothyroidism results from low TSH; the thyroid gland functions well, but no TSH is available to stimulate it. To confuse the picture, the dysfunction may also be completely outside the endocrine axis (e.g., heart failure that causes secondary hyperaldosteronism).

This concept in endocrine gland dysfunction is quite important. Simple blood tests can localize the problem. You may be able to answer a USMLE question simply by reading through the various values for hormones and hormone-releasing factors and figuring out where in the hypothalamus–pituitary–target gland axis the problem lies.

34. What are the signs and symptoms of primary hyperaldosteronism (Conn syndrome)? What are the causes?

Signs: hypertension, hypokalemia, hypernatremia, and edema
Symptoms: weakness and edema

Conn syndrome is caused by an aldosterone-secreting adrenal neoplasm. Because it is a primary disease, renin levels are low; the rest of endocrine axis responds appropriately to gland dysfunction. Conn syndrome can be determined by measuring a plasma aldosterone concentration (PAC) and plasma renin activity (PRA). The PAC/PRA ratio should be greater than 20 with decreased PRA and PAC of 15 or more. Next order a CT of the abdomen to look for an adrenal mass. The treatment is surgical removal of the tumor. Conn syndrome can also be caused by unilateral or bilateral adrenal hyperplasia; in these cases, treat with mineralocorticoid receptor antagonists (spironolactone or eplerenone).

35. What causes secondary hyperaldosteronism?

Secondary hyperaldosteronism is much more common than primary disease. It is due to low perfusion of the kidney, as in congestive heart failure, renal artery stenosis (bruit), dehydration, nephrotic syndrome, and cirrhosis. Other causes include diuretics, renin-secreting tumors, and coarctation of the aorta. The key mechanism

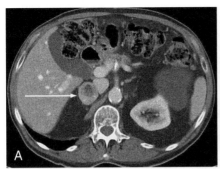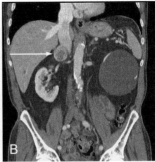

Fig. 10.3 A computed tomographic (CT) scan of the abdomen with intravenous contrast agent of a 71-year-old man with an incidentally discovered right adrenal mass. The fractionated plasma-free metanephrines were abnormal. (A) The axial CT image shows a typical 3.8-cm heterogeneously enhancing right adrenal mass just lateral to the inferior vena cava and consistent with pheochromocytoma *(arrow).* (B) Coronal view shows the location *(arrow)* of the mass superior to the right kidney and inferior and medial to the liver. After alpha- and beta-adrenergic blockade, a pheochromocytoma was removed laparoscopically. (From Kronenberg H, et al. *Williams Textbook of Endocrinology.* 11th ed. Philadelphia: Saunders; 2008 [fig. 15.3].)

is that the kidney senses hypoperfusion and secretes renin, therefore the renin level is high. In secondary hyperaldosteronism, both PAC and PRA are elevated with the PAC/PRA ratio approximately equal to 10. Treatment of the underlying disorder (if possible) resolves the hyperaldosteronism. Potassium levels may be normal or even high. Of note, hyperkalemia may be the cause of increased aldosterone release just as hypocalcemia causes increased release of PTH. Both are normal physiologic responses.

36. Give the classic clinical description of a pheochromocytoma. How is it diagnosed?

Look for wild swings in blood pressure (with some measurements dangerously high), tachycardia, postural hypotension, headaches, sweating, flushing, dizziness, mental status changes, and/or a feeling of impending doom (like a panic attack). A memory aid to remember the common symptoms of a pheochromocytoma is the five paroxysmal Ps: pressure, pain, pallor, palpitations, perspiration. The screening test is a 24-hour urine collection for metanephrines, homovanillic acid, and/or vanillylmandelic acid (catecholamine breakdown products that are abnormally elevated in the urine). An alternative screening test is a plasma fractionated metanephrine assay. If levels are high, order an abdominal CT scan to look for an adrenal mass (Fig. 10.3). Surgical tumor removal is the treatment of choice after stabilization with first alpha-blockers (e.g., phenoxybenzamine) and then beta-blockers.

37. Define diabetes insipidus (DI). What are the two types?

DI is a lack of antidiuretic hormone (ADH or vasopressin) effect in the body. Patients with DI secrete inappropriately dilute urine because of a lack of ADH effect and may urinate up to 25 L of urine per day, resulting in dehydration and hypernatremia. Plasma osmolality is often greater than 295 mOsm/kg. Such patients die rapidly if they are unable to drink water. Normally, when the body is dehydrated, ADH causes urine to become highly concentrated through retention of free water. In DI, the urine remains dilute even though the serum osmolarity is quite high as a result of dehydration. The two types are **central** and **nephrogenic**.

38. What causes central DI?

Central DI is caused by a lack of ADH production by the posterior pituitary. Although it is often idiopathic, look for trauma, neoplasm, sarcoidosis/granulomatous disease, or ischemic encephalopathy as the cause. Order a CT scan or MRI of the head, if indicated.

39. What causes nephrogenic DI?

Nephrogenic DI is due to kidney unresponsiveness to ADH. Look for medications (e.g., lithium and demeclocycline), hypercalcemia, or hereditary mutations as the cause.

40. What diagnostic test can reveal whether DI is central or nephrogenic? How are these conditions treated?

Give the patient a dose of ADH or desmopressin, and measure urine osmolarity. If central DI is the cause, urine osmolarity increases with ADH challenge. In nephrogenic DI, the urine remains inappropriately dilute after the patient is given ADH. Additionally, serum Na^+ can help differentiate between the two. Patients with central DI tend to be hypernatremic, whereas patients with nephrogenic DI are euvolemic. This is because in nephrogenic DI, patients have an intact thirst mechanism, so they have adequate water intake to compensate for the renal loss of water. Treatment for central DI is ADH replacement (desmopressin, given orally or as a nasal spray). Treatment for nephrogenic DI involves stopping any offending drug and giving a thiazide diuretic; ADH does not help. Although giving a diuretic to a patient with DI seems counterintuitive, it has the paradoxic effect of decreasing urine output.

41. Define the syndrome of inappropriate antidiuretic hormone secretion (SIADH). How is it diagnosed?

The name says it all: ADH is released inappropriately. SIADH is a consideration in patients with hyponatremia and normal volume status (euvolemic). In SIADH, serum osmolarity is low, but urine osmolarity is high (inappropriate urine concentration). Look for the values of all electrolytes and lab tests to be low (the classic example is uric acid) because of dilution of the serum with free water secondary to inappropriate ADH.

42. What causes SIADH?

CNS causes: stroke, hemorrhage, infection, trauma

Medications: narcotics, oxytocin (watch for pregnant patients), chlorpropamide, antiepileptic agents, selective serotonin reuptake inhibitors (SSRIs)

Trauma: Pain is a powerful stimulus for ADH. Watch for the postoperative patient who is receiving fluids (and often narcotics) and has pain to develop SIADH.

Lung problems: simple pneumonia or ADH-secreting small cell cancer of the lung

43. How is SIADH treated?

Treat with water restriction. Stop intravenous fluids (as normal saline will worsen hyponatremia due to increased free water retention) and restrict oral fluid intake. For Step 2 purposes, do not give hypertonic saline unless the patient has active seizures before your eyes. You may cause osmotic demyelination syndrome (ODS, formerly called central pontine myelinolysis) from too rapid correction of sodium level (memory aid = "from low to high [sodium], the pons will die"). **Demeclocycline** is sometimes used to treat SIADH if water restriction fails because it induces nephrogenic diabetes insipidus, which allows the patient to get rid of free water.

44. What is cerebral salt wasting (CSW)? How is it different from SIADH?

CSW is a specific form of hyponatremia caused by CNS disease (e.g., hemorrhage, intracranial lesion). Like SIADH, it has high urine osmolality and high urine sodium, but the distinction is that whereas SIADH is euvolemic, CSW is hypovolemic.

45. What is acromegaly? How it is diagnosed and treated?

Acromegaly is caused by excessive secretion of growth hormone (GH) and presents with large hands/feet/brow/jaw, enlarged organs, and glucose intolerance. Additionally, acromegaly leads to concentric myocardial cardiomyopathy, which results in heart failure. It is most commonly caused by a GH-secreting pituitary adenoma. It is first screened with a serum IGF-1 level (elevated) and confirmed with a glucose suppression test, in which glucose fails to suppress GH secretion. Treatment is usually resection, but acromegaly can be medically managed with octreotide (a somatostatin analogue).

ETHICS

CHAPTER 11

1. What are the general principles of ethics?
   - Autonomy: acknowledging and respecting a patient's right to make one's own choices and decisions based on one's values and beliefs
   - Beneficence: acting in the patient's best interests
   - Nonmaleficence: "do no harm," the obligation not to intentionally inflict harm
   - Justice: treating patients equitably

2. True or false: Adult patients of sound mind are allowed to refuse life-saving treatments.
   True. You should not force blood products, antibiotics, or any other treatments on a patient who does not want them.

3. What should you do if a child has a life-threatening condition and the parents refuse a simple, curative treatment (e.g., antibiotics for meningitis)?
   First, try to persuade the parents to change their mind; if this fails, attempt to get a court order to give the treatment. Do not treat until you have talked to the courts unless it is an emergency. Even with Jehovah's Witnesses who do not want their children to receive a blood transfusion, you should seek the court's assistance in getting the transfusion if it is the only treatment option available. However, if the child is in critical condition and cannot wait for the court order, you may begin the transfusion without parental consent.

4. What is the difference between active and passive euthanasia?
   Active euthanasia is the intentional hastening of death, whereas passive euthanasia is withdrawing or opting not to initiate aggressive, "heroic," life-prolonging treatments (e.g., intubation or artificial nutrition) and "letting nature take its course."

5. With whom can you discuss your patient's condition?
   Only with people who need to know because they are directly involved in the patient's care and with people authorized by the patient (e.g., authorized family members). In the case of a patient with a designated health care proxy, information may only be shared if a patient is deemed to lack capacity to make health care decisions, which is when the proxy comes into effect. Do not tell a medical colleague who is uninvolved with the patient's care how that patient is doing, even if the colleague is a friend of yours or of the patient.

6. In what situations are you allowed to breach patient confidentiality?
   Break confidentiality only in the following situations:
   - The patient asks you to do so.
   - Child abuse is suspected (mandated reporting).
   - The courts mandate you to do so.
   - You must fulfill the duty to warn or protect (if a patient talks of suicide or killing another person, you must tell someone, the authorities, or both).
   - The patient has a reportable disease.
   - The patient is a danger to others (e.g., if a patient is blind or has seizures, let the proper authorities know so that they can revoke the patient's license to drive; if the patient is an airplane pilot with paranoid schizophrenia, then authorities need to know).

7. What are the components of informed consent?
   Informed consent involves giving the patient information about the following:
   - Diagnosis (patient's condition and what it means)
   - Prognosis (the natural course of the condition without treatment)
   - Proposed treatment (description of the procedure and what the patient will experience)
   - Risks and benefits of the treatment
   - Alternative treatments
     The patient then must be allowed to make a choice. The documents seen on the wards that patients are made to sign are not technically required or sufficient for informed consent. They are used for medicolegal purposes (i.e., lawsuit paranoia).

8. What should you do if a patient lacks capacity to make decisions?
   A physician can determine capacity for decision making, but courts determine competency. If a patient lacks capacity for decision making, obtain consent from family (spouse, adult children, parents, and then adult siblings) and/or have the courts appoint a guardian (surrogate decision maker or health care power of attorney).

9. True or false: A living will should not be respected if the next of kin asks you not to follow it.
False. Such situations are tricky, but technically (and for the USMLE) living wills or patient-mandated "do-not-resuscitate" orders should be respected and followed if properly documented. The classic board question involves a patient who says in a living will that if he or she is unable to breathe independently, a ventilator should not be used. Do not put the patient on a ventilator, even if the husband, wife, son, or daughter tells you to do so.

10. What should you do if a patient is in critical condition or in a coma and has made no advance directive or living will?
Begin resuscitation of the patient. Contact the family, next of kin, or health care power of attorney, and follow their wishes. In cases of disagreement among family members, suspicion of ulterior motives, or uncertainty, involve the hospital's ethics committee. As a last resort, go to the courts for help.

11. What about depression in the context of end-of-life decisions?
Depression should always be evaluated as a reason for lack of capacity. Patients who are actively suicidal may not have capacity to consent to or refuse life-prolonging treatment.

12. True or false: In some circumstances, patients can be hospitalized against their will.
True. Psychiatric patients may be hospitalized against their will if they are deemed to be a danger to themselves or others or are "gravely disabled," meaning unable to care for themselves by meeting their basic needs of food, clothing, and shelter. Patients can be held only for a limited time (1–3 days) before they must have a hearing before a court official to determine whether they must remain in custody. These decisions are based on the principle of **beneficence** (the principle of doing good for the patient and avoiding harm).

13. True or false: Restraints can be used on patients against their will.
True. Chemical and/or physical restraints can be used on an agitated (e.g., delirious, psychotic) patient if needed, but their use should be brief and reevaluated often (at least once every 24 hours). Be aware that the use of restraints in delirious or demented patients rarely helps prevent falls and may cause injury.

14. When do patients under the age of 18 years not require parental consent for a medical decision?
In general, people under the age of 18 do not require parental consent if they are emancipated (married, living on their own and financially independent, raising children, or serving in the armed forces); have a sexually transmitted disease, want contraception, or are pregnant; want treatment or counseling for substance use disorders; or have psychiatric illness. Some states have exceptions to these rules, but for Step 2 purposes, minors may make their own decisions in such situations.

15. What should you do if a child has a medical emergency and the parents are unavailable for decision making?
Treat the child as you see fit; that is, act in the child's best interest.

16. True or false: It is acceptable to hide a diagnosis from a patient if the family asks you to do so.
False. Do not hide a diagnosis from a patient (including a child) if the patient wants to know (even if the family asks you to do so). Do not lie to any patient because the family asks you to do so. Conversely, you should not force patients to receive information against their will; if they do not want to know the diagnosis, do not tell them.

17. What should you do if a patient requires emergency care but the patient cannot communicate and no family members are available?
Treat the patient as you see fit unless you know that the patient wishes otherwise.

18. True or false: Withdrawing care and withholding care are the same in the eyes of the law.
True. It is important to communicate this principle to family members. The simple fact that a patient is on a respirator does not mean that you cannot turn off the respirator.

19. True or false: In a terminally ill patient with an incurable illness, one of the primary goals is to relieve pain.
True. Opioids are commonly used, even though they may cause respiratory depression. If in keeping with a patient's wishes, it is more important to make the patient comfortable and pain free, even with the risk of respiratory depression in this setting.

20. When is it acceptable to receive gifts from patients or organizations?
As a general rule, gifts from patients and organizations should not be accepted by physicians. When deciding whether accepting a gift from a patient is appropriate, one must consider the cost, timing of the gift, and underlying motivation for giving it. Gifts that are expensive, inappropriate, or are apparently given to secure preferential treatment should not be accepted. The only acceptable gifts from organizations are those of little to no monetary value that directly benefit patient care (e.g., unbiased educational materials). Gifts such as pens or flash drives from pharmaceutical companies do not directly benefit patient care and therefore should not be accepted due to their ability to influence a physician's prescriptions or practices.

CHAPTER 12

GASTROENTEROLOGY

1. Define gastroesophageal reflux disease (GERD). What causes it?

   GERD is stomach acid refluxing into the esophagus. It is due to inappropriate, intermittent relaxation of the lower esophageal sphincter. Patients with a hiatal hernia have a much greater incidence of GERD (see question 4).

2. Describe the classic symptoms of GERD. How is it treated? What are red flag symptoms?

   The main complaint is usually "heartburn," often related to lying supine after eating. GERD may also cause abdominal or chest pain. More rarely, it can cause cough from laryngeal irritation. Initial treatment is behavioral, including elevating the head of the bed and avoiding coffee, alcohol, tobacco, spicy and fatty foods, chocolate, and medications with anticholinergic properties. If this approach fails, antacids, histamine-2 (H2) blockers, and proton-pump inhibitors (PPIs) may be tried. Many patients have already tried over-the-counter remedies before presentation, and many physicians begin empiric treatment at the first visit, since "lifestyle modifications" usually fail. Surgery (Nissen fundoplication) is reserved for severe or refractory cases. Red flag symptoms for GERD include dysphagia/odynophagia, anemia/melena/hematemesis, weight loss, pneumonia, high-risk patients (men age >50 years or those with symptoms lasting >5 years), or no response to PPIs. Patients with these symptoms warrant an upper endoscopy for evaluation.

3. What are the sequelae of GERD?

   Sequelae of GERD include esophagitis, esophageal stricture (which may mimic esophageal cancer), esophageal ulcer, hemorrhage, Barrett esophagus, and esophageal adenocarcinoma (Fig. 12.1).

4. What is a hiatal hernia? How is it different from a paraesophageal hernia?

   A hiatal hernia is a sliding hernia, which means that the entire gastroesophageal junction moves above the diaphragm, pulling the stomach with it. This common and benign finding may predispose to GERD. In a paraesophageal hernia, the gastroesophageal junction stays below the diaphragm, but the stomach herniates through the diaphragm into the thorax. This type of hernia is uncommon but serious; it may become strangulated and should be surgically repaired. Both can be seen on chest x-ray as a round retrocardiac density with air-fluid levels and are often incidental findings.

5. How does peptic ulcer disease (PUD) present?

   PUD classically presents with chronic, intermittent, epigastric pain (burning, gnawing, or aching) that is localized and often relieved by antacids or milk. Look for epigastric tenderness. Other signs and symptoms include occult blood in the stool and nausea or vomiting. PUD is more common in men. The two types of PUD are gastric and duodenal ulcers.

6. Explain the classic differences between duodenal and gastric ulcers

	Duodenal	Gastric
% of cases	75	25
Acid secretion	Normal to high	Normal to low
Main cause	*Helicobacter pylori*	Use of nonsteroidal antiinflammatory drugs (NSAIDs), including aspirin
Peak age	40s	50s
Blood type	0	A
Eating food	Pain gets better, then worse 2–3 hr later	Pain not relieved or made worse

7. What is the diagnostic study of choice for PUD?

   Endoscopy for visualization and biopsy of ulcers is the gold standard (most sensitive test), but an upper gastrointestinal (GI) barium swallow study is cheaper and less invasive. Empiric treatment with medications may be trialed in the absence of diagnostic studies if the symptoms are typical. If endoscopy is done, a biopsy of any gastric ulcer is mandatory to exclude malignancy. Duodenal ulcers do not have to be biopsied initially because malignancy is rare.

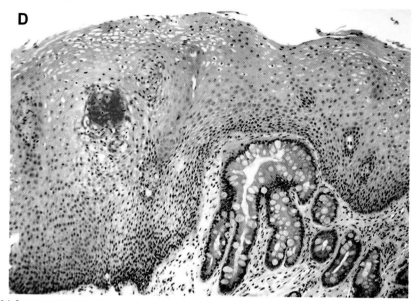

Fig. 12.1 Squamous epithelium of the esophagus overlying developing metaplasia in the crypts *(bottom right)* consistent with early Barrett metaplasia. (From Lisovsky M, Srivastava A. Barrett esophagus: evolving concepts in diagnosis and neoplastic progression. *Surg Pathol Clin.* 2013;6(3):475–496. https://doi.org/10.1016/j.path.2013.05.002. Epub 2013 Aug 6.)

8. **What is the most feared complication of PUD? What should you suspect if an ulcer does not respond to treatment?**
   Perforation is the most feared complication of PUD. Look for peritoneal signs (severe abdominal pain with rebound tenderness and involuntary guarding), history of PUD, and free air on an abdominal radiograph, which can be checked with an abdominal x-ray or computed tomography (CT) scan (Fig. 12.2). Treat with antibiotics that cover enteric organisms (such as ceftriaxone and metronidazole) and laparotomy with repair of the perforation. If ulcers are severe, atypical (e.g., located in the jejunum), or nonhealing, think about stomach cancer or Zollinger-Ellison syndrome (gastrinoma; check gastrin level). PUD is also the most common cause of upper GI bleeding in noncirrhotic patients, which can be severe in some cases.

9. **How is PUD treated initially?**
   First, remember that diet changes are not thought to help heal ulcers, although reduced alcohol and tobacco use may speed healing. Stop all NSAID use. Start treatment with a PPI, test for *Helicobacter pylori* infection (biopsy, stool antigen testing, or urea breath test), and treat with antibiotics if positive. Many regimens exist, but the most commonly used is triple therapy with a PPI, clarithromycin, and amoxicillin. An alternative treatment in areas of high clarithromycin resistance is quadruple therapy: a PPI, bismuth subsalicylate, metronidazole, and tetracycline.

10. **Name the surgical options for ulcer treatment. What complications may occur?**
    Surgical options are generally considered only if medical treatment has failed or if complications are present (perforation, bleeding). Surgical procedures for PUD include antrectomy, vagotomy, and Billroth I or II procedures. After surgery (especially with Billroth procedures), watch for dumping syndrome (weakness, dizziness, sweating, and nausea or vomiting after eating due to emptying of hypertonic gastric contents into the duodenum). Dumping syndrome can be managed with smaller, more frequent meals that are higher in complex carbohydrates, high-fiber foods, and protein-rich foods instead of simple sugars. Patients may also develop hypoglycemia 2 to 3 hours after a meal, which causes recurrence of the same symptoms as well as afferent loop syndrome (bilious vomiting after a meal relieves abdominal pain), bacterial overgrowth (malabsorption, abdominal pain, and altered bowel habits), and vitamin deficiencies (vitamin B_{12} and/or iron, causing anemia).

11. **Define achlorhydria. What causes it?**
    Achlorhydria is absence of hydrochloric acid (HCl) secretion. It is due most commonly to **pernicious anemia**, in which autoantibodies destroy acid-secreting parietal cells, causing achlorhydria and vitamin B_{12} deficiency. Achlorhydria is often associated with other endocrine autoimmune disorders (e.g., hypothyroidism, vitiligo, diabetes, hypoadrenalism). Achlorhydria may also be caused by surgical gastric resection and rarely a VIPoma.

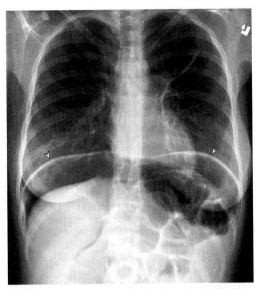

Fig. 12.2 Pneumoperitoneum from bowel perforation on conventional radiographs. Upright radiograph shows the large amount of free intraperitoneal air (lucent area just inferior to the diaphragm). (From Goldman L. *Goldman's Cecil Medicine*. 24th ed. Philadelphia: Saunders; 2011 [fig. 135.1].)

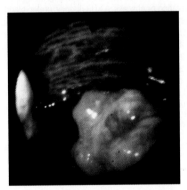

Fig. 12.3 Colonoscopic photograph of a pale colon cancer easily seen against the dark background of pseudomelanosis coli. (From Feldman M, Friedman L, Brandt L. *Sleisenger and Fordtran's Gastrointestinal and Liver Disease*. 9th ed. Philadelphia: Saunders; 2010 [fig. 124.8]. Courtesy Juergen Nord, MD, Tampa, FL.)

12. What are classic differences between upper and lower GI bleeds?

	Upper GI Bleed	*Lower GI Bleed*
Location	Proximal to ligament of Treitz	Distal to ligament of Treitz
Common causes	Gastritis, ulcers, varices, esophagitis	Vascular ectasia, diverticulosis, colon cancer (Fig. 12.3), colitis, inflammatory bowel disease, hemorrhoids
Stool	Tarry, black stool (melena)	Bright red blood seen in stool (hematochezia)
NGT aspirate	Positive for blood	Negative for blood

NGT, Nasogastric tube.

Additionally, an upper GI bleed more commonly presents with an increased blood urea nitrogen (BUN) level as the blood gets digested and absorbed.

13. How is a GI bleed treated?

The first step is to ensure that the patient is stable by checking the ABCs (airways, breathing, circulation) and giving intravenous fluids and blood, if needed, before searching for a cause. Start a PPI intravenously. Other supportive measures include oxygen and bowel rest. **Endoscopy** is usually the first test performed (upper or lower, depending on symptoms and nasogastric tube aspirate). Endoscopically treatable lesions include ulcers, polyps, vascular ectasias, and varices.

14. What radiologic imaging studies can be done to localize a GI bleed? Does surgery have a role?

Radionuclide (i.e., nuclear medicine) scans can detect slow or intermittent bleeds if a source cannot be found with endoscopy. Angiography can detect more rapid bleeds, and embolization of bleeding vessels can be done during the procedure. Surgery is reserved for severe or resistant bleeds and typically involves resection of the affected bowel (usually colon).

15. Define diverticulosis. What are its complications?

Diverticulosis is characterized by saclike mucosal projections through the muscular layer of the colon and/or rectum. It is extremely common, and the incidence increases with age. It is thought to be caused in part by a low-fiber, high-fat diet, which in turn leads to constipation and increased luminal pressure. It is most common in the sigmoid colon. Complications include diverticular GI bleeding (common cause of painless lower GI bleeds and is most commonly found in the right colon) and diverticulitis (inflammation of a diverticulum). Diverticulitis can lead to abscess formation, fistula formation, sepsis, or large bowel obstruction.

16. How do you diagnose and treat diverticulitis? What test should a patient have after a treated episode of diverticulitis?

Signs and symptoms of diverticulitis include left lower quadrant pain or tenderness, fever, diarrhea or constipation, and leukocytosis. The pathophysiology is similar to appendicitis: stool or other debris impacts within the outpouched mucosa (the diverticulum) and causes obstruction, leading to bacterial overgrowth and inflammation. The diagnosis can be confirmed with a CT scan (Fig. 12.4), if needed, which can also help to rule out complications such as perforation or abscess. A KUB (kidney, ureter, bladder x-ray) can be used to assess for ileus or perforation. In the absence of complications, the treatment is antibiotics that cover bowel flora (e.g., a fluoroquinolone plus metronidazole) and bowel rest (i.e., no oral intake). Antibiotics in complicated diverticulitis become more broad spectrum and include piperacillin/tazobactam or one of the penems. Surgery in the form of a bowel resection may be needed when diverticulitis is complicated by perforation or abscess. Percutaneous CT drainage of an abscess is indicated if greater than 3 cm.

After a treated episode of diverticulitis, all patients need colon cancer screening with colonoscopy (colon carcinoma with perforation can mimic diverticulitis clinically and on CT). These studies should be avoided during active diverticulitis, however, due to an increased risk for perforation. Patients should maintain a high-fiber diet.

17. How is diarrhea categorized?

According to etiology:
- Systemic. Any illness can cause diarrhea as a systemic symptom, especially in children (e.g., infection).
- Osmotic
- Secretory
- Malabsorptive
- Infectious
- Exudative
- Altered intestinal transit

18. Define osmotic diarrhea. How can an easy diagnosis be made?

Osmotic diarrhea is caused by nonabsorbable solutes that remain in the bowel, where they retain water (e.g., lactose or other carbohydrate intolerance). It presents with a stool osmolar gap above 50 mOsm/kg, no blood or mucus in stool, and positive fecal fat. The stool osmolar gap is calculated with the following equation: $290 - [2 \times$ (stool Na^+ + stool K^+)]. When the patient stops ingesting the offending substance (e.g., avoidance of milk or a trial of fasting), the diarrhea stops—an easy diagnosis.

19. What causes secretory diarrhea?

Secretory diarrhea results when the bowel secretes too much fluid. It presents with a stool osmolar gap below 50 mOsm/kg, no blood or mucus in stool, and no fecal fat. It is often due to bacterial toxins (cholera, some species of *Escherichia coli*), VIPoma (pancreatic islet cell tumor that secretes vasoactive intestinal peptide), or bile acids (after ileal resection). VIPomas can cause WDHA (watery diarrhea, hypokalemia, achlorhydria) syndrome. Secretory diarrhea persists even when the patient stops eating.

20. What are the common causes of malabsorptive diarrhea?

Celiac disease (look for chronic diarrhea, weight loss, abdominal distention, and dermatitis herpetiformis, and avoid gluten in the diet) (Fig. 12.5), Crohn disease, and postgastroenteritis (due to depletion of brush-border enzymes). Malabsorptive diarrhea improves with bowel rest (i.e., when the patient is not eating).

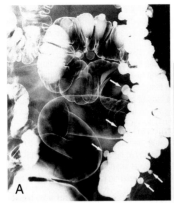
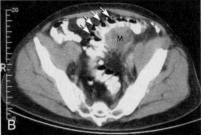

Fig. 12.4 Diverticulosis of the colon is seen on this oblique view of the sigmoid colon (A) during a double-contrast barium enema showing multiple outpouchings *(arrows)* that represent diverticula. Diverticula also can be seen in a computed tomography (CT) scan (B) as outpouchings *(arrows)*, but a developing focal inflammatory mass *(M)* also is compatible with a developing abscess. (From Mettler F. *Essentials of Radiology.* 2nd ed. Philadelphia: Saunders; 2004 [fig. 6.73].)

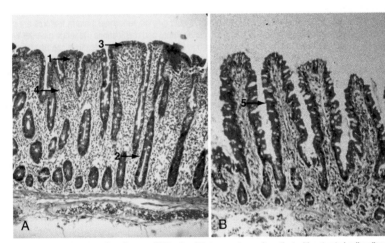

Fig. 12.5 Mucosal pathology in celiac disease. (A) Duodenal biopsy specimen of a patient with untreated celiac disease. The histologic features of severe villus atrophy *(arrow 1)*, crypt hyperplasia *(arrow 2)*, enterocyte disarray *(arrow 3)*, and intense inflammation of the lamina propria and epithelial cell layer *(arrow 4)* are evident. (B) Repeat duodenal biopsy after 6 months on a strict gluten-free diet. There is marked improvement, with well-formed villi *(arrow 5)* and a return of the mucosal architecture toward normal. (From Feldman M, Friedman L, Brandt L. *Sleisenger and Fordtran's Gastrointestinal and Liver Disease.* 9th ed. Philadelphia: Saunders; 2010 [fig. 104.2].)

21. How is celiac disease diagnosed?

It is diagnosed with immunoglobulin A (IgA) antitissue transglutaminase (the preferred test), IgA antiendomysial, or IgG antigliadin (in patients with IgA deficiency, which is a common coexisting condition). Also, an upper endoscopy with biopsy can be performed, which will show atrophic villi and crypt hyperplasia. Celiac disease most often affects the duodenum or proximal jejunum.

22. What are the common clues to infectious diarrhea? What are the common causes?

Look for fever and white blood cells in the stool (only with invasive bacteria such as *Shigella, Salmonella, Yersinia,* and *Campylobacter* species; not found with toxigenic bacteria). Fecal inflammatory markers such as fecal calprotectin or fecal lactoferrin are typically elevated. Differentiating between potential causes of infectious diarrhea is difficult. History plays a role. Travel history (Montezuma's revenge caused by *E. coli*) is also a tip-off. *Shigella* infection tends to present with tenesmus. *Salmonella* is associated with consumption of raw chicken or eggs. *E. coli* O157:H7 infection is often spread via uncooked hamburger meat and often does not present with a fever. *C. perfringens* often presents with predominatly crampy abdominal pain. Hikers and stream-drinkers may have *Giardia* infection, which presents with steatorrhea (fatty, greasy, malodorous stools that float) due to small bowel involvement and unique protozoal cysts in the stool. Treat *Giardia* with metronidazole. Also watch for

Clostridioides difficile diarrhea in patients with a history of antibiotic use. Test the stool for *C. difficile* toxin, and if the result is positive, treat with oral vancomycin (fidaxomicin is another option). Intravenous metronidazole may be added in more severe cases. Fecal microbiota transplantation is employed in recurrent cases.

23. **What causes exudative diarrhea?**

Exudative diarrhea results from inflammation in the bowel mucosa that causes seepage of fluid. Mucosal inflammation is usually due to inflammatory bowel disease (Crohn disease or ulcerative colitis; see question 27) or cancer. Patients commonly have fever as well as white blood cells and other inflammatory markers (e.g., fecal calprotectin) in the stool, as in infectious diarrhea, but a lack of pathogenic organisms, chronicity, and extraintestinal symptoms are clues.

24. **What are the common causes of diarrhea due to altered intestinal transit?**

This type of diarrhea is seen after bowel resections, in patients taking medications that interfere with bowel function, and in patients with thyroid disease (hypo- or hyperthyroidism) or neuropathy (e.g., diabetic diarrhea). Watch for factitious diarrhea, which is caused by secret laxative abuse (endoscopy may reveal pigmented colonic mucosa called melanosis coli). Impaired motility can also occur in autoimmune diseases such as systemic lupus erythematous or amyloidosis.

25. **Define irritable bowel syndrome (IBS). How do you recognize it? How do you treat it?**

IBS is a common cause of GI complaints. Patients may have psychiatric comorbidities and have a history of diarrhea aggravated by stress; bloating; abdominal pain relieved by defecation; and/or mucus in the stool. There is a female-to-male predominance of 3:1, and patients are usually younger. Look for psychosocial stressors in the history and normal exam findings and test results. IBS is diagnosed via the Rome III criteria of abdominal pain plus two of the following: pain related to defecation, pain associated with a change in stool frequency, or pain associated with a change in stool form. You must do at least basic lab tests to rule out inflammatory bowel disease, celiac disease, and infectious causes; endoscopy should only be performed if alarm features are present.

Treatment is a combination of nonpharmacologic management and medications. Depending on the type (predominantly diarrheal [IBS-D], predominantly constipation [IBS-C], or mixed), medications can be chosen. For IBS-C, choices include osmotic laxatives (PEG), lubiprostone (a chloride channel activator), or linaclotide (guanylate cyclase agonists). For IBS-D, loperamide is first-line therapy when nonpharmacologic treatment fails. For the abdominal pain, antispasmodics (i.e., dicyclomine or hyoscyamine) and antidepressants (i.e., TCAs) are used.

26. **What should you do if a patient has diarrhea?**

In all patients with diarrhea, watch for and treat dehydration and electrolyte disturbances, especially metabolic acidosis and hypokalemia. Diarrhea is a common and preventable cause of death in underdeveloped countries. Do a rectal exam, look for occult blood in stool, and examine the stool for bacteria (Gram stain and culture), ova and parasites, fat content (steatorrhea), and white blood cells. If inflammatory bowel disease is suspected, fecal calprotectin is both specific and sensitive.

27. **What should you watch for in children after a bout of diarrhea?**

After bacterial (especially *E. coli* or *Shigella* sp.) diarrhea in children, watch for **hemolytic uremic syndrome**, which is characterized by thrombocytopenia, microangiopathic hemolytic anemia (schistocytes, helmet cells, and fragmented red blood cells on peripheral blood smear), and acute renal failure. Treatment is supportive. Patients may need dialysis and/or transfusions.

28. **Specify the classic differences between Crohn disease and ulcerative colitis**

	Crohn Disease	*Ulcerative Colitis*
Place of origin	Distal ileum, proximal colon	Rectum
Thickness of pathology	Transmural	Mucosa/submucosa only
Progression	Irregular (skip-lesions)	Proximal, continuous from rectum; no skipped areas
Location	From mouth to anus	Involves only colon, rarely extends to ileum
Bowel habit changes	Obstruction, abdominal pain	Bloody diarrhea
Classic lesions	Fistulas/abscesses, cobblestoning, creeping fat, string sign on barium x-ray (Fig. 12.6)	Pseudopolyps, lead-pipe colon on barium x-ray (Fig. 12.7), toxic megacolon
Histology	Noncaseating granulomas	Crypt abscesses
Colon cancer risk	Slightly increased	Markedly increased
Surgery	No (may make worse)	Yes (proctocolectomy with ileoanal anastomosis)

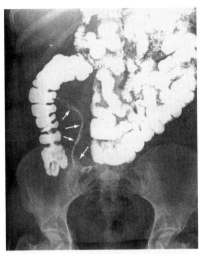

Fig. 12.6 Small bowel follow-through in a patient with Crohn disease that demonstrates a string sign in the right lower quadrant. The classic radiologic string sign *(arrows)* of a markedly narrowed bowel segment amidst widely spaced bowel loops is a result of spasm and edema associated with active inflammation. (From Feldman M, Friedman L, Brandt L. *Sleisenger and Fordtran's Gastrointestinal and Liver Disease.* 9th ed. Philadelphia: Saunders; 2010 [fig. 111.4]. Courtesy Dr. Jack Wittenberg, Boston, MA.)

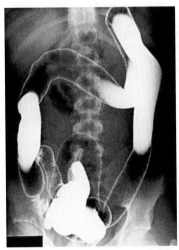

Fig. 12.7 A double-contrast barium enema in a patient with long-standing ulcerative colitis demonstrates a marked loss of haustration. The terminal ileum is normal. (From Feldman M, Friedman L, Brandt L. *Sleisenger and Fordtran's Gastrointestinal and Liver Disease.* 8th ed. Philadelphia: Saunders; 2006 [fig. 109.9].)

29. **Describe the extraintestinal manifestations of inflammatory bowel disease.**
    Both forms of inflammatory bowel disease can cause uveitis, arthritis, ankylosing spondylitis, erythema nodosum, erythema multiforme, primary sclerosing cholangitis, failure to thrive or grow in children, toxic megacolon, anemia of chronic disease, and fever. Toxic megacolon is more common in ulcerative colitis; look for markedly distended colon on abdominal radiograph.

30. **How is inflammatory bowel disease treated?**
    Patients with ulcerative colitis are treated with 5-aminosalicylic acid (5-ASA), with or without a sulfa drug (e.g., sulfasalazine), when stable. For both Crohn disease and ulcerative colitis, steroids and other immune modulators (e.g., azathioprine, cyclosporine, methotrexate) are used during severe disease flare-ups. Maintenance therapy depends on disease severity but often includes biologic agents such as TNF-alpha inhibitors.

31. **What causes toxic megacolon? How is it treated?**
Toxic megacolon is classically seen with inflammatory bowel disease (especially ulcerative colitis) and infectious colitis (especially *C. difficile*). In patients with HIV/AIDS, tissue-invasive cytomegalovirus is the most common cause. It may be precipitated by the use of antidiarrheal medications, for which reason they are usually not given for infectious diarrhea. Most patients have a high fever, leukocytosis, abdominal pain, rebound tenderness, and a dilated segment of colon on abdominal radiograph. Toxic megacolon is an emergency! Start treatment by discontinuing all antidiarrheal medications. Do not allow the patient to eat, place a nasogastric tube, and start intravenous fluids. Give antibiotics to cover bowel flora (such as ceftriaxone and metronidazole). Give steroids if the cause is inflammatory bowel disease. Surgery is required if perforation occurs (free air is seen on abdominal radiograph).

32. **List the common findings of acute liver disease.**
   - Elevated liver function tests (aspartate aminotransferase [AST], alanine aminotransferase [ALT], bilirubin, alkaline phosphatase, and/or prothrombin time and international normalized ratio [INR])
   - Jaundice
   - Dark urine
   - Pale stools
   - Nausea and vomiting
   - Right upper quadrant pain or tenderness
   - Hepatomegaly

33. **List the common causes of acute liver disease.**
   - Alcohol
   - Medications
   - Infection (usually viral hepatitis such as HBV or HCV)
   - Reye syndrome
   - Biliary tract disease
   - Autoimmune disease

   A helpful mnemonic to remember potential causes of liver disease/cirrhosis is **ABCDEFGHI**. This stands for **a**utoimmune hepatitis, hepatitis **B**, hepatitis **C**, **d**rugs/toxins, **e**thanol, **f**atty liver (nonalcoholic steatohepatitis [NASH]), **g**rowths, **h**emodynamic (CHF), **i**ron/copper/A1AT deficiency.

34. **What is the classic abnormality on liver function tests in patients with alcoholic hepatitis?**
An elevated AST that is more than twice the value of ALT, although both may be elevated.

35. **What clues suggest hepatitis A? Describe the diagnostic serology**
Look for outbreaks from a foodborne source, commonly during or after travel. There are no long-term sequelae of infection, although acute liver failure is a remote possibility. IgM antihepatitis A virus (HAV) is positive during jaundice or shortly thereafter. The incubation period for hepatitis A is about 4 weeks, though IgM may be detected by the time symptoms begin. Treatment is supportive. Infection can be prevented with vaccination.

36. **How is hepatitis B acquired? What is the best treatment?**
Hepatitis B is acquired through needles, sex, or perinatal transmission. Transfused blood is now screened for hepatitis B, but this risk of transmission is still about 1/200,000 according to the American Red Cross. A history of transfusion years prior is still a risk factor (screening by blood banks began in 1972 in the United States). Prevention is the best treatment via vaccination. Interferon alfa-2b, peginterferon alfa-2a, adefovir, dipivoxil, entecavir, telbivudine, or tenofovir can be tried in patients with chronic hepatitis and elevated liver enzymes.

37. **Describe the serology of hepatitis B infection, including the surface, core, and e-markers.**
The hepatitis B surface antigen (HBsAg) is positive with any unresolved infection (acute or chronic). The hepatitis B e-antigen (HBeAg) is a marker for infectivity; patients positive for the hepatitis B e-antibody (HBeAb) have a low likelihood of spreading disease. The first antibody to appear is the IgM hepatitis B core antibody (HBcAb), which appears during the "window phase" when both HBsAg and hepatitis B surface antibody (HBsAb) are negative. Positive HBsAb means that the patient is immune (as a result of either recovery from infection or vaccination); HBsAb never appears if the patient has chronic hepatitis.
   Make sure you know and understand Table 12.1 and Fig. 12.8. They are high yield.

38. **What are the possible sequelae of chronic hepatitis B or C?**
Cirrhosis and hepatocellular carcinoma (only with chronic, not acute, infection).

39. **What should be given to persons acutely exposed to hepatitis B?**
Hepatitis B immunoglobulin and hepatitis B vaccination alone have been demonstrated to be effective in preventing transmission after exposure to hepatitis B virus.

40. **Which type of viral hepatitis is the most common cause of chronic hepatitis?**
Hepatitis C. The hepatitis C virus is the most likely cause of hepatitis after a blood transfusion. Although blood is now screened for hepatitis B and C, the hepatitis C test was developed later (screening in the United States began

TABLE 12.1 Serologic Markers at Different Stages of Disease

	HBsAG	HBeAG	HBeAB	HBsAB	HBcAB
Incubation	+	+	-	-	-
Acute stage	+	+	-	-	+
Persistent carrier	+	+/-	-/+	-	+
Recovery (immune)	-	-	+	+	+
Immunization	-	-	-	+	-

The presence of HBeAg and anti-HBe depends on degree of infectivity. *HBcAb*, Hepatitis B core antibody; *HBeAb*, hepatitis B e antibody; *HBeAg*, hepatitis B e antigen; *HBSAb*, hepatitis B surface antibody; *HBsAg*, hepatitis B surface antigen.

Adapted from Cohen J, Powderly WG, Berkley SF, et al. *Infectious Diseases.* 2nd ed. Edinburgh: Mosby; 2004, 2015. With permission.

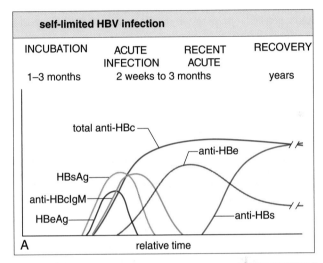

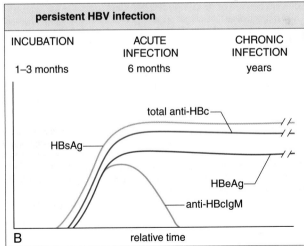

Fig. 12.8 (A) Clinical and virologic course of hepatitis B, with recovery. (B) Clinical and virologic course in a carrier of hepatitis B. (From Goering R, Dockrell H, Wakelin D, et al. *Mims' Medical Microbiology.* 4th ed. Philadelphia: Elsevier; 2007. Redrawn from Farrar WE, Wood MJ, Innes JA, et al. *Infectious Diseases.* 2nd ed. London: Mosby International; 1992.)

in 1972 for hepatitis B and 1992 for hepatitis C). Hepatitis C is also more likely than hepatitis B to progress to chronic hepatitis, cirrhosis, and cancer. Because of the relatively high prevalence in the Baby Boomer generation and lack of symptoms, the Centers for Disease Control and Prevention has recommended that all Americans born between 1945 and 1965 have a one-time screening test for hepatitis C. This recommendation has been updated quite recently, though. The US Preventive Services Taskforce now recommends that all adults age 18 to 79 be screened for hepatitis C.

41. Describe the serology and treatment for hepatitis C.
A positive hepatitis C antibody means that the patient has had an infection in the past but does not mean the infection has been cleared. Most patients become chronic carriers of the virus. A test for hepatitis C virus RNA is available to detect and quantify the viral load. Patients with hepatitis C should also be tested for HIV and hepatitis B. They should be tested for antibodies to hepatitis A and B to determine if vaccination is required.

Treatment of hepatitis C is rapidly evolving since the development of direct-acting antiviral medications. These medications are highly effective and offer the potential to avoid treatment with interferon and sometimes ribavirin. All patients with a detectable hepatitis C viral level over a 6-month period should be considered for treatment. Treatment regimens depend upon the hepatitis C genotype. Genotype 1 is the most common in the United States. Specific treatment regimens are likely beyond the scope of USMLE Step 2 but are included here for thoroughness:
- Ledipasvir-sofosbuvir
- Elbasvir-grazoprevir with or without ribavirin
- Ombitasvir-paritaprevir-ritonavir plus dasabuvir with or without ribavirin
- Simeprevir plus sofosbuvir
- Daclatasvir plus sofosbuvir

A virologic response to treatment is assessed by measuring the viral load at 12 weeks following completion of therapy. A sustained virologic response (SVR) is defined as an undetectable viral load at 24 weeks posttreatment.

42. When is hepatitis D seen? Describe the serology.
Hepatitis D is seen only in patients with hepatitis B. It may become chronic (with hepatitis B coinfection) and is acquired in the same ways as hepatitis B. It can either be acquired in a coinfection with hepatitis B or in a superinfection (hepatitis D infection after hepatitis B infection). The superinfection tends to lead to worse outcomes. IgM antibodies to the hepatitis D antigen demonstrate resolution of recent infection. Presence of the hepatitis D antigen, hepatitis D virus RNA, and high levels of IgM antibodies to hepatitis D indicate chronicity.

43. How is hepatitis E transmitted? What is special about the infection in pregnant women?
Hepatitis E is transmitted like hepatitis A (via food and water; no chronic state). It is often fatal in pregnant women (for unknown reasons).

44. What are the classic causes of drug-induced hepatitis?
Acetaminophen, isoniazid, and other tuberculosis drugs (e.g., rifampin and pyrazinamide), halothane, HMG CoA-reductase inhibitors, and carbon tetrachloride. The first step in treatment is to stop the drug.

45. When should you suspect idiopathic autoimmune hepatitis? What is the serologic marker?
Idiopathic autoimmune hepatitis is classically seen in 20- to 40-year-old women with anti–smooth muscle or antinuclear antibodies and no risk factors or lab markers for other causes of hepatitis. Treat with steroids.

46. What are the usual causes of chronic liver disease?
Alcohol, hepatitis, and metabolic diseases. Watch for the stigmata of chronic liver disease: jaundice, gynecomastia, testicular atrophy, palmar erythema, spider angiomata on skin, asterixis, and ascites.

47. Which species of viral hepatitis can lead to chronic liver disease?
Hepatitis B, C, and D. Hepatitis D can cause infection only in the setting of coexisting hepatitis B (Fig. 12.9).

48. What is nonalcoholic steatohepatitis?
NASH is similar to alcoholic hepatitis but is caused by insulin resistance instead. It is mostly asymptomatic but can present with elevated liver function tests. On ultrasound, it has a hyperechoic texture. Treatment is diet, exercise, and weight loss.

49. Define hemochromatosis. How do you recognize it?
Hemochromatosis, in its primary form, is usually autosomal recessive; look for a family history. Nearly 1 in 250 people in the United States are homozygous for this condition, although penetrance and clinical expression are variable. The pathophysiology is incompletely understood but includes excessive iron absorption by the intestine caused by HFE gene mutations, which prevents transferrin from binding to its receptor, ultimately exposing the blood to excessive iron levels. Excessive iron is deposited in the liver (potentially causing cirrhosis and/or hepatocellular carcinoma), pancreas (potentially causing diabetes), heart (resulting in dilated or restrictive cardiomyopathy), skin (causing hyperpigmentation classically known as **bronze diabetes**), hypogonadism, and joints (arthritis). Men are symptomatic earlier and more often because women lose iron with menstruation. Treat

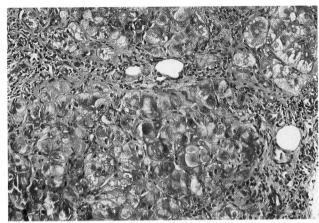

Fig. 12.9 Chronic viral hepatitis. Portal-portal bridging fibrosis is seen in long-standing chronic hepatitis C. (From Odze RD, Goldblum JR. *Surgical Pathology of the GI Tract, Liver, Biliary Tract, and Pancreas.* 2nd ed. Philadelphia: Saunders; 2009 [fig. 38.10].)

with phlebotomy and/or deferoxamine. Secondary iron overload can cause secondary hemochromatosis, which is classically due to an anemia that results in ineffective erythropoiesis (e.g., thalassemia) and excessive iron intake.

50. Define Wilson disease. How do you recognize it? How is it treated?

Wilson disease is an autosomal recessive disease caused by the effects of excessive serum copper. Serum **ceruloplasmin** (a copper transport protein) is usually low or absent, and serum copper may be normal. Biopsy shows excessive copper in the liver. Patients classically have liver disease with central nervous system and psychiatric manifestations (due to copper deposits in the basal ganglia; another name for this disease is hepatolenticular degeneration) and **Kayser-Fleischer** rings in the eye. Treat with penicillamine (copper chelator).

51. What are the clues to a diagnosis of alpha₁-antitrypsin (AAT) deficiency?

The classic description is a young adult who develops cirrhosis and/or emphysema without risk factors for either. AAT deficiency has an autosomal recessive inheritance pattern; look for a positive family history. It is also associated with panniculitis. Diagnosis requires a serum AAT less than 11 μmol/L as well as a severely deficient genotype. Treatment involves intravenous pooled human AAT.

52. What metabolic derangements accompany liver failure?

Coagulopathy: prolonged prothrombin time (PT). In severe cases, partial thromboplastin time (PTT) also may be prolonged. Vitamin K does not resolve the coagulopathy because it cannot be utilized by the damaged liver. Symptomatic patients must be treated with fresh frozen plasma.

Jaundice/hyperbilirubinemia: elevated conjugated and unconjugated bilirubin with hepatic damage (vs. biliary tract disease; see later).

Hypoalbuminemia: the liver synthesizes albumin.

Ascites: due to portal hypertension and/or hypoalbuminemia. Ascites can be detected on physical exam by shifting dullness or a positive fluid wave. A possible complication is **spontaneous bacterial peritonitis** due to infected ascitic fluid that can lead to sepsis. Look for fever and/or change in mental status in a patient with known ascites. Perform a paracentesis, examine the ascitic fluid for elevated white blood cell count (>250 neutrophils is diagnostic), and do Gram stain, culture and sensitivity tests, glucose (low with infection), and protein (<1 g/dL). The usual causes are *E. coli, Streptococcus pneumoniae,* and other enteric bugs. Treat with broad-spectrum antibiotics (cefotaxime is a common choice). A serum ascites albumin gradient (SAAG) of greater than 1.1 implicates portal hypertension as the etiology. Prophylaxis includes diuretics and, in certain cases, fluoroquinolones.

Portal hypertension: seen with cirrhosis (chronic liver disease); causes hemorrhoids, esophageal varices, and caput medusae (engorged veins on the abdominal wall).

Hyperammonemia: the liver clears ammonia. Treat with decreased protein intake (source of ammonia) and lactulose (a laxative that alters luminal pH to disfavor ammonia absorption). The last choice is rifaximin, which kills bowel flora that make ammonia.

Hepatic encephalopathy: mostly due to hyperammonemia; often precipitated by high protein intake, GI bleed, or infection. Look for asterixis (the flapping of outstretched hands) and/or mental status changes. Additionally, it can be precipitated by hypokalemia, metabolic alkalosis, and the placement of a transjugular intrahepatic portosystemic shunt (TIPS). In addition to treating hyperammonemia, look for and treat the underlying cause.

Hepatorenal syndrome: liver failure may cause kidney failure. This portends a poor prognosis. The pathophysiology is complicated, but it is due to portal hypertension causing increased nitric oxide production in the splanchnic circulation. This leads to systemic vasodilation and renal hypoperfusion. The renin-aldosterone-angiotensin system is activated and causes local renal vasoconstriction. It is treated with albumin and splanchnic vasoconstrictors (i.e., octreotide or midodrine).
Hypoglycemia: the liver stores glycogen.
Disseminated intravascular coagulation: activated clotting factors are cleared by the liver.

53. What signs and symptoms suggest biliary tract obstruction as a cause of jaundice?
    - Elevated conjugated bilirubin. Conjugated bilirubin is more elevated than unconjugated bilirubin because the liver still functions and can conjugate bilirubin, but conjugated bilirubin cannot be excreted because of biliary tract disease.
    - Markedly elevated alkaline phosphatase
    - Pruritus
    - Clay-colored stools
    - Dark urine that is strongly positive for conjugated bilirubin. Unconjugated bilirubin is not excreted in the urine because it is tightly bound to albumin.

54. What are the commonly tested types of biliary tract obstructions?
    Bile duct obstruction, cholestasis, cholangitis, primary biliary cholangitis, and primary sclerosing cholangitis.

55. What are the two major causes of common bile duct obstruction? How are they distinguished?
    The most common cause is obstruction with a gallstone (choledocholithiasis). Look for a history of gallstones or the four Fs (female, forty, fertile, and fat). Ultrasound often identifies the stone; if not, use magnetic resonance cholangiopancreatography (MRCP) or endoscopic retrograde cholangiopancreatography (ERCP). ERCP can be therapeutic. Treatment is endoscopic removal of the stone. The second major cause of common bile duct obstruction is cancer. Look for weight loss. Pancreatic cancer is the most common type; look for **Courvoisier sign** (painless jaundice with a palpably enlarged gallbladder). Sometimes cholangiocarcinoma or bowel cancer blocks the common bile duct.

56. What are the two common causes of cholestasis?
    Medications (e.g., birth control pills, trimethoprim-sulfamethoxazole, phenothiazines, androgens) and pregnancy

57. What clues suggest a diagnosis of primary biliary cholangitis (formerly primary biliary cirrhosis)?
    This condition is usually seen in middle-aged women with no risk factors for liver or biliary disease. It causes marked pruritus, jaundice, and positive **antimitochondrial antibodies**. It is also associated with cutaneous xanthomas and osteoporosis. The rest of the workup is negative. Cholestyramine can help with symptoms. Ursodeoxycholic acid can delay progression, but the only treatment is liver transplantation.

58. Who gets primary sclerosing cholangitis? What clues can help with diagnosis?
    Primary sclerosing cholangitis usually occurs in young adults (males > females) with inflammatory bowel disease (usually ulcerative colitis). It presents similarly to bacterial cholangitis. Fever, chills, pruritis, and right upper quadrant abdominal pain are common. Peripheral antineutrophil cytoplasmic antibodies (P-ANCA) can help with diagnosis. On biopsy, concentric bile duct fibrosis in an onion skin–like pattern is seen. Sclerosing cholangitis is associated with ulcerative colitis and cholangiocarcinoma.

59. What usually precipitates acute cholangitis? What is the tip-off to its presence? How is it treated?
    Cholangitis is usually precipitated by a gallstone that blocks the common bile duct with subsequent infection of the bile duct system. The tip-off is the presence of **Charcot triad**: fever, right upper quadrant pain, and jaundice. Treat with antibiotics (e.g., piperacillin-tazobactam), and remove gallstones surgically or endoscopically after the acute infection has resolved. The presence of **Reynold pentad** (Charcot triad plus hypotension and altered mental status) implies a more severe presentation requiring more urgent treatment.

60. What are the classic symptoms of esophageal disease?
    Dysphagia (difficulty in swallowing) and/or odynophagia (painful swallowing). Patients may also have atypical chest pain.

61. Define achalasia. How is it diagnosed and treated?
    Achalasia is caused by incomplete relaxation of a hypertensive lower esophageal sphincter and loss or derangement of peristalsis. It is usually idiopathic but may be secondary to **Chagas disease** (South America; due to *Trypanosoma cruzi*). Patients have intermittent dysphagia for solids and liquids but no heartburn because the lower esophageal sphincter stays tightly closed and does not allow acid reflux. Barium swallow

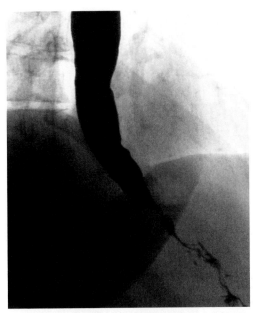

Fig. 12.10 Classic appearances of achalasia. Note the tapered appearance of the gastroesophageal junction with the column of barium above. (From Adam A. *Grainger & Allison's Diagnostic Radiology.* 5th ed. London: Churchill Livingstone; 2008 [fig. 30.21].)

reveals a dilated esophagus with distal bird beak–like narrowing (Fig. 12.10). The diagnosis is often confirmed with esophageal manometry. Treat with calcium channel blockers, nitrates, pneumatic balloon dilatation, or botulinum toxin injection, or in severe cases, peroral endoscopic myotomy or surgical myotomy with fundoplication. Surgery (myotomy) is a last resort. Patients have an increased risk for esophageal carcinoma.

62. What are the signs and symptoms of esophageal spasm? How is it treated?
Both diffuse esophageal spasm (Fig. 12.11) and nutcracker esophagus (best thought of as a special variant of esophageal spasm) are characterized by irregular, forceful, and painful esophageal contractions that cause intermittent chest pain. Diagnose with esophageal manometry (decreased lower esophageal pressure) or barium swallow, which will show a corkscrew–like esophagus. Treat with calcium channel blockers, nitrates, and (if needed) surgery (myotomy).

63. What clues suggest scleroderma as the cause of esophageal complaints?
Scleroderma may cause aperistalsis due to esophageal fibrosis and atrophy of smooth muscle. The lower esophageal sphincter often becomes incompetent, and many patients have heartburn (opposite of achalasia). Look for positive antinuclear antibody and masklike facies (Fig. 12.12) as well as other autoimmune symptoms. Remember also the **CREST** syndrome, which consists of **c**alcinosis, **R**aynaud phenomenon, **e**sophageal dysmotility, **s**clerodactyly, and **t**elangiectasias.

64. What do you need to know about the epidemiology of esophageal cancer?
First, the epidemiology has recently changed, as adenocarcinoma is now more common than squamous cell carcinoma. Adenocarcinoma is due to the long-standing effects of gastric acid reflux and thus occurs in the distal esophagus. Barrett esophagus is the precursor lesion. Squamous cell carcinoma is usually caused by alcohol and tobacco (synergistic effect) and is classically seen in black men over the age of 40 years who smoke and drink alcohol. Patients complain of weight loss and food "sticking" in the chest (progresses solids to liquids). The tumor is usually in the proximal esophagus.

65. What is the relationship between Barrett esophagus and esophageal cancer?
Barrett esophagus, which is usually caused by long-standing GERD, predisposes to esophageal adenocarcinoma. Barrett esophagus describes a columnar metaplasia with goblet cells of the normally squamous cell esophageal mucosa. Once Barrett esophagus is seen on endoscopy and confirmed with endoscopic biopsy, periodic biopsies must be done to monitor for the development of esophageal cancer.

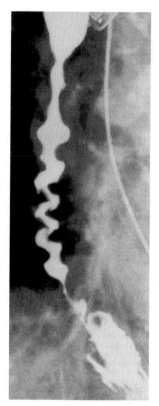

Fig. 12.11 Barium esophagogram showing a corkscrew esophagus in a patient with diffuse esophageal spasm. The patient had dysphagia and chest pain. Upper endoscopy was normal. (From Feldman M, ed. *Gastroenterology and Hepatology: The Comprehensive Visual Reference.* New York: Churchill Livingstone; 1997. With permission.)

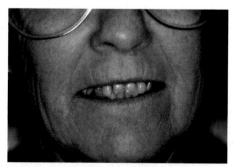

Fig. 12.12 Scleroderma facies. Narrowing of the eyes and masklike restriction of facial movement give a Mona Lisa–like face. (From Scully C. *Handbook of Medical Problems in Dentistry.* Elsevier; 2016 [fig. 5.85].)

66. What causes acute pancreatitis?
    More than 80% of cases are due to alcohol or gallstones. Remember the mnemonic I GET SMASHED:

    I = Idiopathic
    G = Gallstones
    E = Ethanol
    T = Trauma
    S = Steroids
    M = Mumps (and other infections) or Malignancy
    A = Autoimmune

S = Scorpion sting
H = Hypercalcemia or Hypertriglyceridemia
E = ERCP trauma
D = Drugs (e.g., isoniazid, furosemide, simvastatin, steroids, azathioprine)

67. **What are the signs and symptoms of acute pancreatitis?**
Patients classically have epigastric abdominal pain that radiates to the back and decreases when leaning forward, nausea with vomiting that fails to relieve the pain, leukocytosis, and elevated amylase and lipase (more specific) levels. Watch for **Grey Turner sign** (blue-black flanks) and **Cullen sign** (blue-black umbilicus), both of which are due to a hemorrhagic pancreatic exudate and indicative of severe pancreatitis. Remember that perforated ulcers are also associated with elevated amylase and lipase levels and present similarly. However, patients usually have free air on abdominal radiographs and a history of peptic ulcer disease. Diagnosis of acute pancreatitis requires two of the following: characteristic abdominal pain, elevated amylase or lipase three times the upper limit of normal, and characteristic appearance on CT.

68. **How is acute pancreatitis treated?**
Patients are not allowed to eat, a nasogastric tube is often placed, and intravenous fluids and narcotics are given. For pain control, hydromorphone or fentanyl is often used. Other options include meperidine (which has a risk of seizures) or morphine (which causes sphincter of Oddi spasm that increases pancreatitis risk, though clinical evidence of this is lacking).

69. **What are the complications of acute pancreatitis?**
Early complications include ARDS, pleural effusion, and pancreatic ascites. Late complications include pseudocyst formation (drain surgically if symptomatic, persistent for several weeks, or >6 cm), abscess or infection (treat with antibiotics and drainage if needed), and chronic pancreatitis (calcifications of the pancreas may be seen on CT or plain abdominal films).

70. **What causes chronic pancreatitis? How is it treated?**
Chronic pancreatitis in the United States is almost always due to alcoholism and usually results from repeated bouts of acute pancreatitis. Gallstones do not cause chronic pancreatitis. Chronic pancreatitis may lead to diabetes, steatorrhea (excessive fat in the stool due to lack of pancreatic enzymes), calcification of the pancreas (which may be seen on a plain abdominal radiograph), and fat-soluble vitamin deficiencies (due to malabsorption). The incidence of pancreatic cancer is slightly increased in patients with pancreatitis, although smoking is a greater risk factor than alcohol for pancreatic cancer.
    Treat chronic pancreatitis with alcohol abstinence, oral pancreatic enzyme replacement, and fat-soluble vitamin supplements.

71. **Distinguish between Mallory-Weiss and Boerhaave tears in the esophagus. How are they diagnosed?**
Mallory-Weiss tears are superficial erosions in the esophageal mucosa, whereas Boerhaave tears are full-thickness esophageal ruptures. Both may cause a GI bleed and are usually seen with vomiting and retching (alcoholics and bulimic patients) if they are not iatrogenic (due to endoscopy). Diagnosis of a Mallory-Weiss tear is usually made with endoscopy, during which bleeding vessels should be sclerosed, and/or from contrast radiographs. A Boerhaave tear may manifest as pneumothorax, pneumomediastinum, or pleural effusion on chest x-ray. Diagnosis can be made with a Gastrografin-contrast esophagram or CT scan (barium is more inflammatory and should not be used). Findings of a Boerhaave tear include epigastric crepitus (Hamman crunch) on examination. Mallory-Weiss tears usually stop bleeding on their own or with endoscopic treatment, but Boerhaave tears require immediate surgical repair and drainage.

72. **What is the rule about bowel contrast when a GI perforation is suspected?**
For all GI studies, barium is preferred because it provides higher quality-images. However, with suspected GI perforation, do not use barium because it can cause chemical peritonitis or mediastinitis when a perforation/leak is present. Instead, use water-soluble contrast (e.g., Gastrografin). Things get tricky in patients with a significant risk for aspiration, because the lungs tolerate barium well but develop chemical pneumonitis from water-soluble contrast. When in doubt, give water-soluble contrast followed by barium once perforation has been excluded.

73. **What are the common GI malformations in children? How are they distinguished?**

Name*	Presenting Age	Vomit Description	Findings/Key Words
Pyloric stenosis	0–3 mo	Nonbilious, projectile	Males > females; palpable olive-shaped mass in the epigastrium; low Cl/low K metabolic alkalosis
Intestinal atresia	0–1 wk	Bilious	"Double-bubble" sign, Down syndrome

Name*	Presenting Age	Vomit Description	Findings/Key Words
TE fistula†	0–2 wk	Food regurgitation	Respiratory compromise with feeding, aspiration pneumonia, inability to pass a nasogastric tube into the stomach, gastric distention (from air)
Hirschsprung disease	0–1 yr	Feculent	Abdominal distention, obstipation, no nerve ganglia seen on rectal biopsy; males > females
Anal atresia	0–1 wk	Late, feculent	Detected on initial exam in the nursery; males > females
Choanal atresia	0–1 wk	—	Cyanosis with feeding, relieved by crying; inability to pass a nasogastric tube through nose

Cl, Chloride; *K*, potassium; *TE*, tracheoesophageal.
*Treat each of these conditions with **surgical repair**.
†The most common variant (85% of cases) has esophageal atresia with a fistula from the bronchus to the distal esophagus. The result is gastric distention, as each breath transmits air to the GI tract. Be able to recognize a sketch of this most common variant (Fig. 12.13).

74. **What other pediatric GI conditions are commonly found on Step 2? How are they distinguished?**

Name	Presenting Age	Vomit Description	Findings/Key Words
Intussusception	3 mo–2 yr	Bilious	Currant-jelly stools (blood and mucus), palpable sausage-shaped mass, "target sign" on ultrasound; treat with pneumatic or hydrostatic enema guided by fluoroscopy or ultrasound (diagnostic and therapeutic)
Necrotizing enterocolitis	0–2 mo	Bilious	Premature baby, fever, rectal bleeding, air in bowel wall (pneumatosis intestinalis). Treat with NPO, orogastric tube, IV fluids, and antibiotics
Meconium ileus	0–1 wk	Feculent, late	Cystic fibrosis manifestation (as is rectal prolapse)
Midgut volvulus	0–2 yr	Bilious	Sudden onset of pain, distention, rectal bleeding, peritonitis, "bird's beak" on abdominal radiograph; treat with surgery
Meckel diverticulum	0–2 yr	Varies	Rule of 2s*; GI ulceration/bleeding; use Meckel scan to detect; treat with surgery
Strangulated hernia	Any age	Bilious	Physical exam detects bowel loops in inguinal canal

IV, Intravenous, *NPO*, nothing by mouth (no feedings).
*Rule of 2s for Meckel diverticulum: 2% of population affected (most common GI tract abnormality; remnant of omphalomesenteric duct), 2 inches long, within 2 feet of ileocolic junction, presents in the first 2 years of life. Meckel diverticulum can cause intussusception, obstruction, or volvulus.

75. **Which GI malformation primarily causes respiratory problems?**
Diaphragmatic hernia, which is more common in males. Ninety percent are on the left side. The main point to know is that bowel herniates into the thorax through the diaphragmatic defect, compressing the lung and impeding lung development (pulmonary hypoplasia develops). Patients present with respiratory distress and have bowel sounds in the chest and bowel loops in the thorax on chest radiographs (Fig. 12.14). Treat with surgical correction of the diaphragm.

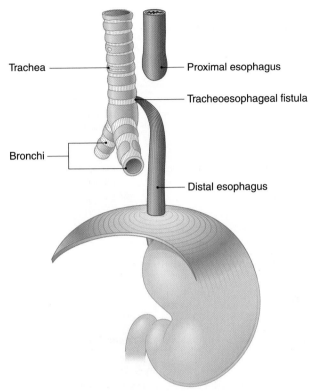

Trachea

Proximal esophagus

Tracheoesophageal fistula

Bronchi

Distal esophagus

Fig. 12.13 Tracheoesophageal fistula. Diagram of the most common type of esophageal atresia and tracheoesophageal fistula. (From Gilbert-Barness E. *Potter's Pathology of the Fetus, Infant and Child.* 2nd ed. St. Louis: Mosby; 2007 [fig. 25.6].)

76. How are omphalocele and gastroschisis differentiated?

   An **omphalocele**, associated with other congenital anomalies, is located in the midline, the sac contains multiple abdominal organs, the umbilical ring is absent, and other anomalies are common. **Gastroschisis** is to the right of the midline, only small bowel is exposed (no true hernia sac), the umbilical ring is present, and other anomalies are rare (Fig. 12.15). An omphalocele is covered in peritoneum, whereas gastroschisis is not.

77. What is Henoch-Schönlein purpura? Why is it mentioned in the GI section?

   Henoch-Schönlein purpura (IgA vasculitis) is a vasculitis that may present with GI bleeding and abdominal pain. Look for a history of upper respiratory infection, characteristic rash (palpable purpura) on the lower extremities and buttocks (Fig. 12.16), swelling in hands and feet, arthritis, and/or hematuria and proteinuria. It is associated with ileoilial intussusception. Treat supportively with hydration, rest, and pain relief. Severe cases may require steroids.

78. What is the most common cause of diarrhea in children?

   As a primary cause, probably viral gastroenteritis (e.g., norovirus, rotavirus). Remember, however, that diarrhea is often a nonspecific sign of any systemic illness (e.g., otitis media, pneumonia, urinary tract infection).

79. True or false: Children may develop inflammatory bowel disease and irritable bowel syndrome.

   True. Abdominal pain may be the result of inflammatory bowel disease or irritable bowel syndrome. Diarrhea, fever, bloody stools, anemia, joint pains, and poor growth are more concerning for inflammatory bowel disease. GI complaints may also be due to anxiety or psychiatric problems as well as behavioral issues (e.g., withholding stool resulting in constipation and abdominal pain). Watch for separation anxiety, children who do not want to go to school, depression, and child abuse.

80. What is the first step in evaluating neonatal jaundice? Why is jaundice of concern in a neonate?

   The first step is to determine whether the jaundice is physiologic or pathologic. Measure total, direct, and indirect bilirubin. The main concern is bilirubin-induced neurologic dysfunction (BIND), which is due to high levels of unconjugated

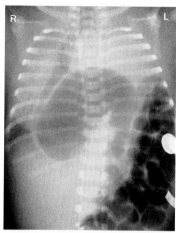

Fig. 12.14 Diaphragmatic hernia shown in a newborn with significant respiratory difficulty. An anteroposterior (AP) view of the chest and abdomen demonstrates opacification of the left hemithorax, with bowel loops pushing up into the opacified left hemithorax. This condition carries a high fatality rate and should be recognized immediately. (From Mettler F. *Essentials of Radiology.* 2nd ed. Philadelphia: Saunders; 2004 [fig. 9.13].)

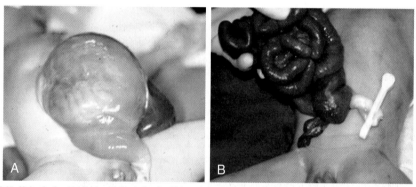

Fig. 12.15 Abdominal wall defects. (A) Omphalocele with intact sac. (B) Gastroschisis with eviscerated multiple bowel loops to the right of the umbilical cord. (From Townsend CM. *Sabiston Textbook of Surgery.* 19th ed. Philadelphia: Saunders; 2012 [fig. 67.20].)

bilirubin with subsequent deposit in the basal ganglia. Kernicterus is the term for the chronic and permanent sequelae of BIND. Look for poor feeding, seizures, flaccidity, opisthotonos, and apnea in the setting of severe jaundice.

81. **What causes physiologic jaundice of the newborn? Who gets it?**
    Physiologic (nonpathologic) jaundice is caused by normal neonatal changes in bilirubin metabolism, which results in increased bilirubin production, decreased bilirubin clearance (low UDP-glucuronyl transferase activity), and increased enterohepatic circulation. These changes result in the low-risk unconjugated (indirect) bilirubinemia that occurs in most newborns and is even more prevalent in premature infants. Bilirubin is mostly unconjugated because of incomplete maturation of liver function. In full-term infants, bilirubin is less than 12 mg/dL, peaks at day 2 to 4, and returns to normal by 2 weeks. In premature infants, bilirubin is less than 15 mg/dL, peaks at day 3 to 5, and may be elevated for up to 3 weeks.

82. **How is severe hyperbilirubinemia recognized?**
    Severe hyperbilirubinemia (sometimes called pathologic jaundice) is suggested by jaundice that is recognized in the first 24 hours of life, total bilirubin that is higher than the hour-specific 95th percentile, a rate of rise is greater than 0.2 mg/dL per hour, jaundice in a term newborn after 2 weeks of age, or a direct bilirubin concentration that is more than 20% of the total bilirubin.

83. **What are the causes of neonatal jaundice?**
    Breastfeeding jaundice: occurs in 1 in 10 breastfed infants and is typically seen in the first week of life. This is essentially an exaggerated physiologic jaundice due to insufficient milk intake (usually due to inadequate

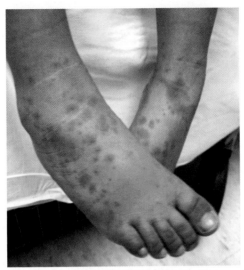

Fig. 12.16 Henoch-Schönlein purpura in a 7-year-old child. Note typical red-purple rash on the lower extremities. (From Marx J. *Rosen's Emergency Medicine*. 7th ed. St. Louis: Mosby; 2009 [fig. 170.10]. Courtesy Marianne Gausche-Hill, MD.)

maternal milk production), which leads to fluid and weight loss and an inadequate number of bowel movements to remove bilirubin from the body.

Breast milk jaundice: typically presents after the first 3 to 5 days of life and has traditionally been defined as the persistence of physiologic jaundice beyond the first week of life. Breast milk jaundice results from a direct effect of breast milk itself, as human milk promotes an increase in intestinal absorption of bilirubin. In contrast to breastfeeding jaundice, breast milk jaundice does not present with signs of dehydration. Bilirubin levels peak within 2 weeks after birth and decline to normal levels by 12 weeks of age. Breastfeeding should continue as long as the hyperbilirubinemia remains in the safe zone.

Illness: infection or sepsis, hypothyroidism, liver insult, cystic fibrosis, and other illnesses may prolong neonatal jaundice and lower the threshold for kernicterus. The youngest, sickest infants are at greatest risk for hyperbilirubinemia and kernicterus. Make sure to obtain blood cultures.

Hemolysis: from Rhesus (Rh) incompatibility or congenital red cell diseases (e.g., hereditary spherocytosis, elliptocytosis, G6PD deficiency) that cause hemolysis in the neonatal period. ABO incompatibility may cause mild jaundice but usually is not clinically significant. Look for anemia, peripheral smear abnormalities, positive family history, and higher levels of unconjugated bilirubin.

Metabolic disorders: Crigler-Najjar syndrome causes severe unconjugated hyperbilirubinemia, whereas Gilbert syndrome causes a mild form. Both are due to problems with UDP-glucuronyl transferase. Rotor and Dubin-Johnson syndromes cause conjugated hyperbilirubinemia. These are due to decreased intrahepatic excretion.

Biliary atresia: full-term infants with clay- or gray-colored stools and high levels of conjugated bilirubin. Treat with surgery.

Medications: avoid sulfa drugs in neonates; they displace bilirubin from albumin and may precipitate kernicterus.

84. How is severe hyperbilirubinemia treated?
Unconjugated hyperbilirubinemia that persists, rises above 15 mg/dL, or rises rapidly is treated with **phototherapy** to convert unconjugated bilirubin to a water-soluble form that can be excreted. A last resort is exchange transfusion, but do not consider this unless the level of unconjugated bilirubin is greater than 20 mg/dL.

85. What should you do if an infant is born to a mother with active hepatitis B?
An infant born to a mother with active hepatitis B should receive the first immunization shot and hepatitis B immune globulin at birth.

CHAPTER 13

GENERAL SURGERY

1. **Define the acute abdomen. What physical exam signs suggest its presence?**
   Acute abdomen generally refers to sudden-onset, severe abdominal pain. The most common causes include pathologies of the gastrointestinal tract such as cholecystitis, appendicitis, pancreatitis, and diverticulitis. Acute abdomen is commonly a sign of an inflamed peritoneum (peritonitis), which is often due to a surgically correctable problem. Patients with an acute abdomen often receive a laparotomy and/or laparoscopy because it signifies a potentially life-threatening condition. The best physical exam confirmations of peritonitis are **rebound tenderness** and **involuntary guarding**. Rebound tenderness is elicited by letting go quickly after deep palpation of the abdomen. Pain occurs in the area of palpation (with generalized peritonitis) or at the location of localized inflammation (e.g., Rovsing sign in appendicitis). Involuntary guarding describes abdominal wall muscle spasm that cannot be controlled. Voluntary guarding (person reflexively or willfully tenses the abdomen during attempted palpation) and tenderness to palpations are softer signs often present in benign diseases.

2. **What should you do if you are not sure whether a stable patient has an acute abdomen?**
   When you are in doubt and the patient is stable, use as-needed pain medications (studies have shown that pain control does not delay diagnosis significantly but does improve the patient's experience), perform serial abdominal exams, and consider computed tomography (CT) scan. If the patient becomes unstable, proceed to laparoscopy and/or laparotomy. You do not need to have a specific diagnosis before, just make sure that you rule out problems that act as mimics of acute abdomen (e.g., gastroesophageal reflux disease [GERD], pulmonary embolism, myocardial ischemia, pneumonia) before proceeding.

3. **Name a few causes of peritonitis that do not require laparotomy or laparoscopy.**
   Pancreatitis, many cases of diverticulitis, renal stones, and spontaneous bacterial peritonitis.

4. **Specify which conditions are associated with pain and peritonitis in the listed abdominal areas.**

Area	Organ (Conditions)
Right upper quadrant	Gallbladder/biliary (cholecystitis, cholangitis) or liver (abscess)
Left upper quadrant	Spleen (rupture with blunt trauma)
Right lower quadrant	Appendix (appendicitis), pelvic inflammatory disease (PID)
Left lower quadrant	Sigmoid colon (diverticulitis), PID
Epigastric area	Stomach (peptic ulcer) or pancreas (pancreatitis)

5. **What are the classic signs and symptoms of gallstone disease?**
   Classic gallstone symptoms include postprandial, colicky pain in the right upper quadrant with bloating and/or nausea and vomiting. The pain usually begins 15 to 60 minutes after a meal (especially a fatty meal). Look for **Murphy sign** (palpation of the right upper quadrant under the rib cage causes arrest of inspiration due to pain) as the main physical exam finding for cholecystitis.

6. **What are the six Fs of cholecystitis? How are the demographics of patients with pigment stones different from those with cholesterol stones?**
   The first five Fs summarize the demographics of people with cholesterol gallstones: fat, forty, fertile, female, and flatulent; the sixth F is febrile, which indicates that such patients have now developed acute cholecystitis. Patients with pigment (i.e., calcium bilirubinate) stones, which are brown in color, are classically young patients with hemolytic anemia (e.g., sickle cell disease, hereditary spherocytosis).

7. **How is a clinical suspicion of cholecystitis confirmed and treated?**
   Ultrasound is the best first imaging study for suspected gallbladder disease (Fig. 13.1). It may show gallstones, a thin layer of fluid around the gallbladder, and/or a thickened gallbladder wall. A more specific ultrasonographic Murphy sign using direct visualization of the gallbladder can be obtained (variant anatomy and significant obesity can create uncertainty). A nuclear hepatobiliary scintigraphic study (e.g., hepatobiliary iminodiacetic acid [HIDA]

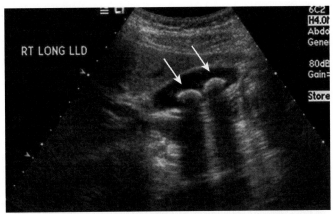

Fig. 13.1 Typical ultrasonographic appearance of cholelithiasis. Two gallstones *(arrows)* are present within the lumen of the gallbladder, casting acoustic shadows. (From Gore RM, Levine MS. *High-Yield Imaging: Gastrointestinal.* Philadelphia, PA: Elsevier; 2010:512-514.)

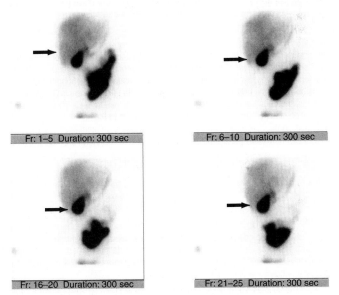

Fig. 13.2 Hepatobiliary iminodiacetic acid (HIDA) scan showing filling of the gallbladder. With gallbladder filling *(arrows),* the diagnosis of acute cholecystitis is effectively eliminated. (From Townsend CM. *Sabiston Textbook of Surgery.* 19th ed. Philadelphia, PA: Saunders; 2012 [fig. 55.13].)

scan) clinches the diagnosis with nonvisualization of the gallbladder (Fig. 13.2). The treatment is pain control and cholecystectomy (antibiotics may be indicated if infection is suspected); a laparoscopic approach is generally preferred over an open procedure.

8. Define cholangitis. How does it differ from cholecystitis? How is it treated?

Cholangitis is an inflammation of the bile ducts, whereas cholecystitis is an inflammation of the gallbladder. Cholangitis is classically due to biliary obstruction with subsequent bile stasis and infection, and it is much more deadly than cholecystitis. Choledocholithiasis (a gallstone in the common bile duct) and malignancy are common causes of obstruction. Autoimmune cholangitis (e.g., sclerosing cholangitis) and primary infection (e.g., *Clonorchis sinensis* and other parasite infections common in some parts of Asia) are other causes. Cholangitis classically presents with **Charcot triad:** (1) right upper quadrant pain, (2) fever or shaking chills, and (3) jaundice. Patients may have a history of gallstones. Start broad-spectrum antibiotics to cover bowel flora (e.g., piperacillin with

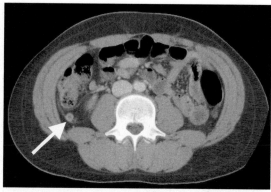

Fig. 13.3 Appendicitis. Retrocecal appendicitis is evident on this computed tomography (CT) scan after intravenous contrast. The appendix *(arrow)* is thick walled, measures 8 mm in diameter, and has adjacent inflammation. (From Teele RL, Helen LM. *Practical Paediatrics.* Philadelphia: Elsevier; 2012:236-250.)

tazobactam), and then manage more definitively depending on the circumstances (e.g., cholecystectomy with evacuation of any common duct stones for gallstone disease, biliary stent placement for unresectable malignant obstruction). If patients becomes sicker, they may develop **Reynold pentad**, which includes Charcot triad plus (4) altered mental status and (5) hypotension.

9. Describe the classic presentation of appendicitis. How is it treated?
   Appendicitis classically presents in 10- to 30-year-olds with a history of crampy, poorly localized periumbilic pain followed by nausea and vomiting. Then the pain localizes to the right lower quadrant, and peritoneal signs develop with worsening of nausea and vomiting. It is said that a patient who is hungry and asking for food does not have appendicitis (called the hamburger sign). A classic clue to the diagnosis is **Rovsing sign:** When you palpate left lower quadrant and then quickly release your hand, the patient feels increased pain in the right lower quadrant. McBurney point, two-thirds of the way from the umbilicus to the anterior superior iliac spine, is the area of maximal tenderness in the right lower quadrant and the site where an open appendectomy incision is made. Ultrasound and CT are increasingly used to confirm the diagnosis before surgery in stable patients (Fig. 13.3).

10. What is the cause of left lower quadrant pain and fever in a patient over 50 years old until proven otherwise? How is it treated?
    Diverticulitis. Treat medically with broad-spectrum antibiotics (e.g., ciprofloxacin plus metronidazole), intravenous (IV) fluids, initial bowel rest with gradual advancement of diet, and a nasogastric tube if nausea and vomiting are present. For disease that recurs or is refractory to medical therapy, consider sigmoid colon resection.

11. What tests should and should not be done to confirm possible cases of diverticulitis? What test does every patient need after a treated episode of diverticulitis?
    Colonoscopy and barium enema should not be performed in the acute setting because colon rupture may occur. However, one of these tests should be done in every patient after treatment to exclude colon carcinoma. Order a CT scan, if necessary, to confirm a diagnosis of diverticulitis.

12. Describe the typical history, physical exam, and lab findings of pancreatitis. How is it treated?
    Look for epigastric pain that radiates to the back in an alcohol abuser or a patient with a history of (or risk factors for) gallstones. Serum amylase and/or lipase should be elevated. If these values are not given, order them! Other common signs include decreased bowel sounds, localized ileus (sentinel loop of bowel on abdominal radiograph), and nausea, vomiting, and/or anorexia.
      Treat pancreatitis supportively; narcotics are often needed for pain control; hydromorphone or fentanyl are common choices these days; meperidine, which has a risk of seizures, has traditionally been favored over morphine because of the concern about sphincter of Oddi spasm, though clinical evidence of this is lacking. Do not feed the patient initially; place a nasogastric tube as needed for nausea and vomiting; and give IV fluids and other supportive care measures. Watch for the complications of pseudocyst and pancreatic abscess, both of which can be diagnosed by CT scan and may require surgical intervention. Also be on the lookout for hemorrhagic pancreatitis, which presents similarly but may be revealed by a decreased hematocrit early on and requires more intensive supportive therapy (i.e., intensive care unit [ICU] care).

13. Describe the usual history of a perforated ulcer. How is it treated?
    Patients often have no history of alcohol abuse or gallstones (pancreatitis risk factors). Abdominal radiographs classically show free air under the diaphragm, and a history of peptic ulcer disease is often included in the patient description. Remember that a perforated bowel can cause increased amylase and lipase levels. Treat with surgery.

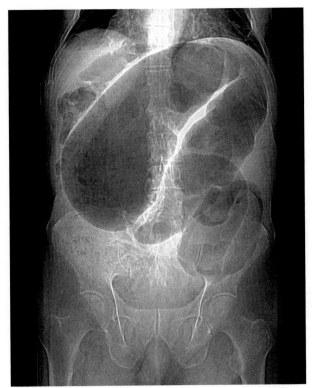

Fig. 13.4 Plain abdominal radiograph of a sigmoid volvulus with a massively distended loop of colon under the left hemidiaphragm. (From Yeo CJ. *Shackelford's Surgery of the Alimentary Tract.* 7th ed. Philadelphia: Saunders; 2012 [fig. 151.2].)

14. What are the hallmarks of small bowel obstruction? How is it treated?

    Small bowel obstruction commonly causes bilious vomiting (early symptom), abdominal distention, constipation, hyperactive bowel sounds (high-pitched, rushing sounds), and usually poorly localized abdominal pain. Radiographs show multiple air-fluid levels. Patients often have a history of previous surgery.

    Start treatment by withholding food, placing a nasogastric tube, and giving IV fluids. If the obstruction does not resolve or if peritoneal signs develop, laparotomy is usually needed. CT scanning can confirm an uncertain diagnosis in stable patients and may reveal the underlying cause of obstruction.

15. What are the common causes of a small bowel obstruction?

    In adults, the most common cause is **adhesions**, which usually develop from prior surgery. Incarcerated hernias, Crohn disease, and malignancy are other common causes. Other causes include Meckel diverticulum and intussusception (both typically seen in children) and meconium ileus in newborns with cystic fibrosis.

16. Describe the signs and symptoms of large bowel obstruction. What causes it? How is it treated?

    Large bowel obstruction usually presents with gradually increasing abdominal pain, abdominal distention, constipation, and feculent vomiting (late symptom). In older adults, the most common causes are diverticulitis, colon cancer, and volvulus (sigmoid most common, followed by cecal). In children, watch for Hirschsprung disease. Treat early by withholding food and placing a nasogastric tube for nausea and vomiting. Sigmoid volvulus (Figs. 13.4 and 13.5) can often be decompressed with an endoscope. Other causes or refractory cases require surgery to relieve the obstruction.

17. List and differentiate the three common types of groin hernias.

    1. **Indirect hernias** are the most common type in both sexes and all age groups. The hernia sac travels through the inner and outer inguinal rings (protrusion begins lateral to the inferior epigastric vessels) and into the scrotum or labia because of a patent processus vaginalis (congenital defect).
    2. **Direct hernias** (no sac) protrude medial to the inferior epigastric vessels because of weakness in the abdominal musculature of Hesselbach triangle. They are less likely to become incarcerated than indirect hernias. They are also uncommon in women.

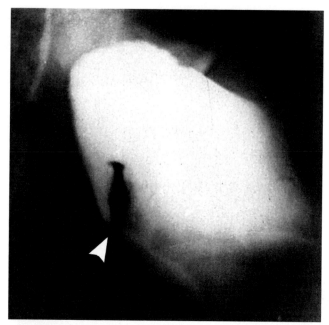

Fig. 13.5 This barium enema shows the characteristic bird's beak sign of volvulus (arrowhead). (From Marx J. Rosen's *Emergency Medicine.* 7th ed. Philadelphia: Mosby; 2009 [fig. 93.3].)

3. **Femoral hernias** are more common than direct or indirect hernias in women (though they are still more common in men). The hernia (no sac) goes through the femoral ring onto the anterior thigh (located below the inguinal ring).

   Of the three types, femoral hernias are the most susceptible to incarceration and strangulation. All three types are treated with elective surgical repair if symptomatic.

18. Define incarcerated and strangulated hernias.

   Incarceration occurs when a herniated organ is trapped and becomes swollen and edematous. Incarcerated hernias are the most common cause of small bowel obstruction in patients who have had no previous abdominal surgery and the second most common cause in patients who have had previous abdominal surgery (Fig. 13.6). Treatment is prompt surgery.

   Strangulation occurs after incarceration when the entrapment becomes so severe that the blood supply is cut off. Strangulation can lead to necrosis and is a surgical emergency. Patients may present with symptoms of small bowel obstruction and shock.

19. True or false: Generally, patients should not eat or drink for 8 or more hours before surgery.

   True. This protocol reduces the chance of aspiration and subsequent pneumonia.

20. What is the best test (other than a good history) for preoperative evaluation of pulmonary function?

   Spirometry, which gives functional vital capacity, forced expiratory volumes, and maximal voluntary ventilation. A good history (e.g., activity level, exercise tolerance) is also useful.

21. What measures help to prevent intraoperative and postoperative deep venous thrombosis and pulmonary embolus?

   Compressive/elastic stockings, intermittent pneumatic compression (IPC), early ambulation, and/or low-dose heparins (unfractionated or low molecular weight).

22. What is the most common cause of fever in the first 24 hours after surgery?

   Atelectasis. Prevent and treat atelectasis with early ambulation, chest physiotherapy/percussion, incentive spirometry, and proper pain control. Too much pain and too many narcotics (both can decrease respiratory effort) increase the risk of atelectasis.

23. What are the other common causes of postoperative fever?

   The five *W*s—**w**ind, **w**ater, **w**alk, **w**ound, and **w**eird drugs—summarize the common causes of postoperative fever in the order that they tend to occur. Wind stands for atelectasis and pneumonia, water for urinary tract

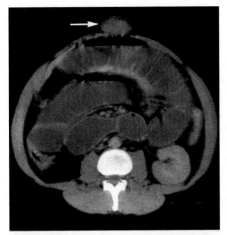

Fig. 13.6 Small intestinal obstruction. A section through the midabdomen from a computed tomography (CT) scan shows dilated, mainly fluid-filled, small intestinal loops. The obstruction was due to an incarcerated paraumbilic hernia, the edge of which can be identified *(arrow)*. (From Adam A, et al. *Grainger & Allison's Diagnostic Radiology*. 5th ed. Edinburgh: Churchill Livingstone; 2008 [fig. 32.37].)

infection (UTI; be sure to remove Foley catheters as soon as possible postoperatively to avoid catheter-associated UTIs), walk for deep venous thrombosis, wound for surgical wound infection, and weird drugs for drug fever. The most common timeline is days 1 to 3 for wind, days 3 to 5 for water, days 4 to 6 for walk, days 5 to 7 for wound, and days 7+ for weird drugs. In patients with daily fever spikes that do not respond to antibiotics, think about an intraabdominal abscess. These most often occur 2 to 3 weeks postoperatively. Order a CT scan to locate and then drain the abscess if one is present.

24. **Define fascial or wound dehiscence. How do you recognize it?**
Fascial or wound dehiscence occurs when the surgical wound opens spontaneously, usually 5 to 10 days postoperatively. Look for leakage of serosanguineous fluid from the wound, particularly after the patient coughs or strains. Frequently the wound is infected. Surgical reclosure of the wound and treatment of infection are required.

25. **Explain the ABCDEs of trauma. How are they used?**
The ABCDEs of trauma are **a**irway, **b**reathing, **c**irculation, **d**isability, and **e**xposure. They are the keys to the initial management of trauma patients. Follow them in order if simultaneous management is not possible. For example, if a patient is bleeding to death and has a blocked airway, address airway management first.

26. **What is the difference between airway and breathing in trauma protocol?**
Airway means provision, protection, and maintenance of an adequate airway at all times. If the patient can answer questions, the airway is fine for now. You can use an oropharyngeal airway in uncomplicated cases and give supplemental oxygen. When you are in doubt or the patient's airway is blocked, intubate. If intubation fails, do a cricothyroidotomy.

   Breathing is similar to airway, but even patients with an open airway may not be breathing spontaneously. The end result is the same. When you are in doubt or the patient is not breathing, intubate. If intubation fails, do a cricothyroidotomy.

27. **Explain circulation, disability, and exposure.**
Circulation refers to circulating blood volume. For practical purposes, it means that if the patient seems hypovolemic (tachycardic, bleeding, weak pulse, pale, diaphoretic, capillary refill >2 seconds), give IV fluids and/or blood products. Initially you should start two large-bore IV lines and give a bolus of 10 to 20 mL/kg (roughly 1 L) of lactated Ringer solution or normal saline. Then reassess the patient after the bolus for improvement. Repeat the bolus, if needed.

   Disability refers to the need to check neurologic function. In practical terms, this translates into doing a Glasgow Coma Scale (GCS) assessment. Intubation is generally recommended for patients with GCS less than 8, as they are usually unable to reliably protect their airway.

   Exposure reminds you to expose and examine the entire body. In other words, remove all of the patient's clothes and "put a finger in every orifice" so that you do not miss any occult injuries.

28. **What imaging films are routinely ordered for most patients with at least moderately severe trauma?**
Cervical spine, chest, and pelvic radiographs.

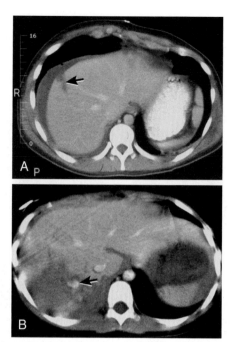

Fig. 13.7 Small and large hepatic lacerations. (A) A computed tomography (CT) scan was obtained through the upper abdomen in this patient after a motor vehicle accident. A small area of low density *(arrow)* is seen in the lateral portion of the right lobe, and blood surrounds the liver. (B) A CT scan in another patient after a motor vehicle accident shows a much larger area of lacerated liver in the posterior aspect of the right lobe. A central area of increased density *(the white area at the tip of the arrow)* indicates acute hemorrhaging at the time of the scan. (From Mettler F. *Essentials of Radiology.* 2nd ed. Philadelphia: Saunders; 2004 [fig. 6.47].)

29. **What is the imaging study of choice for head trauma?**
    Noncontrast CT (better than magnetic resonance imaging for acute trauma).

30. **How do you manage a patient with blunt abdominal trauma?**
    In patients with blunt abdominal trauma, the initial findings determine the appropriate course of action. If the patient is awake and stable and your examination is benign, then observe the patient and repeat the abdominal exam later. You can also do a FAST (focused assessment by sonography in trauma) scan to check for free fluid in the abdomen and pelvis. Meanwhile, perform a CT scan of the abdomen and pelvis with oral and IV contrast.

    If the patient is hemodynamically unstable (hypotension and/or shock that does not respond to fluid challenge), proceed directly to laparotomy.

    If the patient has a positive FAST scan (i.e., there is free fluid, presumably blood, in the abdomen), proceed to laparotomy.

    If the patient has altered mental status, the abdomen cannot be examined, or an obvious source of blood loss explains the hemodynamic instability, order a CT scan of the abdomen and pelvis (Fig. 13.7) with oral and IV contrast (also get a CT scan of the head and cervical spine if altered mental status is present). Diagnostic peritoneal lavage is no longer used because it is nonspecific and less sensitive than CT; it can also alter CT scan results.

31. **How is penetrating abdominal trauma managed?**
    In patients with penetrating abdominal trauma (e.g., gunshot, stab wound), the type of injury and the initial findings determine the course of action. With any gunshot wound that may have violated the peritoneal cavity, proceed directly to laparotomy. With a wound from a sharp instrument, management is more controversial. Either proceed directly to laparotomy (your best choice if the patient is unstable) or perform CT scan if the patient is stable. With nonoperative management, perform serial abdominal exams.

32. **Which six thoracic injuries can be rapidly fatal?**
    1. Airway obstruction
    2. Open pneumothorax
    3. Tension pneumothorax
    4. Cardiac tamponade
    5. Massive hemothorax
    6. Flail chest
       You may be asked to recognize and/or treat any of these six conditions on the USMLE.

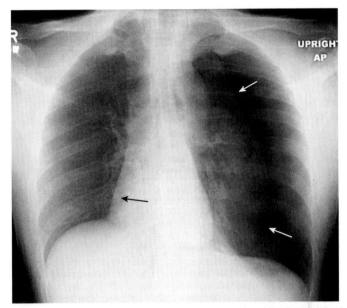

Fig. 13.8 There is a large, left-sided tension pneumothorax *(white arrows)*. The left lung is partially collapsed as the pleural space fills with air. The heart is shifted toward the right *(black arrow)*, which means the pneumothorax is under tension. (From Herring W. *Learning Radiology: Recognizing the Basics.* 4th ed. Philadelphia: Elsevier; 2020:371-372.)

33. **How do you recognize and treat airway obstruction?**
    Patients with airway obstruction have no audible breath sounds, cannot answer questions even if awake, and may be gurgling. Treat with intubation. If intubation fails, do a cricothyroidotomy (or a tracheostomy in the operating room if time allows).

34. **How do you recognize and treat an open pneumothorax?**
    An open pneumothorax presents with an open defect in the chest wall and decreased or absent breath sounds on the affected side. This condition causes poor ventilation and oxygenation. Treat with intubation, positive pressure ventilation, and closure of the defect in the chest wall. To close the defect, use gauze and tape it on three sides only. This approach allows excessive pressure to escape so that you do not convert an open pneumothorax into a tension pneumothorax.

35. **How do you recognize and treat a tension pneumothorax?**
    A tension pneumothorax may occur after blunt or penetrating trauma to the chest. Air forced into the pleural space cannot escape and collapses the affected lung and then shifts the mediastinum and trachea to the opposite side of the chest (Fig. 13.8). Findings include absent breath sounds on the affected side, a hypertympanic percussion sound, and possible tracheal deviation. Hypotension and/or distended neck veins may result from impaired cardiac filling. Treat with needle decompression, followed by insertion of a chest tube.

36. **Describe the presentation of cardiac tamponade. How is it diagnosed and treated?**
    Cardiac tamponade is classically associated with penetrating trauma to the left chest. Patients have hypotension (due to impaired cardiac filling), distended neck veins, muffled heart sounds, **pulsus paradoxus** (exaggerated fall in blood pressure on inspiration), and normal breath sounds. If the patient is unstable, treat with pericardiocentesis; put a catheter through the skin and into the pericardial sac and aspirate blood and fluid. If the patient is stable, you can first do an echocardiogram to confirm the diagnosis.

37. **Define massive hemothorax. How is it diagnosed and treated?**
    Massive hemothorax is defined as a loss of more than 1 L of blood into the thoracic cavity. Patients have decreased (not absent) breath sounds in the affected area, dull note on percussion, hypotension, collapsed neck veins (from blood leaving the vascular tree), and tachycardia. Placement of a chest tube allows the blood to come out. Give IV fluids and/or blood before you place the chest tube if the diagnosis is known in advance. If the bleeding stops after the initial outflow, order a chest radiograph or CT scan to check for remaining blood or pathology. If blood is left behind, the patient is at risk for forming empyema. Treat supportively. If the bleeding does not stop, emergent thoracotomy is required.

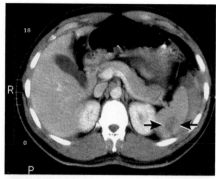

Fig. 13.9 Splenic laceration. This computed tomography (CT) scan done on a patient after a motor vehicle accident shows a dark area near the posterior aspect of the spleen *(arrows)*, which is the laceration. Note also the blood surrounding the spleen. (From Mettler F. *Essentials of Radiology.* 2nd ed. Philadelphia: Saunders; 2004 [fig. 6.60].)

38. **How do you recognize and treat flail chest?**
    Flail chest occurs when several adjacent ribs are broken in multiple places, causing the affected part of the chest wall to move paradoxically during respiration (inward during inspiration, outward during expiration). Almost all patients have an associated pulmonary contusion, which, combined with pain, may make respiration inadequate. When you are in doubt or the patient is not doing well, intubate and give positive pressure ventilation. The patient should also be evaluated for aortic damage.

39. **What is the most common cause of immediate death after an automobile accident or a fall from a great height?**
    Aortic rupture. Look for a widened mediastinum on chest radiograph and an appropriate history of trauma. The most common site of aortic rupture is where the aortic arch meets the descending aorta, where the ligamentum arteriosum tethers to the aorta. Order a CT scan or angiogram if a contained aortic rupture (of those who survive to be admitted to the hospital, 50% will die in the first 24 hours) is suspected. Aortic laceration, traumatic aortic injury, and traumatic pseudoaneurysm all fairly describe the phenomenon seen in initial survivors: an aortic rupture contained by a hematoma or an inadequate amount of surrounding tissue (e.g., adventitia only). Treat with immediate surgical repair.

40. **What do you need to know about splenic rupture?**
    The spleen is the most commonly injured organ in blunt trauma (Fig. 13.9). Patients with splenic rupture, the most severe form of injury, have a history of blunt abdominal trauma, hypotension, tachycardia, shock, and/or **Kehr sign** (referred pain in the left shoulder). Patients with Epstein-Barr virus infection or infectious mononucleosis and splenomegaly should avoid contact sports to prevent rupture. Make sure patients with a history of functional or surgical asplenia have received the pneumococcal, meningococcal, and *H. influenzae* (i.e., encapsulated bugs) vaccines.

41. **What clues suggest a diagnosis of diaphragmatic rupture? How is it treated?**
    Diaphragm rupture usually occurs after blunt trauma and on the left side (because the liver protects the right side of the diaphragm). You may hear bowel sounds when listening to the chest or see bowel that has herniated into the chest on chest radiograph. Treatment is surgical repair of the diaphragm.

42. **What are the three zones of the neck? How is trauma in each of the different zones managed?**
    Zone I is the base of the neck from 2 cm above the clavicles to the level of the clavicles.
    Zone II is the midcervical region from 2 cm above the clavicle to the angle of the mandible.
    Zone III is the top of the neck from the angle of the mandible to the base of the skull.

    With zone I and III injuries, you generally should order an arteriogram before going to the operating room. Zone I injuries also warrant bronchoscopy, esophagoscopy, and contrast swallow study. With zone II injuries, proceed to the operating room for surgical exploration without an arteriogram. In patients with obvious bleeding or a rapidly expanding hematoma in the neck, proceed directly to the operating room, no matter where the injury is.

43. **How should a choking victim be managed?**
    Always leave choking patients alone if they are speaking, coughing, or breathing. If they stop doing all of these, perform the Heimlich maneuver.

44. **What should you do if a tooth is knocked out?**
    Put the tooth back in place with no cleaning (or only saline to rinse it off), and stabilize the tooth in place. The sooner this is done, the better the prognosis for salvage of the tooth.

GENETICS

1. Specify how the following disorders are *usually* transmitted genetically. The choices are autosomal dominant or recessive, X-linked recessive, chromosomal disorder, or polygenic disorder

Disorder	Inheritance Pattern
Von Willebrand disease	Autosomal dominant
Neurofibromatosis type I/II	Autosomal dominant
MEN I/II syndrome	Autosomal dominant
Achondroplasia	Autosomal dominant
Sphingolipidoses (e.g., Tay-Sachs disease, Gaucher disease)	Autosomal recessive
Fabry disease*	X-linked recessive
Hurler disease	Autosomal recessive
Hunter disease	X-linked recessive
Glycogen storage diseases (e.g., McArdle disease)	Autosomal recessive
Cystic fibrosis	Autosomal recessive
Marfan syndrome	Autosomal dominant
Huntington disease	Autosomal dominant
Pyloric stenosis	Polygenic disorder
Cleft lip/palate	Polygenic disorder
Type 2 diabetes	Polygenic disorder
Down syndrome	Chromosomal disorder (trisomy 21)
Familial hypercholesterolemia	Autosomal dominant
Galactosemia	Autosomal recessive
Amino acid disorders (e.g., phenylketonuria)	Autosomal recessive
Edward syndrome	Chromosomal disorder (trisomy 18)
Sickle cell disease	Autosomal recessive
Hemophilia	X-linked recessive
Glucose-6-phosphate dehydrogenase (G6PD) deficiency	X-linked recessive
Patau syndrome	Chromosomal disorder (trisomy 13)
Lesch-Nyhan syndrome	X-linked recessive
Obesity	Polygenic disorder
Neural tube defects	Polygenic disorder
Turner syndrome	Chromosomal disorder (XO)
Schizophrenia	Polygenic disorder

Disorder	Inheritance Pattern
Duchenne muscular dystrophy	X-linked recessive
Wiskott-Aldrich syndrome	X-linked recessive
Bruton agammaglobulinemia	X-linked recessive
Fragile X syndrome	X-linked recessive
Children's polycystic kidney disease	Autosomal recessive
Wilson disease	Autosomal recessive
Alcoholism	Polygenic disorder
Hemochromatosis	Autosomal recessive
Congenital adrenal hyperplasia (e.g., 21-hydroxylase deficiency)	Autosomal recessive
Familial adenomatous polyposis	Autosomal dominant
Adult polycystic kidney disease	Autosomal dominant
Hereditary spherocytosis	Autosomal dominant
Tuberous sclerosis	Autosomal dominant
Myotonic dystrophy	Autosomal dominant

MEN, Multiple endocrine neoplasia.
*Fabry disease is the exception to the rule that the sphingolipidosis disorders are autosomal recessive.

2. What is the likelihood that a mother with an autosomal dominant condition will pass the condition to the child if the father does not have the disease?
50%. The father is not a carrier because autosomal dominant diseases express themselves in carriers, and it is reasonable to assume that the mother has one copy of the diseased gene and one normal gene (unless told otherwise). It is exceedingly rare to find two diseased genes.

3. Genetic testing reveals that both mother and father are carriers of an autosomal recessive condition but do not have the condition themselves. What are the odds that their first child will develop the condition or be a carrier?
The child has a 25% risk of developing the condition, a 50% risk of being a carrier, and a 25% chance of not inheriting the diseased gene at all.

4. The father has an X-linked recessive disorder. What are the chances that he will pass the disease to his son or daughter if the mother does not have the diseased gene?
There is no chance that he will pass the condition to his son; he will give his son a Y chromosome. On the other hand, there is a 100% chance he will pass the diseased gene to his daughter, but because it is X-linked recessive, she has no chance of developing the condition. She will get a diseased X chromosome from the father and a healthy X chromosome from the mother.

5. The mother is a carrier for an X-linked recessive disorder, and the father is healthy. What are the odds that a son or daughter will develop the disease?
There is a 50% chance for a son and no chance for a daughter to develop the disease. However, there is a 50% chance that the daughter will become a carrier.

6. How do you recognize Down syndrome?
Down syndrome (trisomy 21) is the most common cause of intellectual disability in the United States. The biggest risk factor is maternal age (1 in 1500 offspring of 16-year-old mothers and 1 in 25 offspring of 45-year-old mothers). At birth, look for hypotonia, single transverse palmar crease, and characteristic facies (Fig. 14.1). Congenital cardiac defects (especially ventricular septal defects) are common, and affected persons have an increased risk for leukemia, duodenal atresia, and early Alzheimer disease.

7. What is the second most common known cause of inherited intellectual disability?
Fragile X syndrome (X-linked recessive). Affected males often have an elongated face, large ears, and large testicles (macroorchidism).

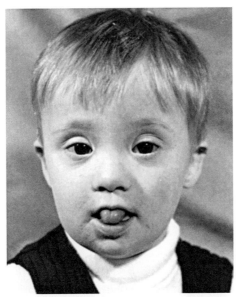

Fig. 14.1 Child with Down syndrome. Note the flat facial profile, flat nasal bridge, protruding tongue, folded ears, slanted palpebral fissures, and epicanthic folds. (From Kliegman R. *Nelson Textbook of Pediatrics*. 19th ed. Philadelphia: Elsevier; 2011 [fig. 76.8A].)

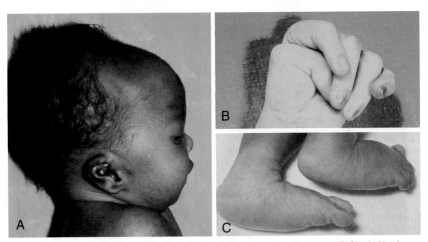

Fig. 14.2 Edwards syndrome. (A) Note the small head, prominent occiput, and low-set, malformed ears. (B) Clenched hand with overlapping fingers. (C) Rocker-bottom feet. (From Kanski JJ. *Clinical Diagnosis in Ophthalmology*. Philadelphia: Elsevier; 2006 [fig. 15.10]. Courtesy B.J. Zitelli and H.W. Davis.)

8. **How do you recognize Edwards syndrome?**
   Edwards syndrome (trisomy 18) affects females more than males. Characteristics include intellectual disability, small size for age, a small head with hypoplastic mandible and low-set ears, and clenched fist with the index finger overlapping the third and fourth fingers (almost pathognomonic) (Fig. 14.2), and rocker-bottom feet.

9. **What is Patau syndrome?**
   Patau syndrome (trisomy 13) presents with intellectual disability, apnea, deafness, holoprosencephaly (fusion of cerebral hemispheres), myelomeningocele, cardiovascular abnormalities, rocker-bottom feet, cleft lip and/or palate, and polydactyly.

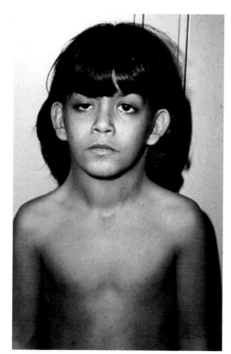

Fig. 14.3 Turner syndrome. This 13-year-old female demonstrates the classic webbed neck and triangular facies of Turner syndrome. She has sexual infantilism and short stature. (From Moshang T. *Pediatric Endocrinology: Requisites.* Philadelphia: Elsevier; 2004 [plate 8-2].)

10. How do you recognize Turner syndrome?

    Patients with Turner syndrome (females with 45,XO) have nuchal lymphedema at birth, short stature, webbed neck, widely spaced nipples, amenorrhea, and lack of breast development (due to primary ovarian failure) (Fig. 14.3). Coarctation of the aorta is common, and you may see a horseshoe kidney or cystic hygroma. A buccal smear classically reveals absent Barr bodies.

11. Describe Klinefelter syndrome

    Patients with Klinefelter syndrome (males who are 47,XXY instead of 46,XY) are tall with small testes (<2 cm in length), gynecomastia, sterility, and a slightly decreased IQ (on average). The classic case on the Step 2 exam is a man who presents with complaints of infertility.

12. What is the hallmark of cri du chat syndrome?

    Cri du chat (French for "cry of the cat") syndrome is due to a deletion on the short arm of chromosome 5. Look for a high-pitched cry that sounds like the cry of a cat, along with severe intellectual disability.

13. What clinical signs suggest galactosemia?

    Congenital cataracts and neonatal sepsis with vomiting after breastfeeding. Patients should avoid galactose- and lactose-containing foods.

14. Describe the clinical findings in tuberous sclerosis

    This autosomal dominant disorder presents with hypopigmented skin macules (ash-leaf spots), seizures, intellectual disability, central nervous system (CNS) and cutaneous hamartomas (tubers), and an increased risk for cardiac rhabdomyomas and renal tumors known as angiomyolipomas. Look for a positive family history.

15. What causes Lesch-Nyhan syndrome? What classic behavior do patients exhibit?

    This syndrome is due to a deficiency of hypoxanthine-guanine phosphoribosyltransferase (HGPRT), which causes congenital hyperuricemia. Patients have intellectual disability and self-mutilating behavior. The classic example is patients who bite their own fingers.

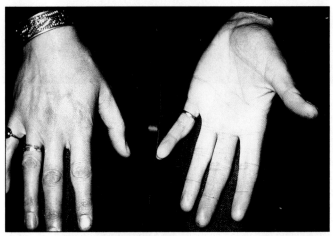

Fig. 14.4 Marfan syndrome. Arachnodactyly in a patient with Marfan syndrome. (From Stamper RL. *Becker-Shaffer's Diagnosis and Therapy of the Glaucomas.* Philadelphia: Elsevier; 2009 [fig. 19.41].)

16. What causes Marfan syndrome? How do you recognize it?

   Marfan syndrome is an autosomal dominant connective tissue disorder caused by abnormal fibrillin-1 protein and associated with ocular, skeletal, and cardiovascular problems. Look for a positive family history. Patients are tall and have arachnodactyly (long, thin fingers) (Fig. 14.4), hyperextensible joints, upward lens dislocation (ectopia lentis), mitral valve prolapse, and aortic dilation with a high risk for thoracic aortic dissection.

1. True or false: Roughly 2% of the population is over the age of 65
   False. Approximately 15% of people are over the age of 65, and this number is increasing.

2. What age group constitutes the most rapidly growing segment of the population?
   Persons over the age of 85.

3. True or false: An 80-year-old person needs more calories than a 30-year-old person
   False. An 80-year-old person has half the lean body mass of a 30-year-old person and thus needs fewer calories. The basal metabolic rate is based on lean body mass. Elderly patients, however, need more vitamin B_{12}, vitamin D (and/or calcium), folate, and nonheme iron than younger patients.

4. True or false: Hearing and vision changes are a normal part of aging
   True. **Presbyopia** (hardening of the lens that decreases the ability to accommodate) becomes almost universal after age 50, thus the common need for reading glasses after age 50. **Presbycusis**, the loss of ability to discriminate between sounds, most markedly at higher frequency, is also part of the normal process of aging. Hearing aids may help.

5. True or false: Older patients require higher doses of most medications
   False. In fact, due to normal age-related changes in pharmacokinetics, including absorption, metabolism, gut transit time, and body fat composition, medications should usually be prescribed at lower doses in the geriatric population. Older patients may also be more susceptible to adverse effects of medication, especially sedating and anticholinergic medications. These medications can lead to confusion, falls, dry mouth, urinary retention and/or incontinence, and constipation, among others. The Beer's list offers consensus guidelines on medications to avoid or use with caution in the geriatric population.

6. What is frailty?
   Frailty is a common geriatric syndrome consisting of poor muscle bulk (sarcopenia) and weakness, osteoporosis, and mobility impairment that predicts lack of resilience to stresses like acute illness or trauma and is associated with poor health outcomes.

7. Why are falls so dangerous for older patients, and how can they be prevented?
   Falls are a significant cause of morbidity and mortality for the elderly, as around 30% of patients over age 65 will fall per year. Falls can lead to fractures, and the 1-year mortality after hip fracture is about 30%. All adults over age 65 should be screened for a history of falls within the past year. Falls are multifactorial but can be prevented by optimizing lighting and vision; removing potential obstacles from the home (e.g., rugs, pets, cords); making bathrooms safer with grab bars and bathing benches or chairs; reviewing medication lists and removing medications that may cause confusion, sedation, blurry vision, or dizziness; and encouraging regular exercise and balance training. Additionally, there is some evidence that vitamin D helps prevent falls in community-dwelling older adults.

8. What is osteoporosis? Who should be screened?
   Osteoporosis is a disease of pathologically decreased bone mineral density, which can lead to bone fractures. It is very common among older patients, especially women. Current recommendations suggest screening all women over age 65 for osteoporosis and younger women with risk factors for secondary osteoporosis with a dual-energy x-ray absorptiometry (DEXA) scan. DEXA scans typically examine bone mineral density in the spine, hip, and radius. The diagnosis is made by a T-score more than −2.5 standard deviations below the reference population of young, healthy women. Additionally, any patient who has an osteoporotic fracture, regardless of the T-score, is considered to have osteoporosis and should be treated.

9. What are the risk factors for osteoporosis? What are the typical therapies for osteoporosis?
   Risk factors for osteoporosis include older age, white or Asian race, low body mass index, and family history of osteoporosis. Other risk factors include testosterone or estrogen deficiency (e.g., through early or iatrogenic menopause), hyper- and hypothyroidism, hyperparathyroidism, Cushing disease, rheumatoid arthritis and other inflammatory arthritides, tobacco use, vitamin D deficiency, long-term glucocorticoid therapy, and malnutrition. Treatment often includes medication therapy with bisphosphonates, encouraging weight-bearing exercise, and minimizing fall risk.

10. Describe the normal changes in male sexual function that occur with aging
    - Increased refractory period (after ejaculation, it takes longer before he can have another erection)
    - Increased amount of time to achieve an erection
    - Delayed ejaculation (an elderly man may ejaculate only one of every three times that he has sex)

11. Describe the normal changes in female sexual function that occur with aging

    Decreased vaginal lubrication (estrogen cream or water-soluble lubricants can be helpful in treating symptoms)
    Dyspareunia (pain with intercourse) due to atrophy of clitoral, labial, and vaginal tissues (treated with estrogen cream)
    Delayed orgasm

12. True or false: Impotence and lack of sexual desire are normal in elderly people
    False. Impotence in men and lack of sexual desire in either sex are not normal and should be investigated and treated. Look for psychiatric disorders (e.g., depression) as well as physical causes, such as medications (selective serotonin reuptake inhibitors [SSRIs] and antihypertensives are notorious culprits), vascular disease (watch for atherosclerosis risk factors), and neurologic disease (especially in diabetics).

13. Describe the normal changes in sleep habits in elderly people
    Elderly persons require less sleep, sleep less deeply, sleep earlier in the evening, wake up more frequently during the night, and awaken earlier in the morning. It also takes longer for elderly persons to fall asleep (longer sleep latency), and they have less stage 3 and 4 and rapid eye movement sleep.

14. What is the best prophylaxis for pressure ulcers in an immobilized patient?
    Frequent turning and the use of special air mattresses.

15. True or false: Brain atrophy is a normal part of aging
    True. Decreased brain weight, enlarged ventricles and sulci, and a slightly decreased ability to learn new material are normal parts of aging.

16. Define pseudodementia. How do you recognize it on the Step 2 exam?
    Depression in the elderly can resemble dementia. Look for a history that would trigger depression (e.g., loss of a spouse, change in living situation or level of independence, terminal or debilitating disease) and other symptoms of depression (e.g., frequent crying, suicidal thoughts).

17. What is the difference between dementia and delirium?
    Dementia is a disease of chronic and progressive cognitive decline. There are many different kinds of dementias, the most common of which is Alzheimer dementia, which has increasing incidence with age. Delirium, by contrast, is an acute state of confusion characterized by waxing and waning mental status, disorientation, changes in arousal, poor attention, abnormal sleep-wake cycle, and/or hallucinations. Delirium usually has an underlying cause, such as severe illness or infection, hospitalization, or medication effects. Delirium can happen to anyone and is very common in intensive care unit patients (even young patients) but is especially common during times of illness in patients who have underlying mild cognitive impairment or dementia. Delirium should improve as the underlying etiology is treated, but supportive care for delirious patients also includes frequent reorientation, removing barriers to communication (e.g., bringing patients' glasses, hearing aids, or dentures to bedside), optimizing sleep-wake cycle by exposing patients to natural light and making sure they have a bed by a window, and avoiding or discontinuing contributing medications. Severe cases can be treated with antipsychotics, though these medications may increase mortality.

18. True or false: Almost 50% of patients over the age of 65 suffer from some type of dementia
    False. Roughly 15% of people over the age of 65 suffer from dementia, but the prevalence increases with age. Roughly 50% of people over age 80 have dementia or mild cognitive impairment. The most common types of dementias are Alzheimer dementia, dementia with Lewy bodies, vascular dementia, Parkinson dementia, and frontotemporal dementia. Other disorders that can cause dementia include HIV and Pick disease. Test for reversible causes of dementia and memory impairment such as electrolyte disturbances (classically hyponatremia), hypothyroidism, depression, neurosyphilis, and vitamin B_{12} deficiency.

19. Describe the characteristics of Alzheimer dementia
    Alzheimer dementia is a neurodegenerative disorder primarily affecting older adults and characterized by memory impairment, particularly short-term memory for facts and events. Memory loss develops insidiously and progresses slowly over time. Language function, visuospatial skills, and executive function tend to be affected early in the disease process, and with progression patients may have difficulty with activities of daily living.

20. Describe the characteristics of dementia with Lewy bodies
    Dementia with Lewy bodies is an increasingly recognized Parkinson plus syndrome characterized by dementia plus two of the three following distinctive clinical features: visual hallucinations (classically involving small animals or small human beings/children), later-onset parkinsonism (in contrast to Parkinson disease, which has later-

onset dementia; bradykinesia, limb rigidity, and gait disorders), and cognitive fluctuations. In contrast to Alzheimer dementia, the memory loss in dementia with Lewy bodies presents later in the course of the disease. Early symptoms include driving difficulties (e.g., getting lost) and impaired job performance. Sleep disorders such as acting out dreams are common in patients with dementia with Lewy bodies.

21. Describe a scenario that would make you suspect vascular dementia
   Look for a patient with vascular risk factors (e.g., hypertension, diabetes, dyslipidemia, coronary artery disease) who presents with dementia of abrupt onset and a stepwise deterioration.

22. True or false: Dementia is common in patients with Parkinson disease
   True. Dementia is a common feature of Parkinson disease. Factors that influence the incidence of dementia include older age, age greater than or equal to 60 years at onset of Parkinson disease, longer duration of Parkinson disease, and severity of parkinsonism.

23. Describe the characteristics of frontotemporal dementia
   Frontotemporal dementia is a characterized by focal deterioration of the frontal and/or temporal lobes, leading to changes in personality or social behavior, with an eventual progression to dementia. Age of onset is typically in the 50s or 60s.

24. True or false: Only 5% of people over the age of 65 live in nursing homes
   True. Watch for the boards to try to push you into old-fashioned stereotypes of the elderly. Not all old people are demented and living in nursing homes.

25. How can advance directives be useful?
   An advance directive is a legal document that specifies a person's wishes regarding one's own health and can guide medical decision making in the event that the person should become incapacitated and unable to make decisions for oneself. Key features of advance directives include designating a proxy decision maker, who may or may not be the person's legal next of kin, and specifying the kinds of treatments or interventions that the person would or would not accept. Often, advance directives are used to communicate a patient's wishes regarding end-of-life care, including wishes around resuscitation, intubation, artificial nutrition, and/or antibiotic therapy. Advance directives come into effect only if the patient is unable to communicate or make decisions for oneself.

CHAPTER 16

GYNECOLOGY

1. Name each of the primary ligaments of female pelvic anatomy and the notable anatomic relationships of each ligament.

Ligament	Relevant Anatomic Structures
Cardinal ligament	Anchors cervix to lateral pelvic wall. Contains uterine blood vessels. Ligated during total abdominal hysterectomy.
Suspensory (infundibulopelvic) ligament	Anchors ovaries to lateral pelvic wall. Contains ovarian vessels. Ligated during oophorectomy. Compromised in ovarian torsion.
Round ligament	Connects each uterine horn to the ipsilateral labia majora. Travels through the inguinal canal.
Broad ligament Mesosalpinx Mesovarium Mesometrium	Connects the lateral pelvic wall to fallopian tubes (mesosalpinx), ovaries (mesovarium), and uterine body (mesometrium).
Ovarian ligament	Connects each ovary to ipsilateral uterine horn.

2. What is the most common cause of preventable infertility in the United States?
   Pelvic inflammatory disease (PID).

3. What is PID? How do you recognize it on the USMLE Step 2 exam?
   PID is typically due to an ascending sexually transmitted infection of the upper female genital tract that may involve the endometrial cavity (endometritis), fallopian tubes (salpingitis), ovaries (oophoritis), parametrial tissues/ligaments (parametritis), and/or peritoneal cavity (peritonitis). Look for a sexually active female aged 13 to 35 years with the following symptoms: (1) abdominal pain, (2) adnexal tenderness, *and* (3) **cervical motion tenderness**. All three criteria must technically be present. In addition, one or more of the following should be present: elevated erythrocyte sedimentation rate (ESR) or C-reactive protein (CRP) level, leukocytosis, fever, or purulent cervical discharge.

4. How is PID treated? What are the common sequelae?
   There are several different regimens recommended by the Centers for Disease Control and Prevention (CDC), but there is one main antibiotic combination used for outpatient PID and two commonly used combinations for inpatient PID. Ceftriaxone plus doxycycline is the typical outpatient combination. For inpatient treatment, consider either cefoxitin or cefotetan plus doxycycline; or consider clindamycin plus gentamicin. Remember these inpatient regimens with the mnemonics *foxy doxy* (ce*fox*itin + *doxy*cycline) or "*gent*ly *clean-da* uterus with *gent*amicin + *clinda*mycin."
   Common sequelae include chronic pelvic pain, increased risk of ectopic pregnancy, infertility due to scarring of the fallopian tubes, and progression to tuboovarian abscess. If suspected PID does not begin to improve after 48 hours, look for an abscess with an ultrasound or computed tomography (CT) scan. Ruptured abscess will present with hemodynamic instability; manage this with emergent laparotomy and excision of the affected tube (for unilateral disease) or total abdominal hysterectomy and bilateral salpingo-oophorectomy (for bilateral disease).

5. Define endometriosis. What are the signs and symptoms?
   Endometriosis is defined as endometrial glands outside the uterus (ectopic). Patients are usually nulliparous and over age 30 with the following symptoms: **dysmenorrhea** (painful menstruation), **dyspareunia** (painful intercourse), **dyschezia** (painful defecation), and/or perimenstrual spotting. The most common site for the ectopic endometrial glands is the ovaries (chocolate cyst appearance); look for tender adnexa in an afebrile patient. Other sites include the broad (uterosacral) ligament and peritoneal surface. Nodularities on the broad ligament are classic findings on physical exam; the classic sequela is a retroverted uterus.

6. **How is endometriosis diagnosed and treated?**
   The gold standard of diagnosis is laparoscopy with visualization of the ectopic tissue showing classic powder-burn lesions. Manage medically with birth control pills (if acceptable to the patient) or second-line agents danazol and gonadotropin-releasing hormone (GnRH) agonists (e.g., leuprolide). Surgery with electrocauterization will definitively destroy the ectopic glands and often improves fertility. In an older patient, consider hysterectomy and bilateral salpingo-oophorectomy for severe symptoms.

7. **What is the most likely cause of infertility in a menstruating woman over the age of 30 without a history of PID?**
   Endometriosis.

8. **Cover the right-hand columns. Specify the findings and treatment for the following vaginal infections.**

Organism	Findings	Treatment
Candida sp.	Cottage cheese–like substance, pseudohyphae on KOH preparation, history of diabetes, antibiotic treatment, or pregnancy	Topical or oral antifungal (e.g., fluconazole)
Trichomonas vaginalis	Pale yellow-green, frothy, watery discharge; strawberry cervix; motile organisms on microscopic inspection; vaginal pH >4.5	Metronidazole
Gardnerella vaginalis	Bacterial vaginosis; malodorous discharge, fishy smell on KOH preparation, clue cells; vaginal pH >4.5	Metronidazole
Human papillomavirus	Venereal warts; koilocytosis on Pap smear; postcoital bleeding	Many (acid, cryotherapy, laser, podophyllin)
Herpesvirus	Multiple shallow, painful ulcers; recurrence and resolution	Acyclovir, valacyclovir
Treponema pallidum (primary syphilis)	Painless chancre; occasional inguinal lymphadenopathy; spirochete on dark-field microscopy	Penicillin
Treponema pallidum (secondary syphilis)	Condyloma lata, maculopapular rash on palms, serology	Penicillin
Treponema pallidum (tertiary syphilis)	Tabes dorsalis, gummas, Argyll-Robertson pupils, CSF fluid examination	Penicillin
Chlamydia trachomatis	Most common STD; dysuria; positive culture and nucleic acid amplification tests (NAAT)	Doxycycline or azithromycin*
Neisseria gonorrhoeae	Mucopurulent cervicitis; growth on chocolate agar; positive NAAT	Ceftriaxone
Molluscum contagiosum	Characteristic appearance of dome-shaped lesions with central umbilication, intracellular inclusions	Curette, cryotherapy, or electrocauterization/coagulation
Pediculosis	Crabs; pruritic; lice can be seen on pubic hairs	Permethrin cream (or malathion)

CSF, Cerebrospinal fluid; *KOH,* potassium hydroxide; *STD,* sexually transmitted disease.
*Chlamydia can be treated with erythromycin if the patient is pregnant. If compliance is a concern (e.g., history of nonadherence, substance abuse, or homelessness), give azithromycin 1 g orally in a single dose so that you can watch the patient take it. Patients with gonorrhea should always be treated for presumed chlamydial coinfection, but *if exclusive Chlamydial infection is confirmed by NAAT,* you do *not* have to treat for potential gonorrheal coinfection (e.g., do *not* give ceftriaxone along with the doxycycline or azithromycin). In clinical practice this distinction is not often made, but that doesn't stop it from appearing on licensing exams. If the NAAT results aren't back yet, treat empirically for both organisms.

9. True or false: With all of the infections listed in the previous table, you should seek out and treat the patient's sexual partners.
False. *Candida* and *Gardnerella* species are not typically sexually transmitted diseases; they are usually caused by disturbances in the normal vaginal flora. You should treat the patient's sexual partners and give counseling (e.g., condoms) for the other infections, which are sexually transmitted.

10. True or false: Patients with gonorrhea should be treated for presumed chlamydial infection.
True. The established treatment strategy for gonorrhea is to give both ceftriaxone (for gonorrhea) and doxycycline (for potential coinfection with chlamydia). However, *if exclusive Chlamydial infection is confirmed by NAAT,* the reverse is not true; do *not* automatically give gonorrhea treatment (e.g., ceftriaxone) to patients with confirmed chlamydial infection. If the NAAT results aren't back yet, treat empirically for both organisms. But if NAAT results show exclusively a chlamydial infection with results negative for gonorrhea, the patient should only receive chlamydial treatment (e.g., either doxycycline or azithromycin *without* ceftriaxone).

11. Define adenomyosis. How does it classically present? What is the treatment?
Adenomyosis is defined as endometrial glands within the uterine musculature. Patients are usually over age 40 with dysmenorrhea and menorrhagia. Look for descriptions of a "large, boggy uterus" on physical exam. Be sure to obtain an endometrial biopsy sample to rule out endometrial cancer. Total abdominal hysterectomy would definitively relieve the symptoms; consider trialing GnRH agonists (e.g., leuprolide) to medically manage symptoms.

12. What are fibroids? How common are they? How often do they become malignant?
Fibroids (i.e., leiomyomas) are benign uterine tumors. They are the most common tumors in women and the most common indication for hysterectomy (when they grow too large or cause symptoms). Up to 40% of women have fibroids by age 40. Malignant transformation is quite rare (<1%).

13. Explain the relationship between uterine leiomyomas and hormones. How do leiomyomas present? What is the treatment?
Leiomyomas of the uterus are estrogen dependent. Therefore you may see rapid growth during pregnancy or the use of estrogen-containing oral contraceptive pills (OCPs) and regression after menopause. Leiomyomas may cause infertility, pain, and menorrhagia or metrorrhagia. Anemia due to leiomyoma is an indication for hysterectomy. Rarely, patients may present with a polyp protruding through the cervix. Dilation and curettage are needed to rule out endometrial cancer in women who present after the age of 35.

The treatment for leiomyoma is usually surgical (the levonorgestrel-releasing intrauterine device is seeing more widespread use, though randomized trials are lacking). Myomectomy can sometimes maintain or even restore fertility. For those no longer desiring pregnancy, total abdominal hysterectomy may be performed.

14. What is the first test to order in any woman of reproductive age with abnormal uterine bleeding?
A pregnancy test.

15. Define abnormal uterine bleeding (AUB). What does the PALM-COEIN classification stand for?
AUB is defined as menstrual flow outside of the normal frequency, duration, volume, or regularity in nonpregnant women of reproductive age. PALM-COEIN classifies abnormal bleeding into the most common causes of AUB as structural causes (PALM: **p**olyp, **a**denomyosis, **l**eiomyoma, **m**alignancy and hyperplasia) and nonstructural causes (COEIN: **c**oagulopathy, **o**vulatory dysfunction, **e**ndometrial dysfunction, **i**atrogenic, **n**ot yet classified).

More than 70% of cases are associated with anovulatory cycles (e.g., unopposed estrogen stimulates continued endometrial proliferation until the tissue finally outgrows its blood supply and randomly begins to slough off). The age of the patient is important because immediately following menarche and immediately before menopause, AUB is common. In fact, AUB during these two transitional times is considered physiologic. Most other women experiencing AUB have polycystic ovary syndrome (PCOS), the most common nonphysiologic cause of AUB.

16. Why is endometrial biopsy recommended in women over age 35 with AUB? What other test should be ordered in all women with AUB (regardless of age)?
Endometrial biopsy in this age range is to rule out endometrial cancer. Hemoglobin and hematocrit (or complete blood count) should be ordered on all women with AUB to make sure that the patient is not anemic from excessive blood loss.

17. How is AUB treated?
Estrogen-progestin OCPs are first-line management for many women with AUB. The levonorgestrel intrauterine device is a highly effective option for treatment of heavy menstrual bleeding (HMB) in women who do not desire pregnancy. Depot medroxyprogesterone acetate (DMPA) may be used for women with AUB who have contraindications to or prefer to avoid estrogen or if they prefer this method of contraception. High-dose oral progestins may be used to treat AUB in women who have contraindications to or prefer to avoid estrogen or

women who are trying to become pregnant. Tranexamic acid is an option for women with HMB who do not desire or should not use hormonal treatment. Nonsteroidal antiinflammatory drugs (NSAIDs) are a nonhormonal, noncontraceptive option for treatment of HMB and reduce the volume of menstrual blood loss by causing a decline in the rate of prostaglandin synthesis in the endometrium, leading to vasoconstriction and reduced bleeding for menorrhagia and AUB if the patient does not desire pregnancy and menstrual cycles are irregular. Monotherapy with progesterone is used for severe bleeding.

18. **Define polycystic ovarian syndrome. How do you recognize it?**
    PCOS is an endocrine imbalance characterized by an excess of androgens in a female patient, often suggested in a clinical vignette by a luteinizing hormone (LH) to follicle-stimulating hormone (FSH) ratio greater than 3:1. On physical exam, look for a combination of hirsutism, significant acne, AUB, and/or infertility in an overweight female. Patients also frequently develop enlarged ovaries with multiple peripherally oriented cysts, which can be seen on ultrasound (Fig. 16.1). However, an ultrasound is not required to make a diagnosis of PCOS. On the Step 2 exam, watch for an overweight woman who has acne, hirsutism, amenorrhea, and/or infertility.

19. **What is the most likely cause for infertility in a woman under age 30 with abnormal menstruation?**
    PCOS.

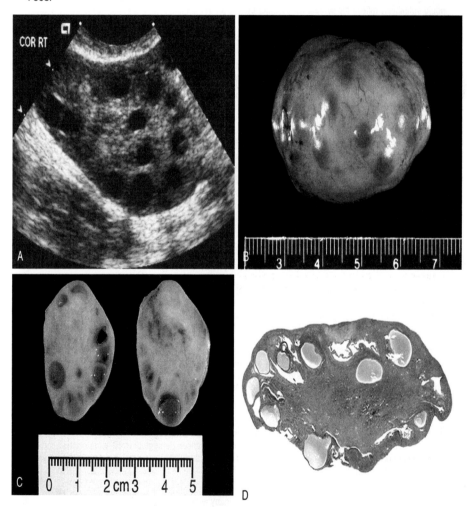

Fig. 16.1 (A) Ultrasonography of polycystic ovaries depicting numerous cysts. (B) Gross appearance of polycystic ovaries. Numerous follicles can be appreciated beneath the capsule. (C) Cross section of B illustrates subcortical cystic follicles. (D) Low-power microphotograph exhibits combination of cystic follicles and fibrotic ovarian cortex. (From Crum CP, Nucci MR, Howitt BE, et al. *Diagnostic Gynecologic and Obstetric Pathology.* 3rd ed. Philadelphia, PA: Elsevier; 2018.)

20. How is PCOS managed? With what risk is PCOS associated?
Manage the dysmenorrhea with OCPs or cyclic progesterone. If the patient desires pregnancy, you can use **letrozole** to induce ovulation. Chronic unopposed estrogen (i.e., not enough progesterone, hence infrequent menses) increases the risk of **endometrial cancer** in patients with PCOS. **Spironolactone** can be used to treat the hirsutism associated with PCOS. Metformin is sometimes used to treat the insulin resistance associated with PCOS and may help restore ovulation. However, metformin is not Food and Drug Administration (FDA)–approved for this use, and OCPs or cyclic progesterone are the preferred agents for endometrial protection.

21. Is infertility usually a male or a female problem?
Two-thirds of cases are due to a female problem, one-third to a male problem.

22. Assuming that the history and physical exam offer no clues, what is the first step in evaluating a couple for infertility?
Investigate the male first by performing semen analysis as it is cheap, easy, and noninvasive.

23. List the relevant characteristics of normal semen analysis.

    Ejaculate volume >1.5 mL
    Sperm concentration >15 million/mL
    Initial forward motility >32% of sperm
    Normal morphology >60% of sperm

24. What is the next step in workup for infertility if semen evaluation returns normal results?
Documentation of ovulation. The history may suggest an ovulatory problem (irregular menstrual cycle length, duration, or amount of flow; lack of premenstrual syndrome symptoms). Monitoring basal body temperature, luteal phase progesterone levels, and/or obtaining an endometrial biopsy during the luteal phase can all be done to check for ovulation.

25. What radiologic test is commonly used to investigate the fallopian tubes and uterine anatomy? What points in the history may lead you to suspect a uterine or tube problem?
A hysterosalpingogram is commonly used to investigate the anatomy of the uterus and fallopian tubes. Clues in the patient's history may suggest a tubal problem (e.g., PID, previous ectopic pregnancy) or a uterine problem (e.g., previous dilation and curettage resulting in intrauterine synechiae; history of fibroids; or symptoms of endometriosis; uterine anomalies such as septate, bicornuate, and didelphys).

26. What study is the last resort in the workup for infertility?
Laparoscopy may be performed as a last resort or with a history suggestive of endometriosis. Lysis of adhesions and destruction of endometriosis lesions often restore fertility.

27. Which two medications can be used to try to restore female fertility? In what situations are they effective?
Medical therapy usually consists of clomiphene citrate to induce ovulation, but this approach requires adequate endogenous production of estrogen. If the woman is hypoestrogenic, use human menopausal gonadotropin (hMG), which is a **combination of FSH and LH**, to increase estrogen production. If medications fail, in vitro fertilization can be attempted.

28. What is the main risk associated with medical induction of ovulation?
Multiple-gestation pregnancies.

29. Distinguish between primary and secondary amenorrhea.
A patient with primary amenorrhea has never experienced menarche, whereas a patient with secondary amenorrhea has a history of normal menstruation, which has now stopped.

30. Until proven otherwise, what is the cause of secondary amenorrhea in a previously menstruating woman of reproductive age?
Pregnancy. Always order a urine pregnancy test to measure human chorionic gonadotropin (hCG) to rule out pregnancy as the first step in your evaluation of secondary amenorrhea.

31. True or false: Excessive exercise may cause amenorrhea.
True. It is not uncommon to find amenorrhea (or hypomenorrhea) in hard-training athletes. The relative energy deficiency in sports (RED-S) syndrome, previously called the female athlete triad, includes low energy availability (eating too little food to support the amount of energy being expended), amenorrhea/oligomenorrhea, and decreased bone mineral density. It results from an exercise-induced depression of GnRH, which reduces the entire hypothalamic-pituitary-gonadal axis. The nonmenstrual components are also seen in males.

32. What are other common causes of secondary amenorrhea?
Additional causes of secondary amenorrhea include:
- PCOS

- Hypothyroidism
- Anorexia nervosa
- Endocrine disorders (headaches, galactorrhea, and visual field defects may indicate a prolactin-secreting pituitary tumor)
- Primary ovarian insufficiency
- Antipsychotics medications (due to increased prolactin)
- History of chemotherapy (causes premature ovarian failure and menopause)

  Although not considered secondary amenorrhea, **menopause** should be kept in mind as a cause for cessation of menstruation in patients beginning at age 45.

33. After ruling out pregnancy, if the cause of secondary amenorrhea is not obvious from the history and physical exam, what is the next step in your evaluation?

Administer progesterone to assess the patient's estrogen status. If vaginal bleeding develops within 2 weeks of completing the progesterone challenge, the patient has sufficient estrogen. In this case, check the LH level. If it is high, consider PCOS. If it is low or normal, check the levels of prolactin and TSH. The high TSH level in hypothyroidism causes high prolactin levels. If the prolactin is high with a normal TSH level, order a magnetic resonance (MR) scan of the brain to rule out pituitary prolactinoma. If the prolactin level is normal, look for low levels of GnRH, which may be induced by drugs, stress, or exercise. In these patients, clomiphene or leuprolide can be used in an attempt to facilitate pregnancy.

34. What if the patient fails to have vaginal bleeding after the progesterone challenge test?

If the patient has no vaginal bleeding, estrogen levels are inadequate. Check the FSH level next. If it is elevated, premature ovarian failure is the problem; check for autoimmune disorders, karyotype abnormalities (e.g., Turner syndrome), and a history of chemotherapy. If the FSH level is low or normal, the problem may be a brain tumor (e.g., craniopharyngioma). Order an MR scan of the brain. Clomiphene would be ineffective in these patients.

35. True or false: Pregnancy can present as primary amenorrhea.

True. Always assess the urine hCG level in the evaluation of any type of amenorrhea.

36. At what age can primary amenorrhea be diagnosed? What is the first step in evaluation?

Primary amenorrhea is defined as the absence of menses at age 15 years in the presence of normal growth and secondary sexual characteristics (e.g., breast development, axillary and pubic hair). If no menses have occurred by age 13 years and there is a complete absence of secondary sexual characteristics such as breast development, evaluation for primary amenorrhea should begin. The first step is to rule out pregnancy.

37. In a patient older than age 13 with no secondary sexual characteristics or thelarche, what is the most likely cause of amenorrhea?

The most likely cause in this setting is a congenital problem. In a phenotypically female patient with normal breast development but no axillary or pubic hair, think of **androgen insensitivity syndrome**. In such patients, the internal female genitalia (e.g., uterus, fallopian tubes, and upper third of the vaginal canal) will be absent. Contrast this against a patient with no breast development and no axillary or pubic hair; these patients are most likely have **5-α-reductase deficiency**.

  In the presence of normal breast development and internal female genitalia, the next step is to measure the serum prolactin level to rule out pituitary adenoma. If the prolactin level is high, order an MR imaging scan of the head. If serum prolactin is normal, administer progesterone and follow the same procedure as in the evaluation of secondary amenorrhea.

38. When in doubt, what is the best way to evaluate any type of amenorrhea?

First, order a pregnancy test. If it is negative, attempt a progesterone challenge test. Further testing depends on whether the progesterone challenge induces withdrawal bleeding or not. Measuring serum levels of TSH and/or prolactin should also be performed.

39. When does menopause occur? What are the signs and symptoms?

The average age of menopause is around 51 years. Patients have irregular cycles or amenorrhea, hot flashes and mood swings, and an elevated FSH level. Amenorrhea for 1 year signals the completion of menopause. Patients also may complain of dysuria, dyspareunia, incontinence, and/or vaginal itching, burning, or soreness. Vaginal symptoms are often due to atrophic vaginitis; expect the vaginal mucosa to be thin, dry, and atrophic with increased parabasal cells on cytology. Topical estrogen improves vaginal symptoms, but other symptoms (e.g., hot flashes) require oral therapy.

40. Describe the current state of hormone replacement therapy.

Hormone replacement therapy is currently recommended short term for the management of moderate-to-severe vasomotor flushing. Long-term use for the prevention of disease (such as osteoporosis or cardiovascular disease) is no longer recommended due to increased risk of venous thromboembolism (VTE) and risk of endometrial cancer.

41. When a woman presents with a nipple discharge, what key pieces of patient history may suggest the underlying etiology?

    A history of using OCPs, hormone therapies, antipsychotic medications (which elevate prolactin), or symptoms suggestive of hypothyroidism all may cause nipple discharge. The color of the discharge and whether the discharge is unilateral or bilateral is also very important. For example, if nipple discharge is bilateral and nonbloody, it is likely galactorrhea due to a prolactinoma (check prolactin level) or endocrine disorder (check a TSH level). Alternatively, when nipple discharge is unilateral and bloody, it may represent an underlying ductal papilloma (benign) or carcinoma (malignant). Perform a core needle biopsy of any breast mass that is discovered on physical exam.

42. What are the most likely causes of a breast mass in a woman under the age of 35?

    Fibrocystic disease: bilateral, multiple, cystic lesions that are tender to the touch, especially premenstrually. This is the most common of all breast diseases. Generally, this is secondary to prior breast trauma and no workup is needed other than routine follow-up. OCPs, progesterone, or danazol may help to relieve symptoms.

    Fibroadenoma: a painless, discrete, sharply circumscribed, unilateral, rubbery, mobile mass. This is the most common benign tumor of the female breast. Patients may be observed for one or more menstrual cycles to see if it regresses spontaneously. Because tumors are estrogen dependent, estrogen-containing OCPs may stimulate growth, whereas menopause causes regression. Excision is curative but not required except for cosmetic reasons.

    Mastitis/abscess: Typically in the first few months postpartum, lactating women may develop a painful, swollen, erythematous breast(s). The nipple may be cracked or fissured. Patients with this presentation *plus a fever* have either mastitis or abscess: To distinguish these two, check for *fluctuance* of the area. If fluctuance is absent, the diagnosis is mastitis. If fluctuance is present, it is an abscess.

43. How does the management of mastitis differ from the management of a breast abscess?

    The patient with mastitis should be treated with analgesics (e.g., acetaminophen, ibuprofen) and antibiotics and instructed to continue breastfeeding with the affected breast(s) even though it is painful. Use a breast pump to empty the breast if needed to prevent further milk duct blockage and potential abscess formation. An antistaphylococcal antibiotic (e.g., dicloxacillin or cephalexin) should be given for more than mild symptoms. If there is risk for methicillin-resistant *Staphylococcus aureus* (MRSA) or if MRSA is cultured, use trimethoprim-sulfamethoxazole or clindamycin. If a fluctuant mass develops or there is no response to antibiotics within a few days, an abscess is likely present and must be drained.

44. True or false: Mammography should be done for any suspicious breast lesion in a woman under age 30.

    False. Mammography is usually not performed on women under age 30 because breast tissue is often too dense to accurately discern a mass. If you are suspicious of breast cancer, which is very rare in this age group, investigate with ultrasound imaging or proceed directly to biopsy.

45. True or false: If a patient is postmenopausal or over age 50 and develops a new breast mass, you should assume it is cancer until proven otherwise.

    True. The risk of breast cancer begins to increase sharply, and the incidence of benign disorders begins to decrease sharply, in this patient population. Most benign disorders are caused by reproductive hormones that women in this age group lack.

46. True or false: Mammography is best used as a tool to evaluate a palpable breast mass.

    False. Mammography is best used as a screening tool to detect nonpalpable breast masses (as a screening tool). A suspicious lesion found on mammography should be followed by a core needle biopsy, even if it seems benign or is nonpalpable on physical exam. Additionally, a clinically suspicious mass should be biopsied unless imaging demonstrates unequivocally benign findings (e.g., a cyst).

47. What causes pelvic relaxation or vaginal prolapse? What are the signs and symptoms?

    Pelvic relaxation is due to a weakening of pelvic supporting ligaments. Look for a history of several vaginal deliveries, a feeling of heaviness or fullness in the pelvis, urinary incontinence, backache, worsening of symptoms upon standing, and resolution of symptoms with lying down.

48. What types of pelvic relaxation are seen clinically? How are they treated?

    Cystocele: The bladder bulges into the upper anterior vaginal wall. Common symptoms include urinary urgency, frequency, and/or incontinence.

    Rectocele: The rectum bulges into the lower posterior vaginal wall. Watch for difficulty with defecation.

    Enterocele: Loops of bowel bulge into the upper posterior vaginal wall.

    Urethrocele: The urethra bulges into the lower anterior vaginal wall. Common symptoms include urinary urgency, frequency, and/or incontinence.

    Conservative treatment for all types of pelvic relaxation involves pelvic and detrusor muscle strengthening exercises and/or a pessary (artificial device to provide support). Surgery is used for refractory or severe cases or patient desire.

49. **Other than abstinence, what are the most effective forms of birth control (when used properly)?**
The most effective forms of birth control, in order of efficacy, are sterilization (e.g., tubal ligation or vasectomy), implants (etonogestrel implant) or an intrauterine device (IUD), injectable hormone depot preparations (progesterone), and birth control pills/patch or a hormonal vaginal ring.

50. **Do IUDs increase the risk of ectopic pregnancy or PID?**
An IUD does not increase a woman's risk of having an ectopic pregnancy; however, if a woman who has an IUD is found to be pregnant, it is more likely to be an ectopic pregnancy than if she didn't have the IUD.
Similarly, IUDs do not increase the risk of PID. If a woman has an IUD in place and is diagnosed with PID, do not remove the IUD unless the organism is *Actinomyces israelii.* Treat with antibiotics with the IUD in place. *Actinomyces* should be treated with penicillin when present.

51. **What is the classic cause of ambiguous genitalia on the USMLE Step 2 exam?**
Adrenogenital syndrome, also known as **congenital adrenal hyperplasia** (CAH). Ninety percent of cases are caused by **21-hydroxylase deficiency**. Patients are typically female because affected males experience precocious sexual development. Patients with 21-hydroxylase deficiency have salt wasting (low sodium), hyperkalemia, hypotension, and elevated 17-hydroxyprogesterone. If salt wasting and hypotension are *absent*, consider **17-hydroxylase deficiency**. Treat with steroids (to induce negative feedback on adrenocorticotropic hormone [ACTH] and suppress androgen production) and administer IV fluids immediately to prevent death.

52. **What should you tell the parents of a child with ambiguous genitalia?**
Tell the parents the truth: You do not know the child's gender. No patient with ambiguous genitalia should be assigned a sex until the workup is complete. A karyotype must be done.

53. **What is indicated by a "bunch of grapes" protruding from a pediatric vagina?**
Sarcoma botryoides, a malignant tumor and a type of embryonal rhabdomyosarcoma.

54. **Define precocious puberty. What causes it? How should it be treated?**
By definition, precocious puberty occurs if the onset of puberty begins in girls younger than 8 years old or boys younger than 9 years old. Premature or precocious puberty is usually idiopathic, but it may be caused by a hormone-secreting tumor (e.g., Leydig cell tumor) or central nervous system disorder (e.g., hamartoma, astrocytoma), both of which must be ruled out. Treat the underlying cause. If the condition is idiopathic, treat with a gonadotropin-releasing hormone analog to prevent premature epiphyseal closure and arrest or reverse puberty until an appropriate age.

55. **What causes vaginitis or discharge in prepubescent girls?**
Most cases are nonspecific or physiologic; however, look for a vaginal foreign body (most common cause of prepubertal vaginal bleeding), sexual abuse (especially if a sexually transmitted disease is present), or *Candida* fungal infection. A candidal infection may be a presentation of diabetes; check the serum glucose level and/or the urine for glycosuria.

56. **How do you recognize and treat an imperforate hymen?**
Imperforate hymen classically presents at menarchal age with primary amenorrhea and hematocolpos (blood in the vagina) that cannot escape, thus the hymen bulges outward. Treatment is surgical opening of the hymen.

57. **What is the usual cause of vaginal bleeding in neonates? How is it treated?**
Vaginal bleeding in neonates is usually physiologic and due to maternal estrogen withdrawal. No treatment is needed; the bleeding will resolve spontaneously.

58. **Which women are candidates for hormone replacement therapy?**
Hormone replacement therapy (i.e., estrogen with or without progesterone) is now controversial and probably best used only as a means of menopause-related symptom relief. Observation during therapy is necessary because estrogen and progesterone are not harmless. Every woman should make the decision on her own after weighing the risks and benefits.

59. **What are the known benefits of estrogen therapy?**
Known benefits of estrogen therapy include:
• Decreased osteoporosis and decreased fractures
• Reduced hot flashes and genitourinary symptoms of menopause (dryness, urgency, atrophy-induced incontinence, frequency)
• Decreased risk of colorectal cancer (according to the Women's Health Initiative, when combined estrogen and progesterone therapy is used)

60. **What are the known risks of estrogen therapy?**
Known risks of estrogen therapy include:
• Increased risk of endometrial cancer (eliminated by coadministration of progesterone)
• Small increase in risk of coronary heart disease with combined estrogen and progesterone therapy, though the risk is not increased in women who are less than 10 years postmenopausal or 50 to 59 years of age
• Increased risk of VTE

- Increased risk of breast cancer (according to the Women's Health Initiative, when combined estrogen and progesterone therapy is used; there was a slightly decreased risk of breast cancer with estrogen only, though this decrease was not statistically significant)
- Increased risk of stroke (according to the Women's Health Initiative, with either estrogen only or combined estrogen and progesterone therapy)
- Increased risk of gallbladder disease

61. What are the most common side effects of estrogen therapy?
Common side effects of estrogen therapy include:
- Endometrial bleeding
- Bloating
- Breast tenderness
- Headaches
- Nausea

62. What are the absolute contraindications to estrogen therapy?
Contraindications to estrogen therapy include:
- Unexplained vaginal bleeding
- Active liver disease
- History of thromboembolism or stroke
- Coronary artery disease
- History of endometrial or breast cancer
- Pregnancy

63. What are the relative contraindications to estrogen therapy?
Relative contraindications to estrogen therapy include:
- Seizure disorder
- Hypertension
- Uterine leiomyomas
- Familial hyperlipidemia
- Migraine headache with aura
- Thrombophlebitis
- Endometriosis
- Gallbladder disease

64. What study is often done before starting estrogen therapy?
Women classically get an endometrial biopsy, ultrasound, or dilation and curettage at the onset of treatment to rule out endometrial hyperplasia and/or cancer and an evaluation of any unexplained bleeding, even while on therapy, unless they have had a normal evaluation within the past 6 months.

65. True or false: Women without a uterus do not need to take progesterone with estrogen.
True. The main reason for giving progesterone with hormone replacement therapy is to eliminate the increased risk of endometrial cancer that accompanies unopposed estrogen therapy. If a woman has no uterus, then she has no need for progesterone.

66. What are the absolute contraindications to combined oral contraceptive pills?
Contraindications to combined OCPs include:
- Acute deep vein thrombosis (DVT)/pulmonary embolism (PE)
- History of DVT/PE, not on anticoagulant therapy
- Known thrombogenic mutations
- VTE, current or past (DVT or PE)
- History of stroke
- Ischemic heart disease
- Moderately or severely impaired cardiac function
- Vascular disease
- Complicated valvular heart disease
- Diabetes with complications (can be a relative contraindication if the complications are not severe)
- Current breast cancer
- Pregnancy
- Decompensated cirrhosis
- Liver tumors (hepatocellular adenoma or hepatoma)
- Migraine with aura at any age or migraine without aura and age greater than or equal to 35 years
- Major surgery with prolonged immobilization
- Age greater than 35 years and smoking 15 or more cigarettes per day
- Hypertension (blood pressure >160/100 mm Hg or with concomitant vascular disease)
- Complicated solid organ transplantation

67. **What are the relative contraindications to combined OCPs?**

Relative contraindications to combined OCPs include:
- Less than 21 days since delivery
- Breastfeeding sooner than 1 month postpartum
- Undiagnosed vaginal or uterine bleeding
- History of breast cancer but no recurrence in past 5 years
- History of DVT/PE with lower risk for recurrence
- Peripartum cardiomyopathy greater than or equal to 6 months
- History of breast cancer with no evidence of current disease for 5 years
- Interacting drugs (certain anticonvulsants, rifampin, ritonavir-boosted protease inhibitors)
- Gallbladder disease (unless asymptomatic or history of cholecystectomy)
- Migraine without aura, and age greater than or equal to 35 years
- Hypertension (well controlled or blood pressure 140–159/90–99 mm Hg)
- Multiple risk factors for arterial cardiovascular disease
- Acute viral hepatitis

68. **What is the relationship between OCPs and hypertension?**

OCPs are one of the most common causes of secondary hypertension. Any patient taking birth control pills who is noted to have an increased blood pressure should discontinue the pills and have her blood pressure rechecked at a later date.

69. **What do you need to know about OCPs and surgery?**

Because of the risks of thromboembolism, OCPs should be stopped 1 month before elective surgery and not restarted until 1 month after surgery.

70. **What are the side effects of OCPs?**

The side effects include glucose intolerance (check for diabetes mellitus annually in women at high risk), depression, edema (bloating), cholelithiasis, **benign liver adenomas**, melasma ("the mask of pregnancy"), nausea, vomiting, headache, hypertension, and drug interactions. Drugs such as rifampin and antiepileptics may induce metabolism of OCPs and reduce their effectiveness.

71. **What is the relationship between OCPs and breast and cervical cancer?**

OCPs have little, if any, effect on the risk of developing breast cancer. Cervical neoplasia may be increased in users of birth control pills.

72. **What is the relationship between OCPs and ovarian and endometrial cancer?**

OCPs have been shown to reduce the incidence of ovarian cancer by 50%; they also reduce the incidence of endometrial cancer.

73. **What are the other beneficial effects of OCPs?**

They decrease the incidence of menorrhagia, dysmenorrhea, benign breast disease, functional ovarian cysts, premenstrual tension, iron-deficiency anemia, ectopic pregnancy, and salpingitis.

CHAPTER 17

HEMATOLOGY

1. Define anemia.
Hemoglobin less than 12 mg/dL in women and less than 14 mg/dL in men.

2. What are the signs and symptoms of anemia?
Signs: tachycardia, pallor (especially of the sclera and mucous membranes), systolic ejection murmurs (from heightened flow), and signs of the underlying cause (e.g., jaundice and/or pigment **gallstones** [Fig. 17.1] in hemolytic anemia, positive stool guaiac with a gastrointestinal [GI] bleed)
Symptoms: fatigue, dyspnea on exertion, light-headedness, dizziness, syncope, palpitations, angina, and claudication

3. What are the important elements of the history when anemia is present?
Important points include medications, blood loss (e.g., trauma, surgery, melena, hematemesis, menorrhagia), chronic diseases (anemia of chronic disease), family history (e.g., hemophilia, thalassemia, sickle cell disease, glucose-6-phosphatase deficiency [G6PD]), and alcoholism (which may lead to iron, folate, and B_{12} deficiencies as well as GI bleeds).

4. What medications can cause anemia? How?
Many medications can cause anemia through various mechanisms. Methyldopa, penicillins, and sulfa drugs can cause red blood cell (RBC) antibodies with subsequent hemolysis; chloroquine and sulfa drugs cause hemolysis in patients with G6PD; phenytoin causes megaloblastic anemia through interference with folate metabolism; and chloramphenicol, cancer drugs, and zidovudine cause aplastic anemia and bone marrow suppression. Other drugs are also implicated, but this list should get you through the USMLE exam.

5. What test should be ordered first to help determine the cause of anemia?
The complete blood count (CBC) with RBC indices. The hemoglobin must be below normal to diagnose anemia. The mean corpuscular volume (MCV) tells you whether the anemia is microcytic (MCV <80), normocytic (MCV = 80–100), or macrocytic (MCV >100).

6. What test should be ordered next?
Peripheral blood smear. There are many "classic" findings that can help make the diagnoses:
- Sickled cells (sickle cell disease) (Fig. 17.2)
- Hypersegmented neutrophils (folate/B_{12} deficiency) (Fig. 17.3)
- Hypochromic and microcytic RBCs (iron deficiency) (Fig. 17.4)
- Basophilic stippling (lead poisoning) (Fig. 17.5)
- Heinz bodies (G6PD) (Fig. 17.6)
- "Bite cells" (classically, G6PD; other hemolytic anemias) (see Fig. 17.6)
- Howell-Jolly bodies (asplenia) (Fig. 17.7)
- Teardrop-shaped RBCs (dacrocytes seen in myelofibrosis) (Fig. 17.8)
- Schistocytes, helmet cells, and fragmented RBCs (intravascular hemolysis) (Fig. 17.9)
- Spherocytes and elliptocytes (hereditary spherocytosis and elliptocytosis) (Fig. 17.10)
- Acanthocytes and spur cells (abetalipoproteinemia) (Fig. 17.11)
- Target cells (thalassemia, liver disease) (Fig. 17.12)
- Echinocytes, including "burr" cells and acanthocytes (uremia, liver disease) (Fig. 17.13)
- Polychromasia (from **reticulocytosis**; should alert you to possibility of hemolysis) (Fig. 17.14)
- Rouleaux formation (multiple myeloma) (Fig. 17.15)
- Parasites inside RBCs (malaria, babesiosis) (Fig. 17.16)
- Iron inclusions (ringed sideroblasts) in RBCs of the bone marrow (sideroblastic anemia) (Fig. 17.17)

7. What are reticulocytes? Why is a reticulocyte count routinely ordered in an anemia workup?
Reticulocytes are immature RBCs. If their count is abnormally decreased in the setting of anemia, the marrow is not responding properly and is thus the site of the problem. A high reticulocyte count should make you think of hemolysis or blood loss as the cause (the marrow is responding properly and is not the problem).

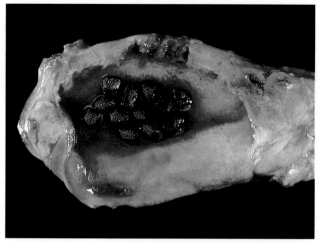

Fig. 17.1 Pigment gallstones within an otherwise unremarkable gallbladder are a marker for hemolytic anemia. (From Kumar V. *Robbins and Kotran Pathologic Basis of Disease, Professional Edition*. 8th ed. Philadelphia: Saunders; 2009 [fig. 18-53].)

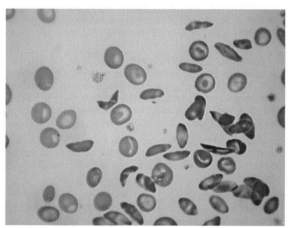

Fig. 17.2 Sickle cells show a sickle or crescent shape resulting from the polymerization of hemoglobin S. This smear also shows target cells and boat-shaped cells with a lesser degree of polymerization of hemoglobin S than in a classic sickle cell. (From Goldman L. *Goldman's Cecil Medicine*. 24th ed. Philadelphia: Saunders; 2011 [fig. 160-7].)

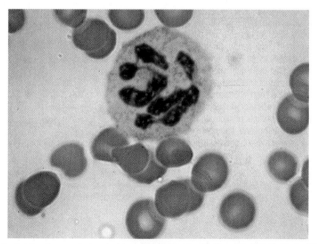

Fig. 17.3 Megaloblastic changes of macrocytosis and a hypersegmented neutrophil. (From Rakel RE. *Textbook of Family Medicine*. 8th ed. Philadelphia: Saunders; 2011 [fig. 39-4]. From the American Society of Hematology Image Bank image #2611. Copyright 1996 American Society of Hematology, used with permission.)

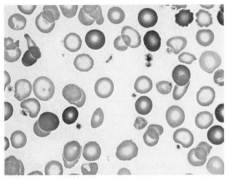

Fig. 17.4 Iron-deficiency anemia. Pale red blood cells with enlarged central pallor. (From McPherson R, Pincus M. *Henry's Clinical Diagnosis and Management by Laboratory Methods.* 21st ed. Philadelphia: Saunders; 2006 [fig. 31-2].)

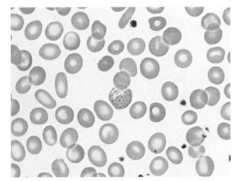

Fig. 17.5 Basophilic stippling. Irregular basophilic granules in red blood cells; often associated with lead poisoning and thalassemia. (From McPherson R, Pincus M. *Henry's Clinical Diagnosis and Management by Laboratory Methods.* 21st ed. Philadelphia: Saunders; 2006 [fig. 29-23].)

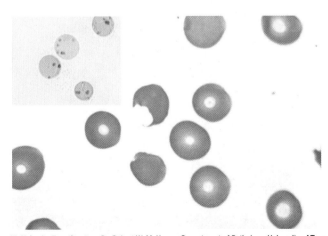

Fig. 17.6 Bite cells with Heinz bodies. (Courtesy Dr. Robert W. McKenna, Department of Pathology, University of Texas Southwestern Medical School, Dallas, TX.)

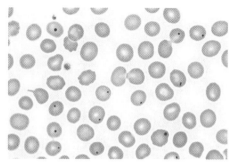

Fig. 17.7 Howell-Jolly bodies in peripheral blood erythrocytes. These nuclear remnants indicate lack of splenic filtrative function. (From Orkin SH, et al. *Nathan and Oski's Hematology of Infancy and Childhood.* 7th ed. Philadelphia: Saunders; 2009 [fig. 14-4].)

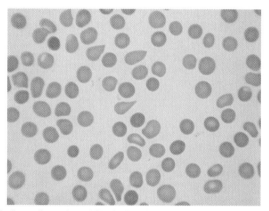

Fig. 17.8 Teardrop red blood cells, usually seen in myelofibrosis. (From Goldman L, Ausiello D. *Cecil Medicine.* 23rd ed. Philadelphia: Saunders; 2008 [fig. 161-13].)

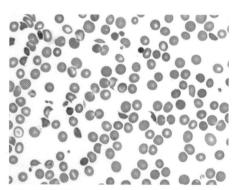

Fig. 17.9 Schistocytes and helmet cells. Red blood cell fragments seen with microangiopathic hemolytic anemia and disseminated intravascular coagulation. (From McPherson R, Pincus M. *Henry's Clinical Diagnosis and Management by Laboratory Methods.* 21st ed. Philadelphia: Saunders; 2006 [fig. 29-19].)

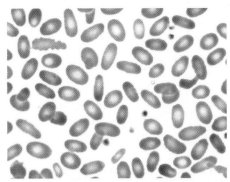

Fig. 17.10 Hereditary elliptocytosis. Blood film reveals characteristic elliptical red blood cells. (From McPherson, Pincus M. *Henry's Clinical Diagnosis and Management by Laboratory Methods.* 22nd ed. Philadelphia: Saunders; 2011 [fig. 30-16].)

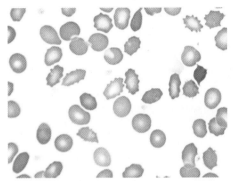

Fig. 17.11 Acanthocytes. Irregularly spiculated red blood cells, frequently seen in abetalipoproteinemia or liver disease. (From McPherson R, Pincus M. *Henry's Clinical Diagnosis and Management by Laboratory Methods.* 21st ed. Philadelphia: Saunders; 2006 [fig. 29-20].)

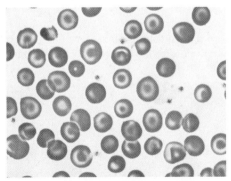

Fig. 17.12 Target cells are frequently seen in hemoglobin C disease and liver disease. (From McPherson R, Pincus M. *Henry's Clinical Diagnosis and Management by Laboratory Methods.* 21st ed. Philadelphia: Saunders; 2006 [fig. 29-18].)

8. Which test comes next?

At this point, it depends. If you have a complete history and results of the other three tests (CBC with RBC indices, peripheral smear, and reticulocyte count), most possibilities will be eliminated, and you can order a confirmatory test. If the answer is still not clear, consider a bone marrow biopsy. For the Step 2 exam, biopsy is unlikely to be necessary unless malignancy is the cause of the anemia.

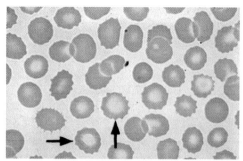

Fig. 17.13 Echinocytes, or burr cells, are the hallmark of uremia. (From Hoffman R, et al. *Hematology: Basic Principles and Practice.* 5th ed. London: Churchill Livingstone; 2008 [fig. 156-1].)

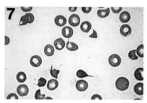

Fig. 17.14 Microangiopathic hemolytic anemia demonstrating red blood cell fragments, anisocytosis, polychromasia, and decreased platelets. (From Johns Hopkins. *The Harriet Lane Handbook.* 19th ed. Philadelphia: Elsevier; 2011 [plate 7].)

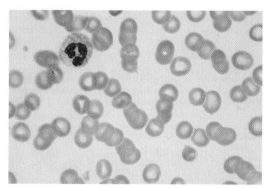

Fig. 17.15 Rouleaux formation of stacked red blood cells seen in multiple myeloma. (From Goldman L, Ausiello D. *Cecil Medicine.* 23rd ed. Philadelphia: Saunders; 2008 [fig. 161-19].)

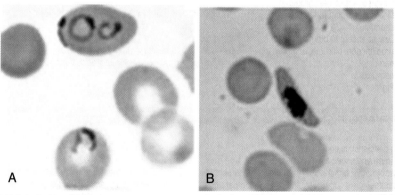

Fig. 17.16 Malaria. Peripheral blood smears showing (A) early trophozoite and (B) crescent-shaped gametozyte. (Garcia LS. Malaria. *Clin Lab Med.* 2010;30[1]:93-129.)

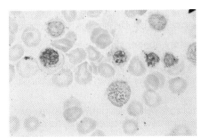

Fig. 17.17 Ringed sideroblasts seen in sideroblastic anemia. (From Goldman L, Ausiello D. *Goldman's Cecil Medicine.* 23rd ed. Philadelphia: Saunders; 2008 [fig. 163-5].)

9. What are the classic causes of microcytic, normocytic, and anemia? Which of these tends to have an inappropriately low reticulocyte count?

Microcytic	Normocytic
With normal or elevated reticulocyte count	*With normal or elevated reticulocyte count*
Thalassemia/hemoglobinopathy (e.g., sickle cell disease)	Acute blood loss Hemolysis (multiple causes) Medications (antibody-causing)
With low reticulocyte count	*With low reticulocyte count*
Lead poisoning Sideroblastic anemia Anemia of chronic disease (some cases) Iron deficiency	Cancer/dysplasia (e.g., myelophthisic anemia, acute leukemia) Anemia of chronic disease (some cases) Aplastic anemia/medications causing bone marrow suppression Endocrine failure (thyroid, pituitary) Renal failure

Macrocytic (All Types Have Low Reticulocyte Count)
Folate deficiency
Vitamin B_{12} deficiency
Medications (methotrexate, phenytoin)
Alcohol abuse (interferes with folate metabolism)
Cirrhosis, liver disease

10. What clues point to hemolysis as the cause for anemia?
    - Elevated lactate dehydrogenase (LDH)
    - Elevated bilirubin (unconjugated as well as conjugated if the liver is functioning)
    - Jaundice
    - Low or absent haptoglobin (intravascular hemolysis only)
    - Urobilinogen, bilirubin, and hemoglobin in urine (only conjugated bilirubin shows up in the urine, and hemoglobin shows up in the urine only when haptoglobin has been saturated, as in brisk intravascular hemolysis)
    - Pigmented gallstones or history of cholecystectomy (usually at a young age)

11. What is the most common cause of anemia in the United States?
    Iron-deficiency anemia.

12. Why do people get iron deficiency?
    Iron deficiency is common in women of reproductive age because of menstrual blood loss. In all patients over age 40 (men and especially postmenopausal women), it is important to rule out colon cancer as a cause of chronic, asymptomatic blood loss. Increased requirements may also lead to iron deficiency in children and pregnant or breastfeeding women. Give iron-containing formula or iron supplements to all infants except full-term infants who are exclusively breastfed. Start iron supplementation (iron-fortified cereal or daily iron supplement) at 4 to 6 months for full-term infants and at 2 months for preterm infants. Giving cow's milk before 1 year of age may lead

to anemia by causing GI bleeding, so avoidance of cow's milk in the first year is essential. Iron supplements also are commonly given during pregnancy and lactation (because of the increased demand).

13. **What are the classic laboratory abnormalities in iron-deficiency anemia? What weird cravings may occur with iron deficiency?**
Look for low iron and low ferritin levels, elevated total iron-binding capacity (TIBC; also known as transferrin), and low TIBC saturation. Rare patients may develop a craving for ice (pagophagia) or dirt/clay (**pica**).

14. **What is Plummer-Vinson syndrome?**
A triad of unknown etiology: esophageal web resulting in dysphagia; iron-deficiency anemia; and glossitis. It is associated with squamous cell carcinoma of the esophagus and pharynx.

15. **How is iron deficiency treated?**
First you must determine the cause. In a menstruating woman, a presumptive diagnosis of menstrual blood loss is often made. In patients over 40 years, be sure to test the stool for occult blood and strongly consider colonoscopy to detect colon cancer. Postmenopausal vaginal bleeding may also cause anemia and warrants screening for gynecologic cancer. Treat with iron supplements for 3 to 6 months in uncomplicated cases to replete body iron stores.

16. **What causes folate deficiency? In what patient populations is it commonly seen?**
Folate deficiency is commonly seen in alcoholics (poor intake) and pregnant women (increased need). All women of reproductive age should take folate supplements (ideally before pregnancy occurs) to prevent neural tube defects in their offspring. Rare causes of folate deficiency include poor diet (e.g., "tea and toast" diet), methotrexate, prolonged therapy with trimethoprim-sulfamethoxazole, anticonvulsant therapy (especially phenytoin), and malabsorption. Look for macrocytes and **hypersegmented neutrophils** with no neurologic signs or symptoms and low folate levels in serum or red blood cells. Treat with oral folate.

17. **What is the most common cause of vitamin B_{12} deficiency?**
Pernicious anemia. This megaloblastic anemia is caused by **antiparietal cell antibodies.** Remember the physiology of B_{12} absorption with intrinsic factor secretion by parietal cells and absorption of the B_{12}—intrinsic factor complex in the ileum. Achlorhydria (no stomach acid secretion and elevated stomach pH) and antibodies to parietal cells are generally present in pernicious anemia.

18. **What else may cause vitamin B_{12} deficiency? How is B_{12} deficiency diagnosed?**
Gastrectomy, terminal ileum resection or disease (e.g., Crohn disease), strict vegan diet, chronic pancreatitis, and the infamous *Diphyllobothrium latum* (fish tapeworm) infection. The peripheral smear looks the same as in folate deficiency (macrocytes, hypersegmented neutrophils), but patients have **neurologic deficits** (e.g., loss of sensation and position sense, paresthesias, ataxia, spasticity, hyperreflexia, positive Babinski sign, dementia). Diagnosis is clinched by a low serum B_{12} level. The presence of antiintrinsic factor antibodies is confirmatory for pernicious anemia. The Schilling test is of historical interest but is no longer commonly used in the diagnosis of B_{12} deficiency.

19. **How is vitamin B_{12} deficiency treated?**
Vitamin B_{12} supplements are given. The usual replacement is via parenteral (intramuscular) injection or high-dose oral replacement. Because of the potential for erratic absorption, oral replacement may be best utilized after levels have been normalized via the parenteral route. Supplementation may be required for life.

20. **How is thalassemia differentiated from iron deficiency?**
Both cause microcytic, hypochromic anemia, but thalassemia must be differentiated from iron deficiency because iron levels are normal in thalassemia. Iron supplementation is contraindicated in patients with thalassemia because it may cause iron overload. Look for elevations in hemoglobin A2 or hemoglobin F (beta thalassemia only); target cells, nucleated RBCs, and diffuse basophilia on peripheral smears; skull radiograph with "crew-cut" appearance; extramedullary hematopoiesis (Fig. 17.18); splenomegaly; and positive family history. Thalassemia is more common in blacks, Mediterraneans, and Asians.

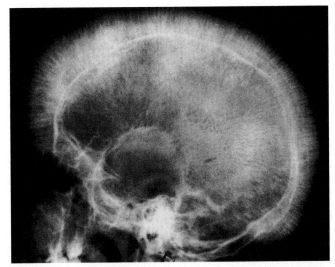

Fig. 17.18 Thalassemia. X-ray film of the skull showing new bone formation on the outer table, producing perpendicular radiations resembling a crewcut. (From Kumar V. *Robbins and Cotran Pathologic Basis of Disease, Professional Edition.* 8th ed. Philadelphia: Elsevier; 2009 [fig. 14-13]. Courtesy Dr. Jack Reynolds, Department of Radiology, University of Texas Southwestern Medical School, Dallas, TX.)

21. What diagnostic test confirms a diagnosis of thalassemia? How is it treated?
    Diagnosis is made by hemoglobin electrophoresis. There are four gene loci for the alpha chain of hemoglobin but only two for the beta chain. Patients with four affected loci produce no alpha globulin (hemoglobin Barts) and die in utero (hydrops fetalis), while patients with three affected loci (hemoglobin H) are symptomatic at birth or early childhood. Patients with beta thalassemia are not symptomatic until 6 months of age.

    No treatment is required for minor thalassemia. Patients are often asymptomatic because they are used to living with a lower level of hemoglobin. Thalassemia major is more symptomatic and severe. Treat with transfusions as needed and iron chelation therapy to prevent secondary hemochromatosis.

22. What two clues on the Step 2 exam often point to a diagnosis of sickle cell disease?
    Peripheral smear and race. Eight percent of blacks are heterozygous for sickle cell trait. Know what sickled RBCs look like. Patients usually have a high percentage of reticulocytes (8%–20%).

23. What are the clinical manifestations and complications of sickle cell disease?
    - Aplastic crises (due to parvovirus B19 infection)
    - Bone pain (due to infarcts; the classic example is avascular necrosis of the femoral head)
    - Dactylitis (also known as hand-foot syndrome, seen in children)
    - Renal papillary necrosis
    - Splenic sequestration crisis
    - Autosplenectomy (increased infections with encapsulated bugs such as *Pneumococcus, Haemophilus,* and *Neisseria* species)
    - Acute chest syndrome (mimics pneumonia)
    - Pigment cholelithiasis
    - Priapism
    - Stroke

24. How is sickle cell disease diagnosed and treated?
    Diagnosis is made by hemoglobin electrophoresis. Screening is done at birth, but symptoms usually do not appear until around 6 months of age because of the lack of adult hemoglobin production. Treat with prophylactic penicillin until at least 5 years of age and perhaps longer, beginning as soon as the diagnosis is made. Proper vaccination includes the pneumococcal, meningococcal, and *H. influenzae* type B vaccines (given to all children anyway), as well as yearly influenza vaccination. Other strategies include folate supplementation, early treatment of infections, and adequate hydration.

A sickle cell crisis involves severe pain in various sites due to RBC sickling. Treat with oxygen, lots of intravenous fluids, and analgesics (do not be afraid to use narcotics). Consider transfusions if symptoms and/or findings are severe.

25. **What findings help you in the setting of acute blood loss as a cause of anemia?**
The important point is that immediately after blood loss the hemoglobin may be normal; it takes at least 3 to 4 hours, often more, for reequilibration. Look for obvious bleeding; pale, cold skin; tachycardia (often the first sign of acute anemia); and hypotension (a late sign of hypovolemic shock, especially in younger patients with better hemodynamic reserve). Transfuse if indicated, even with a normal hemoglobin in the acute setting. Consider internal hemorrhage in the setting of trauma and abdominal aortic aneurysm in patients with a pulsatile abdominal mass. Consider evaluation with an ultrasonographic FAST (focused assessment with sonography in trauma) exam.

26. **What are the commonly tested causes of autoimmune hemolytic anemia?**
    - Systemic lupus erythematosus (or medications that cause lupuslike syndromes, such as procainamide, hydralazine, and isoniazid) and other autoimmune disorders
    - Drugs (the classic example is methyldopa, but penicillins, cephalosporins, sulfa drugs, and quinidine also have been implicated)
    - Leukemia or lymphoma
    - Infection (the classic examples are mycoplasmosis, Epstein-Barr virus, and syphilis)

27. **What lab test is often positive in patients with autoimmune anemia?**
The **Coombs test** is positive in most autoimmune anemias. You may also see spherocytes on peripheral smear because of incomplete macrophage destruction (extravascular hemolysis) of RBCs.

28. **What clues point to lead poisoning as a cause of anemia?**
Lead poisoning causes a hypochromic, microcytic anemia, almost always in a child. With acute lead poisoning, look for vomiting, ataxia, colicky abdominal pain, irritability (aggressive behavior, behavioral regression), and encephalopathy, cerebral edema, or seizures. Usually, however, poisoning is chronic and low level with minimal nonspecific symptoms. Watch for basophilic stippling on peripheral smear, elevated free erythrocyte protoporphyrin or lead level, and consider risk factors for lead exposure (a child who eats paint chips or lives in an old, run-down building).

29. **True or false: Children with risk factors should be screened for lead poisoning.**
True. Screening all asymptomatic children with a serum lead level at 1 and 2 years old regardless of risk is becoming controversial. However, in children with risk factors, screening is very important because chronic low-level exposure may lead to permanent neurologic sequelae. Screening should start at 6 months in children with risk factors, such as pica (especially paint chips and dust in old buildings that may have lead paint), residence in an old or neglected building, and/or residence near or with family members who work at a lead-smelting or battery-recycling plant. Screen and measure symptomatic exposure with serum lead levels (normal value: <10 µg/dL).

30. **How is lead poisoning treated?**
Treat initially with decreased exposure (best strategy) as well as lead chelation therapy, if needed. Use succimer in children and dimercaprol in adults; in severe cases, use dimercaprol plus ethylenediamine tetraacetic acid (EDTA) for children or adults.

31. **How can sideroblastic anemia be recognized on the Step 2 exam? Should the presence of sideroblastic anemia raise concern about other conditions?**
The typical description is a microcytic, hypochromic anemia with increased or normal iron, ferritin, and total iron-binding capacity (transferrin). This description should immediately steer you away from iron deficiency. Look for polychromatophilic stippling and the classic "ringed sideroblast" in the bone marrow (know what it looks like). Sideroblastic anemia may be related to myelodysplasia or future blood dyscrasia. Although you will probably not be asked about management, treatment is supportive. In rare cases, the anemia responds to **pyridoxine**. Do not give iron.

32. **How do you recognize anemia of chronic disease?**
First, look for the presence of a disease that causes chronic inflammation (e.g., rheumatoid arthritis, systemic lupus erythematosus, cancer, tuberculosis). The anemia is either normocytic or microcytic. Serum iron is low, but so is total iron-binding capacity. Thus the percent saturation may be near normal. Serum ferritin is elevated (because ferritin is an acute-phase reactant, the level should be increased). Treat the underlying disorder to correct the anemia. Do not give iron.

33. **Describe the hallmarks of spherocytosis.**
This normochromic, normocytic anemia is associated with spherocytes on peripheral smear, positive family history (autosomal dominant), splenomegaly, positive osmotic fragility test, and an increased **mean corpuscular hemoglobin concentration** (the only occasion on which this RBC index is useful for the Step 2 exam). Treatment often involves splenectomy. Spherocytes may also be seen in extravascular hemolysis, but the osmotic fragility test is normal.

34. **Why do chronic renal disease patients develop anemia? How do you treat it?**
All patients with chronic renal failure develop a normocytic, normochromic anemia with decreased reticulocyte count due to decreased erythropoietin production. If necessary, give erythropoietin to correct the anemia.

35. **What clues point to a diagnosis of aplastic anemia?**
Although aplastic anemia may be idiopathic, on the Step 2 exam watch for chemotherapy, radiation, malignancy affecting the bone marrow (especially leukemias), benzene, and implicated medications (e.g., chloramphenicol, carbamazepine, sulfa drugs, zidovudine, gold). Decreased white blood cells (WBCs) and platelets accompany the anemia. Treat first by stopping any possible causative medication; then try antithymocyte globulin, colony-stimulating factors (such as erythropoietin, sargramostim, filgrastim, pegfilgrastim), or bone marrow transplant.

36. **Define myelophthisic anemia. What clues on the peripheral smear suggest its presence?**
Myelophthisic anemia is due to a space-occupying lesion in the bone marrow. The common causes are malignant invasion that destroys bone marrow (most common) and myelodysplasia or myelofibrosis. On the peripheral smear, look for marked anisocytosis (different size), poikilocytosis (different shape), nucleated RBCs, giant and/or bizarre-looking platelets, and **teardrop-shaped** RBCs (dactocytes). A bone marrow biopsy may reveal no cells ("dry tap" if the marrow is fibrotic) or malignant-looking cells.

37. **How do you recognize glucose-6-phosphate dehydrogenase deficiency on the USMLE?**
This genetic disorder is X-linked recessive, affecting males. It is most common in blacks and Mediterraneans. Look for sudden hemolysis or anemia after exposure to fava beans or certain drugs (antimalarials, salicylates, sulfa drugs) or after infection. You may see **Heinz bodies** and "bite cells" on peripheral smear. The diagnosis is made with a RBC enzyme assay, which should not be done immediately after hemolysis because of the potential for a false-negative result (all of the older RBCs already have been destroyed, and the younger RBCs are not affected in most patients). Treat with avoidance of precipitating foods and medications; discontinue the triggering medication first.

38. **Name some other causes of anemia.**
   - Endocrine failure (especially pituitary and thyroid; look for endocrine symptoms)
   - Mechanical heart valves (hemolyzed RBCs)
   - Disseminated intravascular coagulation (DIC), thrombotic thrombocytopenic purpura, and hemolytic uremic syndrome (look for schistocytes and RBC fragments on smear and other appropriate findings)
   - Other hemoglobinopathies (the hemoglobin C and E varieties are fairly common)
   - Paroxysmal nocturnal or cold hemoglobinuria
   - *Clostridium perfringens* infection, malaria, and babesiosis (causes intravascular hemolysis and fever)
   - Hypersplenism (associated with splenomegaly and often with low platelets and WBCs)

39. **When is transfusion indicated for anemia (at what hemoglobin level)?**
Always transfuse on clinical grounds; observe the symptoms. In other words, treat the patient, not the lab value. There is no such thing as a "trigger value" for transfusion. Having said this, hemoglobin level less than 7 g/dL is typically an indication for transfusion.

40. **What are the indications for the use of various blood products?**
Whole blood: used only for rapid, massive blood loss or exchange transfusions (poisoning, thrombotic thrombocytopenic purpura).
Packed RBCs: used for routine transfusions.
Washed RBCs: free of traces of plasma, WBCs, and platelets; good for IgA deficiency as well as allergic or previously sensitized patients.
Platelets: given for symptomatic thrombocytopenia (usually <10,000/μL).
Granulocytes: used on rare occasions for neutropenia.
Fresh frozen plasma (FFP): contains all clotting factors; used for bleeding diathesis when you cannot wait for vitamin K to take effect (e.g., DIC, severe warfarin poisoning) or when vitamin K will not work (liver failure).
Cryoprecipitate: contains fibrinogen and factor VIII; used in hemophilia, von Willebrand disease, and DIC.

41. **What blood type can be given in an emergency to avoid a transfusion reaction?**
Type O negative blood can be used to avoid a reaction when you cannot wait for blood typing or when the blood bank does not have the patient's blood type.

42. **Describe the signs and symptoms of a blood transfusion reaction.**
Look for **febrile reaction** (e.g., chills, fever, headache, back pain) from antibodies to WBCs; **hemolytic reaction** (e.g., anxiety or discomfort, dyspnea, chest pain, shock, jaundice) from antibodies to RBCs; or **allergic reaction** (e.g., urticaria, edema, dizziness, dyspnea, wheezing, and anaphylaxis) to an unknown component in donor serum. Oliguria may be an associated finding.

43. **What should you do if you suspect a transfusion reaction?**
The first step is to stop the transfusion. If oliguria is present, treat with intravenous fluids and diuresis (mannitol or furosemide).

44. **What are the other risks of transfusion?**

    There is a small but real risk of infection (usually viral infections such as hepatitis B and C, human immunodeficiency virus, and cytomegalovirus), development of noncardiogenic pulmonary edema (transfusion-associated circulatory overload or transfusion-related acute lung injury), and hyperkalemia (from hemolysis). With large transfusions (>5 units of packed RBCs), bleeding diathesis may result from dilutional thrombocytopenia and citrate (a blood preservative and calcium chelator that prevents clotting). Look for oozing from puncture or IV sites. With massive transfusion, there is a possibility of developing hypocalcemia due to citrate preservative binding to calcium.

45. **What are the most common causes of disseminated intravascular coagulation?**

    The most common cause is pregnancy and obstetric complications (roughly 50% of cases), followed by malignancy (33%), sepsis, and trauma (especially head trauma, prostate surgery, and snake bites).

46. **How do you recognize and treat DIC in a classic at-risk patient?**

    DIC usually manifests with bleeding diathesis but may have thrombotic tendencies. Look for the classic oozing or bleeding from puncture and IV sites; prolonged prothrombin time (PT), partial thromboplastin time (PTT), and bleeding time (BT). DIC is the only disorder on the Step 2 exam that prolongs all three tests. Other clues include positive D-dimer, increased fibrin degradation products, thrombocytopenia, decreased fibrin, and decreased clotting factors (including factor VIII).

    Treat the underlying cause (e.g., evacuate the uterus, give antibiotics). You may need to give transfusions with fresh frozen plasma or, in rare cases, heparin (only if thrombosis occurs).

47. **With what conditions is eosinophilia associated?**
    - Allergic or atopic diseases (allergic rhinitis, asthma, allergic bronchopulmonary aspergillosis, eczema, urticaria, atopic dermatitis, milk-protein allergy, drug reactions)
    - Parasitic infections
    - Fungal infections
    - HIV infection
    - Malignancies (lymphoma, leukemia, lung cancer, gastric cancer, pancreatic cancer, colon cancer, ovarian cancer)
    - Connective tissue/autoimmune diseases (Churg-Strauss vasculitis, rheumatoid arthritis, lupus, scleroderma, eosinophilic fasciitis, Dressler syndrome, inflammatory bowel disease)
    - Granulomatous disorders (sarcoidosis)
    - Skin disorders (psoriasis, pemphigus)
    - Immune disorders (Wiskott-Aldrich syndrome, hyper-IgE syndrome, IgA deficiency, thymoma)
    - Adrenal insufficiency
    - Pulmonary eosinophilia (Löffler syndrome)
    - Cirrhosis
    - Atheroembolic disease
    - Familial eosinophilia
    - Eosinophilia-myalgia syndrome (from using L-tryptophan)

48. **With what conditions is basophilia associated?**

    Allergies or neoplasm/blood dyscrasia.

49. **True or false: The lupus anticoagulant causes a clotting tendency.**

    True. Although the lupus anticoagulant may cause a prolonged PTT, the patient has a tendency toward thrombosis. Look for associated lupus symptoms, positive results on the Venereal Disease Research Laboratory (VDRL) or rapid plasma reagin (RPR) tests for syphilis, or a history of recurrent miscarriages to help you recognize this condition.

50. **What genetic and acquired causes of an increased tendency toward clot forming may appear on the Step 2 exam?**

    The list keeps growing. Watch for factor V Leiden mutation (or activated protein C resistance), prothrombin G20210A mutation, hyperhomocysteinemia, elevated factor VIII level, deficiencies in protein C, protein S, or antithrombin III as genetic causes of an increased tendency toward thrombosis. Acquired causes include antiphospholipid syndrome (lupus anticoagulant and anticardiolipin antibody), hyperhomocysteinemia, pregnancy, cancer, and estrogen-containing medications. Note that hyperhomocysteinemia can be genetic or acquired. All are treated with anticoagulant therapy to prevent deep venous thrombosis and pulmonary embolus. Suspect these conditions if a patient develops recurrent clots or develops a clot in the absence of risk factors for clot development. Women desiring contraception should not use oral estrogen-containing contraceptives, which increase thrombotic risk; favor nonhormonal methods such as an intrauterine device.

51. **Which clotting tests measure which portions of the coagulation cascade? Which medications affect these tests?**

    Prothrombin time measures the function of the extrinsic clotting pathway (prolonged by warfarin), activated partial thromboplastin time measures the function of the intrinsic clotting pathway (prolonged by heparin), and bleeding time measures platelet function (prolonged by aspirin).

52. How do specific diseases affect clotting tests? What are the main differential points?

Disease	PT	PTT	BT	Platelet Count	RBC Count	Other
von Willebrand disease	Normal	High	High	Normal	Normal	Autosomal dominant (look for family history)
Hemophilia A/B	Normal	High	Normal	Normal	Normal	X-linked recessive, A = low factor VII, B = low factor IX
Hemophilia C	Normal	High	Normal	Normal	Normal	Autosomal recessive, low factor XI
DIC	High	High	High	Low	Normal/ low	Appropriate history, low level of factor VIII
Liver failure	High	High	Normal	Normal/ low	Normal/ low	Jaundice, normal factor 8 level; do not give vitamin K (ineffective); use FFP
Heparin	Normal	High	Normal	Normal/ low	Normal	Watch for thrombocytopenia and thrombosis
Warfarin	High	Normal	Normal	Normal	Normal	Vitamin K antagonist (factors II, VII, IX, and X)
ITP	Normal	Normal	High	Low	Normal	Watch for preceding URI
TTP	Normal	Normal	High	Low	Low	Hemolysis (smear), CNS symptoms (hallucinations, altered mental status, headache, stroke); treat with plasmapheresis; do not give platelets!
Scurvy	Normal	Normal	Normal	Normal	Normal	Fingernail and gum hemorrhages, bone hemorrhages; caused by vitamin C deficiency

BT, Bleeding time; *CNS,* central nervous system; *DIC,* disseminated intravascular coagulation; *FFP,* fresh frozen plasma; *ITP,* idiopathic thrombocytopenic purpura; *PT,* prothrombin time; *PTT,* partial thromboplastin time; *RBC,* red blood cell; *TTP,* thrombotic thrombocytopenic purpura; *URI,* upper respiratory infection.

53. **What are the common causes of thrombocytopenia? What kinds of bleeding problems are caused by low platelet counts?**
Common causes of thrombocytopenia include purpura (idiopathic or thrombotic), hemolytic uremic syndrome, DIC, HIV, splenic sequestration, heparin (including heparin-induced thrombocytopenia; treat by first stopping heparin), other medications (especially quinidine and sulfa drugs), autoimmune disease, and alcohol. Bleeding from thrombocytopenia is in the form of petechiae, nosebleeds, and easy bruising.

54. **What causes petechiae or "platelet-type" bleeding in the setting of normal platelets?**
Vitamin C deficiency (scurvy) causes bleeding similar to that seen with low platelets (splinter and gum hemorrhages, petechiae); perifollicular and subperiosteal hemorrhages are unique to scurvy. Patients have a poor dietary history (the classic example is hot dogs and soda or tea and toast), myalgias and arthralgias, and capillary fragility (bleeding is due to collagen problems in the vessels). Treat with oral vitamin C.
    Other causes include uremia (results in platelet dysfunction), inherited connective tissue disorders (Ehlers-Danlos syndrome, Marfan syndrome), and chronic corticosteroid use (causes capillary fragility).

CHAPTER 18

HYPERTENSION

1. Define hypertension

   "Hypertension" was redefined in the updated American College of Cardiology/American Heart Association (ACC/AHA) guidelines, published in 2017. There are now four blood pressure categories for adults, based on systolic blood pressure (SBP) and diastolic blood pressure (DBP):

   - **Normal**: SBP <120 mm Hg **and** DBP <80 mm Hg
   - **Elevated**: SBP between 120 and 129 mm Hg **and** DBP <80 mm Hg
   - **Hypertension stage 1**: SBP between 130 and 139 mm Hg **or** DBP between 80 and 89 mm Hg
   - **Hypertension stage 2**: SBP ≥140 mm Hg **or** DBP ≥90 mm Hg
        Note that patients with SBP and DBP in two separate categories are considered to be in the higher of the two categories.

2. What is the "two-measurement" rule in the diagnosis of hypertension?

   Blood pressure should be measured on two separate office visits before the diagnosis of hypertension can be made. However, if asked, recommend nonpharmacologic measures after the first abnormal measurement.

3. What causes hypertension?

   Roughly 90% to 95% of cases are idiopathic, multifactorial, or essential (primary) hypertension. Only about 5% to 10% of hypertension is secondary to a known or identifiable medical condition.

4. How often should you screen for hypertension?

   According to the 2017 ACC/AHA guidelines, adults with no prior history of hypertension should be screened on an annual basis. It is recommended that patients with risk factors such as obesity (e.g., body mass index [BMI] ≥30) be screened every 6 months.

5. What is the target blood pressure for patients with hypertension?

   A BP *below* 130/80 mm Hg is the target for all hypertensive adults, according to the 2017 ACC/AHA guidelines. This includes patients with comorbidities such as atherosclerotic or cardiovascular disease, diabetes mellitus, chronic kidney disease, heart failure, and peripheral artery disease.

6. What are the conservative (i.e., nonpharmacologic) treatments for hypertension? When should you recommend these interventions?

   A healthy diet with regular exercise is the mainstay of nonpharmacologic therapy. Dietary recommendations include reduced sodium intake (e.g., <1500 mg/day), enhanced potassium intake (3500–5000 mg/day), moderate alcohol intake (men ≤2 drinks/day; women ≤1 drink/day), and adoption of the DASH diet (little-known fact: DASH is an acronym for Dietary Approaches to Stop Hypertension). Regular exercise should include 90 to 150 minutes per week of aerobic or dynamic resistance activity, aiming to lose weight until the patient achieves a BMI of 27 or below. This is the first-line treatment for patients in the "elevated" category, but should also be recommended to patients with hypertension stages 1 and 2 even if planning to begin pharmacotherapy.

7. What are the primary pharmacologic treatments for hypertension?

   The 2017 ACC/AHA guidelines split pharmacotherapies into two categories: **primary** and **secondary** agents. Primary agents include thiazide diuretics, angiotensin-converting enzyme inhibitors (ACEIs), angiotensin receptor blockers (ARBs), or calcium channel blockers (CCBs; both dihydropyridine and nondihydropyridine).

8. What are the secondary pharmacologic treatments for hypertension?

   Secondary agents include loop diuretics, potassium-sparing diuretics, aldosterone antagonist diuretics, direct renin inhibitors, beta-blockers, alpha-blockers, and direct vasodilators.

9. In patients with hypertension stage 1, how do you decide when to treat with pharmacotherapy versus nonpharmacologic intervention alone?

   Pharmacotherapy should be initiated in patients with hypertension stage 1 who also have one of the following comorbidities: diabetes mellitus, chronic kidney disease, or history of atherosclerotic cardiovascular disease such as a prior myocardial infarction (MI), acute coronary syndrome (ACS), peripheral artery disease (PAD), transient ischemic attack (TIA), stroke, prior revascularization procedure, stable angina, or serum low-density lipoprotein (LDL) greater than 190 mg/dL. These patients should be reevaluated in 1 month to assess response to pharmacotherapy. Patients with hypertension stage 1 without these comorbidities should begin with nonpharmacologic therapy alone and be reevaluated in 3 to 6 months.

10. Which thiazide diuretic is preferred for first-line pharmacotherapy? Why?
Chlorthalidone is preferred due to its prolonged half-life and evidence of superior reduction in left ventricular hypertrophy compared to other agents.

11. How do thiazide diuretics affect serum levels of sodium, potassium, calcium, and uric acid?
Thiazide diuretics will lower the serum levels of sodium and potassium and will raise the serum levels of calcium and uric acid. Monitor your patients for clinical signs of hyponatremia, hypokalemia, and hyperuricemia when starting a thiazide. Thiazide-related hypokalemia may be managed by adding a potassium-sparing diuretic (e.g., amiloride, triamterene).

12. In which two clinical scenarios should you be cautious about administering a thiazide diuretic?
Be cautious when administering a thiazide in patients with a history of gout or who are currently taking lithium for a mood disorder. Thiazides may induce a hyperuricemic gouty attack or lithium toxicity due to reduced renal excretion.

13. Which diuretic medications are preferred over thiazides to treat hypertension in patients with heart failure or chronic kidney disease?
Loop diuretics (e.g., furosemide, bumetanide, torsemide). Besides these two clinical scenarios, loop diuretics are considered secondary antihypertensive agents.

14. Which primary agents may precipitate acute renal failure in hypertensive patients with bilateral renal artery stenosis? Why?
ACEIs, due to their vasodilatory effect on the efferent glomerular arterioles that causes further reduction in the glomerular filtration rate (GFR).

15. Which hypertensive medications should not be combined with ACEIs? Why?
ARBs (sartans) and direct renin inhibitors (aliskiren), due to similar mechanisms of action.

16. What is the most significant electrolyte change to watch for in patients starting an ACEI?
Hyperkalemia, which may also be caused by ARBs or aliskiren.

17. Which life-threatening condition must you watch for when starting an ACEI? If this occurs, how is it managed?
Watch for life-threatening angioedema when starting a patient on an ACEI. Patients experiencing angioedema should immediately discontinue the ACEI, allow 6 weeks to pass, then begin an ARB.

18. In which clinical situations are ACEIs the preferred antihypertensive medication?
ACEIs are preferred to control hypertension in patients with stable heart failure, history of MI, proteinuric chronic kidney disease, or albuminuric diabetes mellitus. ACEIs are the only antihypertensive medication proven to reduce mortality associated with congestive heart failure as well as reduce the progression to nephropathy and neuropathy in diabetic patients.

19. Name two dihydropyridine and two nondihydropyridine CCBs used to treat hypertension
Two major dihydropyridine CCBs used to treat hypertension are amlodipine and nifedipine. Two major nondihydropyridine CCBs are verapamil and diltiazem.

20. In which patient population could you consider CCBs as first-line hypertensive monotherapy?
In the general black population, including those with diabetes, initial antihypertensive monotherapy should include either a thiazide diuretic or CCB.

21. In which clinical situation should antihypertensive CCBs be avoided? Why?
Heart failure with reduced ejection fraction (HFrEF), as CCBs may reduce cardiac output by decreasing cardiac contractility and heart rate, thereby exacerbating the existing heart failure. Watch out for clinical signs of heart failure such as pedal edema in patients taking CCBs, especially dihydropyridines (e.g., amlodipine, nifedipine).

22. Which antihypertensive agents may also improve the effects of Raynaud syndrome?
Dihydropyridine CCBs (e.g., amlodipine).

23. Coadministration of which antihypertensive agent should be avoided in patients taking nondihydropyridine CCBs? Why?
Beta-blockers, due to the increased risk of bradycardia or heart block.

24. Which antihypertensive medications should be considered in patients with comorbid atrial fibrillation or atrial flutter?
Nondihydropyridine CCBs **or** beta-blockers; although remember not to give these medications together.

25. True or False: Beta-blockers may be used as monotherapy in hypertensive patients with no additional medical conditions

   False. Beta-blockers have proven to be either ineffective or inferior to primary antihypertensive agents when used as monotherapy in patients with no additional medical conditions.

26. In which clinical situations might you consider a beta-blocker as first-line antihypertensive pharmacotherapy?

   Beta-blockers may be considered first-line antihypertensive pharmacotherapy in patients with atrial fibrillation or flutter, hyperthyroidism, migraines, and essential tremor. Beta-blockers may also be used as first-line treatment in patients with heart failure or with history of ischemic heart disease, although ACEIs are also considered first line in these conditions. On your exam, you are unlikely to be asked to choose between an ACEI and a beta-blocker.

27. Which antihypertensive medications may exacerbate preexisting asthma or COPD? Why?

   Noncardioselective beta-blockers (e.g., propranolol), due to the bronchoconstrictive effects of blocking beta$_2$-receptors in smooth muscle along the airway.

28. Which antihypertensive medication is associated with gynecomastia and the risk of impotence?

   Spironolactone, an aldosterone antagonist diuretic.

29. Which antihypertensive medications are contraindicated during pregnancy?

   ACEIs, ARBs, and aliskiren are contraindicated during pregnancy.

30. Which medications are recommended for women of reproductive age and pregnant women with hypertension?

   Labetalol, hydralazine, and alpha-methyldopa are safe during pregnancy. If preeclampsia is present (e.g., new-onset hypertension with frequent headaches, vision problems, or end-organ damage), remember that magnesium sulfate can be used to lower the mother's BP.

31. Which medical condition is a contraindication for the use of methyldopa?

   Liver disease.

32. Which antihypertensive medication is associated with drug-induced lupuslike syndrome?

   Hydralazine, a direct vasodilator.

33. How is hypertension managed in patients experiencing an acute ischemic stroke?

   First, determine if the patient is a candidate for intravenous (IV) thrombolytic therapy (e.g., <4.5 hours have passed since the patient's last-known well time). If so, the patient's BP must be lowered to *below* 185/110 mm Hg before the thrombolytic may be administered, **and** the patient's BP must then be maintained below 180/105 for the next 24 hours. If the patient is *not* a candidate for IV thrombolytic therapy but their BP is *above* 220/110, reduce BP by 15% over the next 24-hour period. If the patient is not a candidate for IV thrombolytics and their BP is *below* 220/110, managing their hypertension is not your next step. Continue the workup for acute ischemic stroke and consider mechanical thrombectomy if indicated.

34. Define hypertensive urgency. How is it distinguished from hypertensive emergency?

   Hypertensive urgency and hypertensive emergency both present with blood pressure greater than 180/120 mm Hg. The key difference is that hypertensive **emergency** also includes evidence of end-organ damage, while hypertensive **urgency** does not. Examples of the end-organ damage that may be seen in hypertensive emergencies include acute renal failure, acute ischemic stroke, intracerebral hemorrhage, dissecting aortic aneurysm, acute left ventricular failure (presenting with pulmonary edema), unstable angina, acute myocardial infarction, or encephalopathy. When considering encephalopathy, watch for headaches, confusion, retinal hemorrhages, papilledema, mental status changes, vomiting, blurry vision, dizziness, and/or seizures.

35. How does the management of hypertensive urgency differ from the management of hypertensive emergency?

   The principal differences in management are whether to initiate oral vs parenteral antihypertensive medication and whether to hospitalize the patient or not. A patient with hypertensive urgency may be started on an oral antihypertensive agent (or have the current pharmacotherapy intensified) and discharged home to follow up with the primary care physician. In hypertensive emergency, however, every minute counts and the patient's BP has to be reduced *now* or risk further and potentially irreversible end-organ damage. Admit this patient to the intensive care unit (ICU), begin parenteral antihypertensive therapy, and monitor end-organ damage. Despite the need for immediate intervention, **be careful not to reduce BP by more than 25% in the first hour**. There are three exceptions to this rule, discussed next.

36. In which three clinical conditions should systolic blood pressure during hypertensive emergency be reduced to below 140 mm Hg within the first hour?
According to the 2017 ACC/AHA guidelines, these three conditions are pheochromocytoma crisis, aortic dissection, and eclampsia/severe preeclampsia.

37. Which parenteral medications are most commonly used during hypertensive emergencies?
Dihydropyridine CCBs (e.g., nicardipine), nitric-oxide vasodilators (e.g., sodium nitroprusside or nitroglycerin), and beta-blockers (e.g., labetalol or esmolol) are the most common parenteral medications used to manage a hypertensive crisis. IV phentolamine may also be used to rapidly lower BP during a pheochromocytoma crisis.

38. What are the most common causes of secondary hypertension?
In younger adults, a common cause of secondary hypertension is excessive alcohol intake. In younger women specifically, birth control pills may be the cause of their apparent hypertension. Renovascular disease (classically seen in young women with fibromuscular dysplasia) may cause secondary hypertension and can be identified by auscultating an abdominal bruit. Obstructive sleep apnea and primary aldosteronism are also common causes of secondary hypertension.

39. List the less common (but commonly tested) causes of secondary hypertension
Pheochromocytoma. Look for paroxysmal spikes in blood pressure associated with acute diaphoresis, headache, flushing, and confusion. As a screening test, order a 24-hour urine collection to assess catecholamine products (metanephrines, vanillylmandelic acid, homovanillic acid). The definitive treatment for pheochromocytoma requires surgical intervention.
Renal artery stenosis (RAS). Unlike young patients with fibromuscular dysplasia, elderly patients typically have RAS due to atherosclerosis. A renal artery bruit is classically present (although not sensitive); magnetic resonance imaging (MRI) or conventional angiography makes the definitive diagnosis. Remember that giving ACEIs to patients with bilateral RAS may precipitate acute renal failure. RAS is definitively treated with angioplasty or stenting.
Polycystic kidney disease (PCKD). Look for a palpable flank mass, positive family history (autosomal dominant pattern of inheritance), and elevations in serum creatinine and blood urea nitrogen when suspecting PCKD.
Cushing syndrome. Look for classic stigmata of Cushing syndrome on physical exam (e.g., central obesity, moon facies, striae, proximal muscle weakness, buffalo hump). Order a 24-urine collection to assess free cortisol or a dexamethasone suppression test. Treat with surgical resection of the tumor.
Conn syndrome. The cause is an aldosterone-secreting adrenal neoplasm. Look for high aldosterone levels despite low renin levels, hypernatremia, hypokalemia, metabolic alkalosis, and/or an adrenal mass seen on abdominal computed tomography (CT). The screening test of choice is the plasma aldosterone to plasma renin activity ratio; a ratio of greater than 30 is indicative of primary hyperaldosteronism. Definitive treatment is surgical resection of the tumor.
Coarctation of the aorta. Look for hypertension *in the upper extremities only*, with unequal pulses, radiofemoral delay, and rib notching on chest radiograph. In a female patient, it may be associated with Turner syndrome. MRI or angiography makes a definitive diagnosis. Treat with surgical repair of the coarctation.
Renal failure from any cause. In children, think poststreptococcal glomerulonephritis or hemolytic uremic syndrome.

40. What is the clinical value of lowering blood pressure?
Lowering BP decreases the risk of stroke, heart disease, MI, atherosclerosis, renal failure, and dissecting aortic aneurysm. Hypertension is the number-one modifiable risk factor for stroke.

41. What is the most common cause of death among patients with untreated hypertension?
The same as for the general population—coronary artery disease.

42. Which tests should be ordered for every patient with a diagnosis of hypertension? Why?
1. **Electrocardiogram:** to assess for cardiac arrhythmias or structural changes (e.g., left ventricular hypertrophy).
2. **Chemistry 7 panel** (i.e., basic metabolic panel): investigate for possible signs of secondary hypertension (e.g., electrolyte disturbances in Conn syndrome) and evaluate for diabetes.
3. **Urinalysis:** investigate for possible signs of secondary hypertension (e.g., red blood cell casts in poststreptococcal glomerulonephritis) and assess for kidney damage (proteinuria).
4. **Hemoglobin and hematocrit:** to evaluate for anemia or polycythemia.
5. **Lipid panel:** to evaluate for dyslipidemia, which may suggest an underlying atherosclerotic disease.

CHAPTER 19

IMMUNOLOGY

1. List the four classic types of hypersensitivity reactions.
   - Anaphylactic (type I)
   - Cytotoxic (type II)
   - Immune complex mediated (type III)
   - Cell mediated/delayed (type IV)

2. What causes type I hypersensitivity? Give the classic clinical examples.
   Type I (immediate) hypersensitivity is due to preformed immunoglobulin E (IgE) antibodies that cause release of vasoactive amines (e.g., histamine, leukotrienes) from mast cells and basophils. Examples are anaphylaxis, angioedema, atopy, allergic rhinitis, urticaria, and some forms of asthma. Anaphylaxis may be due to bee stings, food allergy (especially peanuts and shellfish), medications (especially penicillins and sulfa drugs), or latex allergy.

3. Describe the clinical findings with chronic type I hypersensitivity.
   Look for eosinophilia, elevated IgE levels, positive family history, and seasonal exacerbations. Patients may also have allergic "shiners" (bilateral infraorbital edema) and a transverse nasal crease ("allergic salute sign") due to frequent nose rubbing. Pale, bluish, edematous nasal turbinates with many eosinophils in clear, watery nasal secretions are also classic.

4. How do you recognize and treat true anaphylaxis?
   Look for the classic triggers mentioned earlier just before the patient becomes tachycardic, hypotensive, and flushed and develops itching or hives (urticaria), facial swelling (angioedema), and difficulty breathing. Symptoms tend to develop rapidly and dramatically. Nausea, vomiting, and abdominal pain are also concerning for anaphylaxis, since similar receptors are present in the gut wall.
   Treat immediately by securing the airway (laryngeal edema may prevent intubation, in which case do a cricothyroidotomy, if needed). Give intramuscular epinephrine, H1 and H2 receptor blockers, and corticosteroids. If symptoms continue or hypotension develops, consider pressor support and intravenous epinephrine.

5. What usually causes hereditary angioedema?
   A deficiency of **C1 esterase inhibitor** (complement) is the usual cause of hereditary angioedema. Patients have diffuse swelling of the lips, eyelids, and possibly the airway, unrelated to allergen exposure. The disease is autosomal dominant; look for a positive family history. C4 complement levels are low. Some benefit has been shown with administration of fresh frozen plasma to replace C1 esterase. Androgens are used for long-term treatment because they increase liver production of C1 esterase inhibitor.

6. What type of testing can identify an allergen if it is not obvious?
   Skin or patch testing (Fig. 19.1).

7. What causes type II hypersensitivity? List some classic clinical examples.
   Type II (cytotoxic) hypersensitivity is due to preformed IgG and IgM antibodies that react with the antigen and cause secondary inflammation. Examples include the following:
   - Autoimmune hemolytic anemia (classically caused by methyldopa, penicillins, or sulfa drugs) or other cytopenias caused by antibodies (e.g., idiopathic thrombocytopenic purpura)
   - Transfusion reactions
   - Erythroblastosis fetalis (Rh incompatibility)
   - Goodpasture syndrome (identified by linear immunofluorescence on kidney biopsy)
   - Myasthenia gravis
   - Graves disease
   - Pernicious anemia
   - Pemphigus vulgaris
   - Hyperacute transplant rejection (as soon as the anastomosis is made at transplant surgery, the transplanted organ deteriorates in front of the surgeon's eyes)

8. What lab test is usually positive with a type II hypersensitivity that causes anemia?
   Coombs test (usually the direct Coombs test).

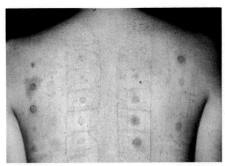

Fig. 19.1 Patch testing. A battery of common and suspected allergens is applied to the back with a patch for 48 hours and then removed. The skin is then examined at 96 hours. Irritant reactions disappear, allergic ones do not. This patient has many positive reactions of varying intensity. (From Habif TP. *Clinical Dermatology.* 5th ed. Philadelphia: Mosby; 2009 [fig. 4-30].)

9. **What causes type III hypersensitivity? List some classic clinical examples.**
   Type III (immune complex mediated) hypersensitivity is due to antigen-antibody complexes that deposit in vessels and cause an inflammatory response. Examples include serum sickness, systemic lupus erythematosus (SLE), rheumatoid arthritis, polyarteritis nodosa, cryoglobulinemia, and certain types of glomerulonephritis (e.g., from chronic hepatitis).

10. **What causes type IV hypersensitivity? How is it related to tuberculosis (TB) testing?**
    Type IV (cell mediated/delayed) hypersensitivity is due to sensitized T lymphocytes that release inflammatory mediators. The TB skin test (purified protein derivative [PPD]) exploits this immune system reaction. Other examples include contact dermatitis (especially poison ivy, nickel earrings, cosmetics, and medications), chronic transplant rejection, diabetes mellitus type 1, and granulomas (e.g., sarcoidosis).

11. **What sexually transmitted infectious infection should be considered when a patient presents with a sore throat and mononucleosis-like syndrome?**
    Acute human immunodeficiency virus (HIV) infection, because initial seroconversion usually presents as a mononucleosis-like syndrome (e.g., fever, malaise, pharyngitis, rash, lymphadenopathy). Also consider gonococcal pharyngitis in sexually active young persons with severe pharyngitis and nontender cervical lymphadenopathy.

12. **How is HIV diagnosed? How long after exposure does the HIV test become positive?**
    Most organizations now recommend that screening be performed with a fourth-generation combination immunoassay for the p24 antigen and HIV-1/2 antibodies with confirmatory testing via a HIV-1/2 antibody differentiation immunoassay. It takes 3 weeks for antibodies to develop in the majority of patients. Antibodies are present by 6 months in 95% of patients. Therefore, if a patient requests testing because of recent high-risk sexual behavior or if a known exposure has occurred, Centers for Disease Control and Prevention (CDC) guidelines call for testing at 4 weeks, 12 weeks, and 24 weeks if third-generation (ELISA) testing is used, or at 16 weeks if fourth-generation testing is used. If the exposure occurred within the last 72 hours, postexposure prophylaxis (PEP) should be offered. PEP consists of taking a fully active three-drug regimen (tenofovir/emtricitabine plus raltegravir) for 28 days.
    Rapid tests, which usually produce results within a few minutes to hours, are available, but as the positive predictive value varies with the prevalence of HIV infection in the population, preliminary positive tests require confirmatory testing with ELISA and Western blot. Negative test results are reliable unless the patient is in the window period, which is generally considered to be 3 weeks with the third-generation tests and about 16 days with fourth-generation tests incorporating p24 antigen. If acute HIV infection is suspected, it is necessary to send HIV viral load in addition to HIV antibody.

13. **Are control tests needed when a PPD test is done in HIV-positive patients?**
    Most authorities no longer recommend control (also known as anergy) testing when a PPD test is done in HIV-positive patients; however, serum testing with interferon-gamma release assays (IGRAs; e.g., QuantiFERON Gold) is becoming increasingly popular for the diagnosis of latent TB infection in both HIV-positive patients and in the general population.

14. **How do you recognize and treat *Pneumocystis jirovecii* pneumonia (PCP)?**
    For the Step 2 exam, think of PCP first in any patient with HIV and pneumonia, even though community-acquired pneumonia is more common even in patients with acquired immunodeficiency syndrome (AIDS). Look for severe hypoxia with normal radiographs or diffuse, bilateral interstitial infiltrates (Fig. 19.2). Patients usually present with a dry, nonproductive cough and dyspnea. PCP may be detected with silver stains (Wright-Giemsa, Giemsa, or methenamine silver) applied to induced sputum; if not, you can use bronchoscopy with bronchoalveolar

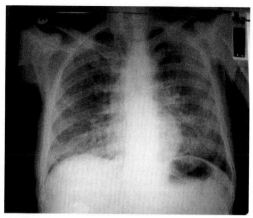

Fig. 19.2 Chest radiograph showing bilateral perihilar shadowing in a patient with *Pneumocystis* pneumonia. (From Kumar P. *Kumar & Clark's Cases in Clinical Medicine*. Edinburgh: Saunders; 2013:325–381.)

lavage and brush biopsy to make the diagnosis. High levels of lactate dehydrogenase (LDH) are suspicious in the appropriate setting. PCP is now occasionally treated presumptively (typically with trimethoprim-sulfamethoxazole with corticosteroids if severe hypoxia is present), with diagnostic testing reserved for those in whom the diagnosis is unclear or initial treatment fails. Alternative treatment includes monotherapy with atovaquone or pentamidine or combination therapy with clindamycin plus primaquine or trimethoprim plus dapsone.

If the patient's CD4 count is greater than 200, the patient is considered immune competent, and AIDS-related diseases such as PCP are very unlikely.

15. How do you recognize and treat disseminated histoplasmosis?
For Step 2, think of disseminated histoplasmosis in patients with a history of travel to the Ohio and Mississippi river valleys. Patients will have systemic signs, weight loss, pulmonary symptoms, and reticuloendothelial symptoms (i.e., hepatosplenomegaly and lymphadenopathy). A common triad of lab findings includes pancytopenia, transaminitis, and increased LDH/ferritin. Initial treatment is amphotericin B, which is then followed with maintenance therapy of itraconazole for at least a year.

16. What are common causes of diarrhea in HIV? How can they be differentiated?
There are four common causes: *Cryptosporidium*, *Microsporidium/Isosporidium*, *Mycobacteria avium* complex (MAC), and cytomegalovirus (CMV). *Cryptosporidium* infection most commonly occurs with a CD4 count under 180/mm^3 and presents with severe, watery diarrhea, low-grade fever, and weight loss. *Microsporidium/Isosporidium* infection most commonly occurs with a CD4 under 100/mm^3 and presents with crampy abdominal pain and watery diarrhea. Fever is rare. MAC and CMV infections occur with a CD4 count under 50/mm^3. The former presents with watery diarrhea and high fever (often >39°C) while the latter presents with frequent, small-volume, bloody diarrhea and abdominal pain.

17. What is the most common primary immunodeficiency? How do you recognize it?
IgA deficiency, which causes recurrent respiratory and gastrointestinal infections. IgA levels are always low, and levels of IgG subclass 2 may be low. Do not give immunoglobulins, which may cause anaphylaxis due to development of anti-IgA antibodies. Alternatively, if any patient develops anaphylaxis after immunoglobulin exposure or blood transfusion, you should think of IgA deficiency.

18. How do you recognize Bruton agammaglobulinemia?
Bruton agammaglobulinemia (X-linked agammaglobulinemia) is an X-linked recessive disorder with low or absent B cells due to no B-cell maturation. It is caused by a defect in the *BTK* gene. Infections begin after 6 months when maternal antibodies disappear. Look for recurrent lung or sinus infections with *Streptococcus* and *Haemophilus* species and absent/scanty lymph nodes and tonsils. Therapy includes immunoglobin replacement therapy and prophylactic antibiotics in certain situations.

19. What causes DiGeorge syndrome? How do you recognize it?
DiGeorge syndrome is caused by hypoplasia of the third and fourth pharyngeal pouches due to a deletion to 22q11. Look for hypocalcemia and tetany (from hypocalcemia due to absent parathyroid glands) in the first 24 to 48 hours of life. The thymus may also be absent or hypoplastic, and congenital heart defects and typical facies are often present. A useful mnemonic to remember the features of DiGeorge is CATCH-22: **c**ardiac anomalies (truncus arteriosus, tetralogy of Fallot), **a**bnormal facies, **t**hymic aplasia, **c**left palate, **h**ypoparathyroidism/**h**ypocalcemia, microdeletion in chromosome **22**.

20. **What is the classic cause of severe combined immunodeficiency (SCID)? How does it present?**
SCID may be autosomal recessive or X-linked. The classic cause is **adenosine deaminase deficiency** (autosomal recessive), though X-linked is the most common cause of SCID (i.e., a defect in the interleukin-2 receptor gamma chain). Patients have B- and T-cell defects and severe infections in the first few months of life. Other symptoms include failure to thrive, cutaneous anergy, chronic diarrhea, and absent or dysplastic thymus and lymph nodes. Treatment is stem cell transplant.

21. **What triad indicates the diagnosis of Wiskott-Aldrich syndrome?**
Wiskott-Aldrich deficiency is an X-linked recessive disorder. The classic triad consists of eczema, thrombocytopenia (look for bleeding), and recurrent infections (usually respiratory). A mnemonic to remember this disease is WATER: **W**iskott-**A**ldrich, **t**hrombocytopenia, **e**czema, and **r**ecurrent pyogenic infections.

22. **How do you recognize Chediak-Higashi syndrome?**
Chediak-Higashi syndrome is an autosomal recessive disorder characterized by giant granules in neutrophils, pyogenic infections, and often oculocutaneous albinism. The underlying defect is abnormal organellar protein trafficking due to a mutation in the *CHS1/LYST* gene, resulting in impaired phagocytosis.

23. **Describe the pathophysiology of chronic granulomatous disease.**
Chronic granulomatous disease (CGD) is usually an X-linked recessive disorder that affects males. Because of a defect in the activity of the enzyme nicotinamide adenine dinucleotide phosphate (NADPH) oxidase, patients have recurrent infections with catalase-positive organisms (e.g., *Staphylococcus aureus*, *Pseudomonas* sp., *Aspergillus*, *Candida*). Diagnosis is clinched if the question mentions deficient nitroblue tetrazolium (NBT) dye reduction by granulocytes. This test measures the respiratory burst, which patients with CGD lack. The patient will have a yellow/colorless NBT test (a positive test is blue and means that the respiratory burst is intact). On the USMLE, if you see "CGD" then look for "NBT" in the answer choices. Another test that might be mentioned is the dihydrorhodamine test, which is essentially flow cytometry.

24. **Cover the right-hand column, then answer the questions about HIV management on the left.**

Question	Answer
After HIV diagnosis, how often do you check the CD4 count?	Every 3–4 mo initially, then every 6–12 mo for patients who are adherent to therapy with sustained viral suppression and stable clinical status for more than 2–3 yr.
When do you start antiretroviral therapy?	Since 2011, the CDC has recommended HIV treatment with highly active antiretroviral therapy (HAART) regardless of CD4 count. However, HAART is contraindicated in the setting of a preexisting opportunistic infection due to potential for immune reconstitution inflammatory syndrome (IRIS).
What are the AIDS-defining illnesses?	*Pneumocystic jirovecii* pneumonia (PCP) Esophageal or other invasive candidiasis Wasting syndrome Kaposi sarcoma Disseminated *Mycobacterium avium* infection Tuberculosis Cytomegalovirus disease Disseminated histoplasmosis Progressive multifocal leukoencephalopathy (PML) HIV-associated dementia or encephalopathy Recurrent bacterial pneumonia Toxoplasmosis Immunoblastic lymphoma Chronic or extrapulmonary cryptosporidiosis Burkitt lymphoma Invasive cervical cancer Chronic herpes simplex Chronic intestinal isosporiasis Recurrent *Salmonella* infection
When do you start PCP prophylaxis?	When the CD4 count is <200/mm^3

Question	Answer
What is the drug of choice for PCP prophylaxis?	Trimethoprim-sulfamethoxazole (Bactrim)
What other agents are used in patients with allergy or intolerance to Bactrim?	Dapsone, aerosolized pentamidine, and atovaquone
When should you start *Mycobacterium avium complex* (MAC) prophylaxis?	MAC prophylaxis with a macrolide had been common practice with a CD4 count <50/mm^3, but this is no longer routine in the era of effective antiretroviral therapy.
True or false: Once the CD4 is <200/mm^3, the patient is automatically considered to have AIDS (even without opportunistic infections).	True
True or false: Give the measles-mumps-rubella vaccine.	True (CD4 count must be >200/mm^3)
True or false: Give the varicella vaccine.	True, if patient does not have evidence of immunity to varicella (CD4 count must be >200/mm^3)
True or false: Do not give annual influenza vaccines.	False (give every year to all HIV-infected patients)
True or false: Pneumococcal vaccine should be given.	True. It should be given to all HIV-infected patients, and revaccination every 5 years should be considered.
True or false: Give hepatitis A vaccine.	True, if the patient has chronic liver disease or is at increased risk for hepatitis A infection
True or false: Give hepatitis B vaccine.	True
True or false: PPD testing should be done annually.	True, if the initial test is negative and the patient is high risk
True or false: Oral polio vaccine should be given to patients who are at risk of exposure through travel or work.	False (use inactive polio vaccine injection)
The risk of which cancer is increased on the skin and in the mouth?	Kaposi sarcoma
The risk of which type of blood cell cancer is increased?	Non-Hodgkin lymphoma (usually primary B-cell lymphomas of central nervous system [CNS])
What do positive India ink preparations of the cerebrospinal fluid indicate?	*Cryptococcus neoformans* meningitis
What do ring-enhancing lesions in the brain on CT or MR scans usually indicate?	Toxoplasmosis, cysticercosis/*Taenia solium*, or primary CNS lymphoma
True or false: HIV may cause thrombocytopenia.	True
True or false: HIV can cause dementia.	True
True or false: HIV protects against peripheral neuropathies.	False. HIV can cause them.
True or false: HIV-positive mothers may breastfeed their infants.	False. HIV can be transmitted through breast milk.
First-choice agent for cytomegalovirus retinitis	Valganciclovir

Question	Answer
Second-choice agents for cytomegalovirus retinitis	Ganciclovir, foscarnet, or cidofovir
True or false: Pregnant patients should receive antiretroviral therapy.	True. Three-drug therapy is currently recommended (no different for the pregnant female; earlier administration is best).
True or false: Low-risk infants born to HIV-positive mothers should take zidovudine (ZDV).	True (for at least 6 wk after delivery). There are separate guidelines for high-risk infants, who take a three-drug regimen akin to PEP.
True or false: Cesarean section increases maternal HIV transmission.	False. Cesarean section is the recommended mode of delivery for HIV+ women with viral load >1000 copies to prevent perinatal transmission. Women with viral load <1000 copies may be offered vaginal delivery if appropriate.
Most likely cause of pneumonia in HIV+ patient	*Streptococcus pneumoniae*
Most likely cause of opportunistic pneumonia in HIV+ patient	*Pneumocystis jirovecii*
Stain used on sputum to detect PCP	Silver (Wright-Giemsa or Giemsa)
Two pathogens that cause chronic diarrhea only in AIDS	*Cryptosporidium* and *Isospora* spp.
True or false: Herpes-zoster infection in young adults = possible HIV infection.	True (suggests immunodeficiency)
True or false: Thrush in young adults may mean HIV infection.	True (also associated with diabetes, leukemia, and steroids)
True or false: A positive HIV antibody test in a newborn is unreliable.	True. Maternal antibodies in the neonate can give a false-positive result for the first 4–6 mo and is considered unreliable in neonates; definitive testing is done with HIV DNA PCR.

25. Complement deficiencies of C5 through C9 cause recurrent infections with which genus of bacteria?
    Neisseria species.

26. Define chronic mucocutaneous candidiasis.
    Chronic mucocutaneous candidiasis is a cellular immunodeficiency specific for candida infection. Patients have thrush and candidal infections of the scalp, skin, and nails as well as anergy to *Candida* sp. with skin testing. It is often associated with hypothyroidism. The rest of the immune function is intact; no other types of infections are present.

27. Give the classic description of hyper-IgE syndrome (Job-Buckley syndrome).
    Patients with hyper-IgE syndrome have recurrent staphylococcal infections (especially of the skin) and extremely high IgE levels. They also commonly have fair skin, coarse facial features, eczema, retained primary teeth, and recurrent fractures.

CHAPTER 20

INFECTIOUS DISEASES

1. Cover the middle and right-hand columns, and specify which organisms are associated with each type of infection and what type of empiric antibiotic should be used while waiting for culture results.

Condition	Main Organism(s)	Empiric Antibiotics
Urinary tract infection	Escherichia coli	Nitrofurantoin (avoid in the elderly and those with decreased renal function), trimethoprim-sulfamethoxazole, fosfomycin, amoxicillin-clavulanate, cephalosporins, quinolones
Bronchitis	Viruses, Haemophilus influenzae, Mycoplasma, Chlamydia pneumonia, Moraxella spp.	Usually no benefit from antibiotics. May consider macrolides or doxycycline (in cases such as a purulent cough >1-wk duration)
Pneumonia (classic)	Streptococcus pneumoniae, H. influenzae	Azithromycin, third-generation cephalosporin, levofloxacin
Pneumonia (atypical)	Mycoplasma, Chlamydia spp., Legionella	Macrolide antibiotic, doxycycline
Osteomyelitis	Staphylococcus aureus, Salmonella spp., Pseudomonas aeruginosa	Vancomycin, ceftazidime, piperacillin/tazobactam; oxacillin, nafcillin, and cefazolin for MSSA
Cellulitis	Staphylococci, Streptococci,	Cephalexin, dicloxacillin, trimethoprim-sulfamethoxazole, doxycycline, or clindamycin are often used as first-line agents due to the emergence of MRSA.
Erysipelas	Staphylococci, Streptococci	Penicillin, amoxicillin for uncomplicated cases, otherwise treat like cellulitis.
Meningitis (neonate)	Streptococci B, E. coli, Listeria spp.	Ampicillin + aminoglycoside (usually gentamicin). An expanded spectrum third-generation cephalosporin (cefotaxime) should be added if a gram-negative organism is suspected.
Meningitis (child/adult)	S. pneumoniae, Neisseria meningitidis*	Cefotaxime or ceftriaxone + vancomycin
Endocarditis (native valve)	Staphylococci, streptococci	Vancomycin
Endocarditis (prosthetic valve)	Numerous different organisms	Vancomycin + gentamicin + cefepime or a carbapenem
Sepsis	Gram-negative organisms, streptococci, staphylococci	Third-generation penicillin/cephalosporin + aminoglycoside, or imipenem
Septic arthritis‡	S. aureus Gram-negative bacilli Gonococci	Vancomycin Ceftazidime or ceftriaxone Ceftriaxone, ciprofloxacin, or spectinomycin

†Examples: oxacillin, nafcillin.

*H. influenzae is no longer as common a cause of meningitis in children because of widespread vaccination. In a child with no history of immunization, H. influenzae is the most likely cause of meningitis.

‡Think of staphylococci if the patient is monogamous or not sexually active. Think of gonorrhea for younger adults who are sexually active.

MRSA, methicillin-resistant Staphylococcus aureus; MSSA, methicillin-sensitive Staphylococcus aureus

2. Cover the right-hand columns, and specify the empiric antibiotic of choice for each organism.

Organism*	Antibiotic	Other Choices
Streptococcus A or B	Penicillin, cefazolin	Erythromycin
S. pneumonia	Third-generation cephalosporin (ceftriaxone) + vancomycin	Fluoroquinolone (levofloxacin)
Enterococcus	Penicillin or ampicillin + aminoglycoside (gentamicin)	Vancomycin + aminoglycoside
Staphylococcus aureus	Antistaphylococcus penicillin (e.g., methicillin)	Vancomycin, trimethoprim-sulfamethoxazole, doxycycline, clindamycin, daptomycin, or linezolid for MRSA
Gonococcus†	Ceftriaxone	Cefixime or high-dose azithromycin followed by test of cure in 1 wk
Meningococcus	Cefotaxime or ceftriaxone	Chloramphenicol or penicillin G if proven to be penicillin susceptible
Haemophilus	Second- or third-generation cephalosporin	Amoxicillin
Pseudomonas	Antipseudomonal penicillin (ticarcillin, piperacillin) +/− beta lactamase inhibitor (clavulanate, tazobactam)	Ceftazidime, cefepime, aztreonam, imipenem, ciprofloxacin
Bacteroides	Metronidazole	Clindamycin
Mycoplasma	Erythromycin, azithromycin	Doxycycline
Treponema pallidum	Penicillin	Doxycycline
Chlamydia	Doxycycline, azithromycin	Erythromycin, ofloxacin
Lyme disease (*Borrelia* spp.)	Cefuroxime, doxycycline, amoxicillin	Erythromycin

*Always use culture sensitivities to guide therapy once available.
†With genital infections, always treat for presumed *Chlamydia* coinfection with azithromycin or doxycycline.

3. Cover the right-hand column, then specify what each Gram stain most likely represents.

Gram Stain Result	Meaning
Blue/purple color	Gram-positive organism
Red color	Gram-negative organism
Gram-positive cocci in chains	Streptococci
Gram-positive cocci in clusters	Staphylococci
Gram-positive cocci in pairs (diplococci)	*Streptococcus pneumoniae*
Gram-negative coccobacilli (small rods)	*Haemophilus* sp.
Gram-negative diplococci	*Neisseria* sp. (sexually transmitted disease, septic arthritis, meningitis) or *Moraxella* sp. (lungs, sinusitis)
Plump gram-negative rod with thick capsule (mucoid appearance)	*Klebsiella* sp.
Gram-positive rods that form spores	*Clostridium* sp., *Bacillus* sp.
Pseudohyphae	*Candida* sp.
Acid-fast organisms	*Mycobacterium* (usually *M. tuberculosis*), *Nocardia* sp.

Gram Stain Result	Meaning
Gram-positive with sulfur granules	*Actinomyces* sp. (pelvic inflammatory disease in intrauterine device users; rare cause of neck mass/cervical adenitis)
Silver staining	*Pneumocystis jirovecii,* Cryptococcus, Candida, Legionalla, *H. pylori,* Treponema, and *Bartonella henselae* (cat-scratch disease)
Positive India ink preparation (thick capsule)	*Cryptococcus neoformans*
Spirochete	*Treponema* sp., *Leptospira* sp. (both seen only on dark-field microscopy), *Borrelia* sp. (seen on regular light microscope)

4. What is the gold standard for diagnosis of pneumonia?
   Sputum culture. Try to get the culture before starting antibiotics, though many physicians treat empirically without culture in routine cases. Get blood cultures, too, because bacteremia is common with pneumonia.

5. What is the most common cause of pneumonia? How does it classically present?
   Streptococcus pneumoniae. Look for rapid onset of shaking chills after 1–2 days of upper respiratory infection symptoms (sore throat, runny nose, dry cough), followed by fever, pleurisy, and productive cough (yellowish-green or rust-colored from blood), especially in older adults. Chest radiograph shows lobar consolidation (Fig. 20.1), and the white blood cell count is high with a large percentage of neutrophils. Treat with a macrolide (e.g., azithromycin, clarithromycin), doxycycline, third-generation cephalosporin plus a macrolide or doxycycline, or a fluoroquinolone that provides atypical pathogen coverage (e.g., levofloxacin, moxifloxacin).

6. What is the best prevention against *S. pneumoniae*?
   Vaccination. Give pneumococcal vaccine to all children as well as adult patients over 65 years old, asplenia (splenectomized patients, patients with sickle cell disease who have autosplenectomy, or splenic dysfunction), immunocompromised patients (human immunodeficiency virus [HIV], malignancy, organ transplant), and all patients with chronic disease (e.g., diabetes, cardiac disease, asthma and other pulmonary disease, renal disease, liver disease, or tobacco use).

7. How do you recognize and treat *Haemophilus influenzae* pneumonia?
   H. influenzae is now uncommon in children due to vaccination, but it is still an important cause of pneumonia in the elderly and in those with underlying lung disease such as chronic obstructive pulmonary disease (COPD). It often resembles pneumococcal pneumonia clinically, but look for gram-negative coccobacilli on sputum Gram stain. Treat with amoxicillin or a second- or third-generation cephalosporin.

8. Describe the hallmarks of *Staphylococcus aureus* pneumonia.
   S. aureus tends to cause hospital-acquired (nosocomial) pneumonia and pneumonia in patients with cystic fibrosis (along with *Pseudomonas* sp.), intravenous (IV) drug abusers, and patients with chronic granulomatous disease (look for recurrent lung abscesses). Empyema and lung abscesses are relatively common with *S. aureus* pneumonia. *S. aureus* pneumonia can be a complication of influenza.

9. In what clinical situations do you tend to see gram-negative pneumonias?
   Pseudomonas infection is classically associated with cystic fibrosis. *Klebsiella* infection is associated with people with alcohol use disorder and people who are homeless (watch for classic description of currant jelly sputum). Enteric gram-negative organisms (e.g., *Escherichia coli*) are associated with aspiration, neutropenia, and hospital-acquired pneumonia. These types of pneumonias often have a high mortality rate because of the types of patients affected and the severity of the pneumonia (abscesses are common). Treat empirically with an antipseudomonal penicillin (e.g., ticarcillin, piperacillin) with or without a beta lactamase inhibitor (e.g., clavulanate, tazobactam). Alternatives include ceftazidime or ciprofloxacin.

10. How do you recognize *Mycoplasma* pneumonia?
    Mycoplasma infection is most common in adolescents and young adults (the classic patient is a college student or soldier who lives in a dormitory/barracks and has sick contacts). It is one of the atypical pneumonias because it presents differently from a typical pneumonia due to *Streptococcus pneumoniae*. For example, it has a long prodrome with gradual worsening of malaise, headaches, dry nonproductive cough, and sore throat; the fever tends to be low grade. Chest radiograph shows a patchy, diffuse bronchopneumonia and classically looks terrible, although the patient often does not feel that bad (which is why it is sometimes called "walking pneumonia"). Look for positive **cold-agglutinin antibody titers**, which may cause hemolysis or anemia. Atypical pneumonia is treated empirically with a macrolide antibiotic (azithromycin), doxycycline, or broad-spectrum fluoroquinolone (e.g., levofloxacin or moxifloxacin).

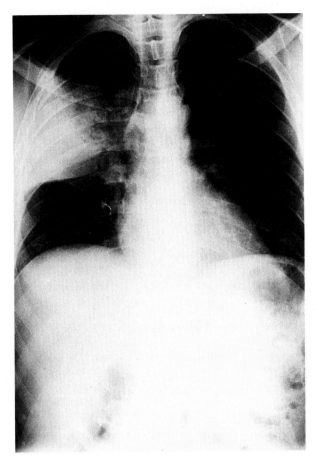

Fig. 20.1 Pneumonia. Right middle lobe infiltrate. (From Au-Yong I, Au-Yong-A. *On-Call X-Rays Made Easy.* Edinburgh: Churchill Livingston Elsevier;2010:48-57.)

11. **What about chlamydial pneumonia?**
    Chlamydia sp. is second only to *Mycoplasma* sp. as the cause of atypical pneumonia in adolescents and young adults. It presents similarly but has negative cold-agglutinin antibody titers. Treat with erythromycin in children under 8 years of age and either azithromycin or doxycycline in children over 8 years of age, adolescents, and adults.

12. **In what setting do you see *Pneumocystis jirovecii* pneumonia (PCP) and cytomegalovirus (CMV) pneumonia?**
    HIV-positive patients with CD4 counts less than 200/mm³ (acquired immunodeficiency syndrome [AIDS]) and other severely immunosuppressed patients (e.g., organ transplant recipients taking powerful immunosuppressants or patients on cancer chemotherapy) are susceptible to PCP. In patients with AIDS, PCP is the most common opportunistic pneumonia and may require bronchoalveolar lavage for diagnosis. PCP can be seen with silver stains and typically causes bilateral interstitial lung infiltrates. Chest x-ray may show a "bat wing" appearance, which represents bilateral interstitial infiltrates. Lactate dehydrogenase (LDH) may be elevated, and arterial blood gas (ABG) may show an increased A-a gradient. Treat with trimethoprim-sulfamethoxazole plus corticosteroids. CMV pneumonia is characterized by intracellular inclusion bodies. Treat with ganciclovir or valganciclovir.

13. **What is the best time to treat PCP?**
    Before it happens. PCP is acquired when the CD4 count is below 200/mm³. At that point you should institute PCP prophylaxis with trimethoprim-sulfamethoxazole. Alternatives include dapsone or atovaquone.

14. Cover the two right-hand columns. Specify the organism after looking at the scenario associated with it.

Scenario	Organism(s)	Comments
Stuck with thorn or gardening	*Sporothrix schenckii*	Treat with itraconazole.
Aplastic crisis in sickle cell disease	Parvovirus	B19
Sepsis after splenectomy	*S. pneumoniae, H. influenzae, N. meningitis* (encapsulated bugs)	Encapsulated organisms
Pneumonia in the southwestern United States (California, Arizona)	*Coccidioides immitis*	Treat with itraconazole or fluconazole, amphotericin B for severe disease.
Pneumonia after cave exploring or exposure to bird droppings in Ohio and Mississippi river valleys	*Histoplasma capsulatum*	Majority are self-limited and do not require treatment.
Pneumonia after exposure to a parrot or exotic bird	*Chlamydia psittaci*	Treat with doxycycline or azithromycin.
Fungus ball/hemoptysis after tuberculosis or cavitary lung disease	*Aspergillus* sp.	Treat with voriconazole.
Pneumonia in a patient with silicosis	*Mycobacterium tuberculosis*	
Diarrhea after hiking/drinking from a stream	*Giardia lamblia*	Stool cysts; treat with metronidazole.
Pregnant woman with cats	*Toxoplasma gondii*	Treat infected pregnant women with pyrimethamine and sulfadiazine.
B_{12} deficiency and abdominal symptoms	*Diphyllobothrium latum* (intestinal tapeworm)	
Seizures with ring-enhancing brain lesion on CT	*Taenia solium* (cysticercosis) or toxoplasmosis	Treat neurocysticercosis with albendazole or praziquantel, usually with steroids. Consider anticonvulsants.
Squamous cell bladder cancer in Middle East or Africa	*Schistosoma haematobium*	
Worm infection in children	*Enterobius* sp.	Positive tape test, perianal itching. Treat with mebendazole or albendazole.
Fever, muscle pain, eosinophilia, and periorbital edema after eating raw meat	*Trichinella spiralis* (trichinosis)	
Gastroenteritis in young children	Rotavirus, Norwalk virus	
Food poisoning after eating reheated rice	*Bacillus cereus*	Infection is usually self-limited.
Food poisoning after eating raw seafood	*Vibrio parahaemolyticus*	
Diarrhea after travel to Mexico	*E. coli* (Montezuma revenge)	ETEC. Treat with ciprofloxacin.

Scenario	Organism(s)	Comments
Diarrhea after antibiotics	*Clostridioides difficile*	Use oral vancomycin or fidaxomicin. Oral metronidazole may be used in settings where access to vancomycin or fidaxomicin is limited for an initial episode of nonsevere *C. diff* infection.
Baby paralyzed after eating honey	*Clostridioides botulinum*	Toxin blocks acetylcholine release.
Genital lesions in children in the absence of sexual abuse or activity	Molluscum contagiosum	
Cellulitis after cat/dog bites	*Pasteurella multocida*	Treat animal bite wounds with prophylactic amoxicillin-clavulanate.
Slaughterhouse worker with fever	*Brucella* spp. (brucellosis)	
Pneumonia after being in hotel or near air conditioner or water tower	*Legionella pneumophila*	May have diarrhea and hyponatremia. Treat with azithromycin or levofloxacin.
Burn wound infection with blue/green color	*Pseudomonas* sp.	*S. aureus* is also a common burn infection, but it lacks blue-green color.

15. How is syphilis diagnosed?
    Screen for syphilis with a rapid plasma reagin (RPR) or Venereal Disease Research Laboratory (VDRL) test. Confirm a positive test with a fluorescent treponemal antibody absorbed (FTA-ABS) or microhemagglutination (MHA-TP) test because false positives occur with the RPR and VDRL tests, classically in patients with antiphospholipid syndrome (or systemic lupus erythematosus with antiphospholipid antibodies). Once syphilis is treated, the RPR and VDRL tests become negative, whereas the FTA-ABS and MHA-TP tests often remain positive for life. You can also scrape the base of a genital chancre or condyloma latum and look for spirochetes on dark-field microscopy.

16. Which group of patients should always be screened for syphilis?
    Pregnant women. Early treatment can prevent birth defects.

17. How is syphilis treated?
    With penicillin. Use doxycycline for penicillin-allergic patients.

18. Describe the three stages of syphilis.
    Primary stage: Look for painless chancre that resolves on its own within 8 weeks.
       Secondary stage: Roughly 6 weeks to 18 months after infection; look for condyloma lata, maculopapular rash (classically involves palms and soles of feet) (Fig. 20.2), and lymphadenopathy.
          Tertiary stage: Years after initial infection (between the secondary and tertiary stages is the latent phase, in which the disease is quiet and asymptomatic). Look for gummas (granulomas in many different organs), neurologic symptoms and signs (e.g., neurosyphilis, Argyll-Robertson pupil, dementia, paresis, tabes dorsalis, Charcot joints), and thoracic aortic aneurysms.

19. How do you recognize measles (rubeola) infection in a child?
    Pathognomonic Koplik spots (tiny white spots on buccal mucosa) are seen 3 days after high fever, cough, runny nose, and conjunctivitis with or without photophobia. On the next day, a maculopapular rash begins on the head and neck and spreads downward to cover the trunk (cephalocaudal progression). Look for a history of lack of immunization. Treat supportively. Patients are contagious until several days after the rash first appears. Don't forget to contact the health department regarding cases of measles.

20. Describe the complications of measles.
    Complications include giant cell pneumonia, especially in very young and immunocompromised patients; otitis media; and encephalitis, either acute or late (**subacute sclerosing panencephalitis**, which usually occurs years later).

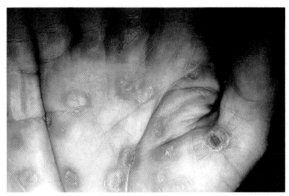

Fig. 20.2 Palmar lesions of secondary syphilis. (From Mandell GL, Bennett, JE, Dolin R. *Mandell, Douglas, and Bennett's Principles and Practice of Infectious Diseases.* 7th ed. London: Churchill Livingstone; 2009 [fig. 238-5].)

21. **Why is rubella infection (German measles) an important disease?**
    Infection in pregnant mothers can cause severe birth defects in the fetus. Screen all women of reproductive age, and immunize those without evidence of rubella antibodies before pregnancy to avoid this complication. Remember, however, that the vaccine is contraindicated in pregnant women.

22. **How do you recognize a rubella infection in children? What are the complications?**
    Rubella is milder than measles. Signs and symptoms include low-grade fever, malaise, and tender swelling of the suboccipital and postauricular nodes; arthralgias are common. After a 2- to 3-day prodrome, a faint maculopapular rash appears on the face and neck and spreads to the trunk (cephalocaudal progression), just as in measles. Complications include encephalitis and otitis media.

23. **How do you recognize roseola infantum (exanthem subitum)? What causes it?**
    Roseola infantum is often easy to recognize because of the progression: high fever (may be higher than 40°C) with no apparent cause for 4 days, which may result in febrile seizures, followed by an abrupt return to normal temperature just as a diffuse macular/maculopapular rash appears on the chest and abdomen. It may be associated with lymphadenopathy, erythematous tympanic membranes, and sterile pyuria. It is caused by human herpesvirus type 6 (a DNA herpes family virus). The diagnosis is clinical, and treatment is supportive. The disease is rare in children older than 3 years.

24. **How do you recognize erythema infectiosum (fifth disease) in children? What causes it?**
    Look for the classic "slapped-cheek" rash (Fig. 20.3). Confluent erythema over the cheeks looks like someone slapped the child across the face accompanied by mild constitutional symptoms (e.g., low fever, malaise). One day later, a maculopapular rash appears on the arms, legs, and trunk. The disease is caused by parvovirus B19, the same virus that causes aplastic crisis in sickle cell disease. Parvovirus can have serious consequences during pregnancy, including fetal demise via hydrops fetalis (high output heart failure and anasarca).

25. **How do you recognize chickenpox? What causes it?**
    The description and progression of the rash should lead you to the diagnosis: discrete, intensely pruritic macules (usually on the trunk) turn into papules, which turn into vesicles that rupture and crust over. Such changes occur within 1 day. Because the lesions appear in successive crops, the rash will be in different stages of progression in different areas. It is caused by the varicella-zoster virus.

26. **How can you make a definitive diagnosis of chickenpox? At what point is a patient with chickenpox no longer infectious?**
    A Tzanck smear of tissue from the base of a vesicle shows multinucleated giant cells. A presumptive diagnosis can be made if the rash is classic. Infectivity ceases only when the last lesion crusts over. The virus, however, remains dormant in the dorsal root ganglion for possible future reactivation.

27. **What are the complications of chickenpox?**
    A complication is infection of the lesions with streptococci or staphylococci, which can cause impetigo, erysipelas, cellulitis, and/or sepsis. The patient should be instructed to keep clean to avoid infection. Other complications include pneumonia (especially in very young children, adults, and immunocompromised patients), encephalitis, and **Reye syndrome**. Do not give aspirin to a child with a fever unless you have a diagnosis that requires its use (e.g., Kawasaki disease). The varicella-zoster virus can reactivate years later from its dormant state to cause herpes zoster (also known as shingles) (Fig. 20.4), a painful vesicular rash that develops in a dermatomal distribution, often with preceding pain and paresthesias. A child who has not been immunized or exposed to chickenpox can catch the disease from someone with shingles.

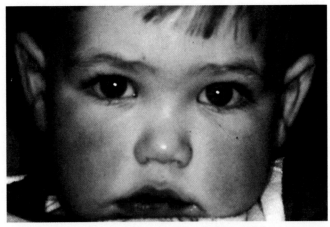

Fig. 20.3 "Slapped cheek" appearance of erythema infectiosum. (From Baren JM, Rothrock SG, Brennan J, et al. *Pediatric Emergency Medicine.* 1st ed. Philadelphia, PA: Saunders; 2007 [fig. 123-5].)

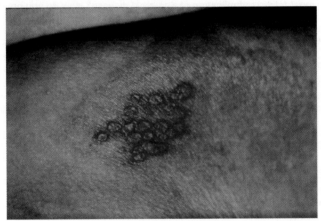

Fig. 20.4 Herpes zoster. Grouped vesicopustules on an erythematous base. (From Marx J, Hockberger R, et al. *Rosen's Emergency Medicine.* 7th ed. Philadelphia: Mosby; 2009 [fig. 118-28]. Courtesy of David Effron, MD.)

28. **Describe the treatment and prophylaxis for chickenpox**
    No treatment other than supportive care (e.g., acetaminophen, fluids, avoidance of infecting others) is needed in most cases. Acyclovir can be used in severe cases. Routine vaccination with the varicella vaccine is now recommended for all children in the United States. Varicella zoster immune globulin is available for prophylaxis in patients with debilitating illness (e.g., leukemia, AIDS) if you see them within 4 days of exposure and for newborns of mothers with chickenpox. IV immunoglobulin can be given if varicella zoster immune globulin is not available.

29. **What is scarlet fever? What causes it? How is it recognized and treated?**
    Scarlet fever is a febrile illness with a rash caused by certain *Streptococcus* species. Look for a history of untreated streptococcal pharyngitis. Note that only streptococcal species that produce erythrogenic toxin can cause scarlet fever. Pharyngitis is followed by a sandpaper-like rash on the abdomen and trunk with classic circumoral pallor and strawberry tongue. The rash tends to desquamate once the fever subsides. Oral penicillin V is the treatment of choice for streptococcal pharyngitis to prevent rheumatic fever. Alternative therapies include amoxicillin, cephalosporins, macrolides, or clindamycin.

30. **What are the diagnostic criteria for Kawasaki disease (mucocutaneous lymph node syndrome)?**
    Fever for more than 5 days (mandatory for diagnosis); bilateral conjunctival injection; changes in the lips, tongue, or oral mucosa (e.g., strawberry tongue, fissuring, injection); changes in the extremities (e.g., skin desquamation, edema, erythema); polymorphous truncal rash, which usually begins 1 day after the fever starts; and cervical lymphadenopathy (Fig 20.5). Also look for arthralgia or arthritis. This is a rare disease seen in patients under 5 years old.

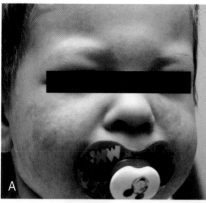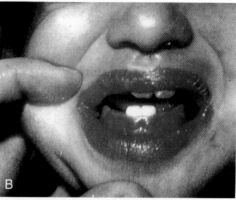

Fig. 20.5 Facial features of Kawasaki disease with (A) morbilliform rash and nonsuppurative conjunctivitis and (B) red, chapped lips. (From Marcdante K, Kliegman R. *Nelson Essentials of Pediatrics*. Philadelphia: Elsevier;2019:347-349.)

31. **What is the most feared complication of Kawasaki disease? How do you prevent it?**
Complications involving the heart (coronary artery aneurysms, congestive heart failure, arrhythmias, myocarditis, and even myocardial infarction [MI]). Follow the child with echocardiography to detect heart involvement. Include Kawasaki disease in the differential diagnosis of any child who has an MI. If Kawasaki disease is suspected, give aspirin and IV immunoglobulins. Both have been proven to reduce cardiac morbidity. Kawasaki disease is one of the few indications for aspirin in a child.

32. **Describe the classic findings of Epstein-Barr virus (EBV) infection (infectious mononucleosis).**
Fatigue, fever, pharyngitis, and cervical lymphadenopathy in a young adult. The signs and symptoms are similar to those of streptococcal pharyngitis, but malaise tends to be prolonged and pronounced in EBV infection. To differentiate from streptococcal pharyngitis, look for the following:
- Splenomegaly (patients are at increased risk of splenic rupture and should avoid contact sports and heavy lifting)
- Hepatomegaly
- Atypical lymphocytes (bizarre forms that may resemble leukemia) with lymphocytosis, anemia, or thrombocytopenia
- Positive serology (heterophile antibodies [e.g., Monospot test]) or specific EBV antibodies (viral capsid antigen, Epstein-Barr nuclear antigens)

33. **What is an important differential diagnosis of EBV infection or influenza infection?**
Acute HIV infection, which can cause a mononucleosis-type syndrome.

34. **What is the association between EBV and cancer?**
EBV is associated with nasopharyngeal cancer, African Burkitt lymphoma, and posttransplant lymphoproliferative disorder.

35. **Describe the classic clinical vignette for Rocky Mountain spotted fever. What causes it? What is the treatment?**
Look for history of a tick bite (especially in a patient on the East Coast) 1 week before the development of high fever/chills, severe headache, and prostration or severe malaise. A rash appears roughly 4 days later on the palms/wrists and soles/ankles and spreads rapidly to the trunk and face (unique pattern of spread). Patients often look quite ill (e.g., disseminated intravascular coagulation, delirium). The infection is caused by *Rickettsia rickettsii*. Treat with doxycycline; chloramphenicol is a second choice.

36. **How do you recognize and treat the rash of impetigo? What causes it?**
Impetigo is a superinfection of a break in the skin (e.g., previous chickenpox, insect bite, scabies, cut). Impetigo is caused by *Streptococcus* and *Staphylococcus* species. The rash starts as thin-walled vesicles that rupture and form yellowish crusts (Fig. 20.6). The skin classically is described as "weeping." Typical lesions appear on the face and tend to be localized. The rash is infectious; look for a history of sick contacts. Treat with dicloxacillin, cephalexin, or clindamycin to cover both *Streptococcus* and *Staphylococcus* species. Topical mupirocin also may be used.

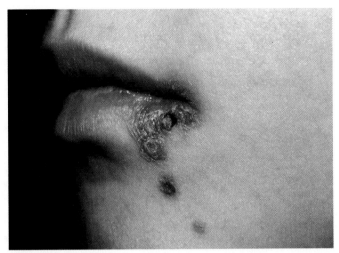

Fig. 20.6 Impetigo. Multiple crusted and oozing lesions. (From Kliegman RL, Stanton B, Behrman R, et al. *Nelson Textbook of Pediatrics.* 19th ed. Philadelphia, PA: Saunders; 2011 [fig. 657-1].)

37. Describe the two clinical types of endocarditis. What are the causative organisms?
    - **Acute** (fulminant) endocarditis, which typically affects normal heart valves and most commonly is caused by *Staphylococcus aureus.*
    - **Subacute**, which has an insidious onset and typically affects previously damaged or prosthetic valves. The most common cause is viridans streptococci, but other streptococcal and staphylococcal species also may cause endocarditis (e.g., *Staphylococcus epidermis, Streptococcus bovis,* and enterococci). Suspect colon cancer if *S. bovis* turns up on blood culture.

38. How is endocarditis diagnosed and treated?
    The diagnosis is generally made by blood cultures. Empiric treatment is begun until the culture and sensitivity results are known. An antistaphylococcal penicillin (such as oxacillin or nafcillin) plus an aminoglycoside is a good choice for native valve endocarditis. A third-generation penicillin or cephalosporin plus an aminoglycoside is a reasonable choice. Empiric treatment for prosthetic valve endocarditis is vancomycin plus gentamicin plus either cefepime or a carbapenem.

39. What are the classic signs and symptoms of endocarditis?
    Look for general signs of infection (e.g., fever, tachycardia, malaise) plus new-onset heart murmur, embolic phenomena (stroke and other infarcts), **Osler nodes** (painful nodules on tips of fingers), **Janeway lesions** (*nontender,* erythematous lesions on palms and soles), **Roth spots** (round retinal hemorrhages with white centers), and septic shock (more likely with acute than subacute disease).

40. What elements of the history point to endocarditis?
    Look for patients who are more likely to be affected by endocarditis:
    - IV drug abusers, who usually have right-sided lesions (Left-sided lesions are much more common in the general population.)
    - Patients with abnormal heart valves (e.g., prosthetic valves, rheumatic valvular disease, congenital heart defects such as ventricular septal defects or tetralogy of Fallot)
    - Postoperative patients (especially after dental surgery)
    - Immunocompromised patients

41. What are the recommendations for endocarditis prophylaxis?
    The 2008 American Heart Association recommendations conclude that only an extremely small number of cases of infective endocarditis might be prevented by antibiotic prophylaxis for dental procedures. Cardiac conditions for which prophylaxis with dental procedures is recommended include prosthetic cardiac valve, previous infectious endocarditis, congenital heart disease, and cardiac transplant recipients who develop valvulopathy. Antibiotic prophylaxis is no longer recommended for genitourinary or gastrointestinal procedures.
    If a prophylactic antibiotic is indicated, it should be administered in a single dose before the procedure. Amoxicillin is the preferred choice for oral therapy. Cephalexin, clindamycin, azithromycin, or clarithromycin may be used in patients with penicillin allergy. Ampicillin, cefazolin, ceftriaxone, or clindamycin may be used for patients unable to take oral medication.

42. What is the classic age group for meningitis? Describe the physical findings.
Neonates are the classic age group for meningitis; 75% of all cases occur in children younger than 2 years. Deciding when to do a lumbar tap is difficult, because patients often do not have classic physical findings (Kernig sign and Brudzinski sign). Look for lethargy, hyper- or hypothermia, poor muscle tone, bulging fontanelle, vomiting, photophobia, altered consciousness, and signs of sepsis (e.g., hypotension, jaundice, respiratory distress). Seizures may also be seen, but simple febrile seizures are common in the absence of meningitis if the patient is between 5 months and 6 years old. The maximum height of a fever, as opposed to the rate of rise, is felt to be the main determinant of risk in febrile seizures.

43. What should you do if you suspect meningitis?
In the absence of trauma, do a lumbar puncture immediately and begin broad-spectrum antibiotics and IV fluids. Do *not* wait for culture or other results to start antibiotics.

44. What is the most common neurologic sequela of meningitis?
Hearing loss. All pediatric and many adult patients need formal hearing evaluation after recovering from meningitis. Vision testing is also recommended. Other sequelae include intellectual disability, motor deficits/paresis, epilepsy, and learning/behavioral disorders. Dexamethasone may help reduce the incidence of hearing loss in patients with meningitis.

45. What are the common viral (aseptic) causes of meningitis in children?
Mumps and measles meningitis may be seen in children who are not immunized. The best treatment is prevention via immunization. Watch for neonatal herpes encephalitis (HSV-2) if the mother has genital lesions of herpes simplex virus at the time of delivery. Other children and adults can develop HSV-1 herpes encephalitis, which classically affects the **temporal lobes** on a head computed tomography (CT) or magnetic resonance imaging (MRI) scan. Give IV acyclovir.

46. Which types of bacterial meningitis require antibiotic prophylaxis in contacts?
N. meningitidis and *H. influenzae*. If a case of meningitis is due to *Neisseria,* give all contacts rifampin, ciprofloxacin, ceftriaxone, or azithromycin as prophylaxis; rifampin is used for *H. influenzae* meningitis prophylaxis.

47. What are the "big three" respiratory infections in patients younger than 5 years?
Croup, epiglottitis, and respiratory syncytial virus infection (bronchiolitis). These three diseases are high yield on the USMLE.

48. How do you recognize croup (acute laryngotracheitis)? Describe the cause and treatment.
The disease begins with symptoms of viral upper respiratory infection (e.g., rhinorrhea, cough, fever). Roughly 1 to 2 days later, patients develop a "barking" cough, hoarseness, and inspiratory stridor. The **steeple sign** (reflects subglottic narrowing of the trachea) (Fig. 20.7) is classic on a frontal radiograph of the chest or neck. Look for a child 1 to 2 years of age. Croup usually occurs in the fall or winter. Fifty percent to 75% of cases are due to infection with parainfluenza virus; the other common causative agent is influenza virus. Treat with dexamethasone, racemic epinephrine, and humidified oxygen.

49. How do you recognize epiglottitis? Describe the cause and treatment.
Epiglottitis usually occurs in children 2 to 5 years old. The main cause is *Haemophilus influenzae* type b; thus widespread vaccination has significantly reduced the incidence of this condition. *Staphylococcus aureus, S. pyogenes,* and *S. pneumoniae* are other potential causes. Look for little or no prodrome, with rapid progression to high fever, toxic appearance, drooling, and respiratory distress with no coughing (the three *Ds*—drooling, dysphagia, and distress) in unvaccinated children less than 2 to 5 years old. The **thumb sign** (describes a swollen, enlarged epiglottis) (Fig. 20.8) is classic on lateral radiographs of the neck. Do not examine the throat or irritate the child in any way. You may precipitate airway obstruction. When a case of epiglottitis is diagnosed, the first step is to be prepared to establish an airway (intubation and, if needed, tracheostomy). Treat with a combination of oxacillin or cefazolin or clindamycin or vancomycin plus cefotaxime or ceftriaxone.

50. Describe the classic clinical vignette for bronchiolitis. What is the cause? How is it treated?
Bronchiolitis generally affects children aged 0 to 18 months and usually occurs in the fall or winter. More than 75% of cases are caused by respiratory syncytial virus (RSV); other causes are parainfluenza and influenza viruses. Patients first develop symptoms of viral upper respiratory infection, followed 1 to 2 days later by rapid respirations, intercostal retractions, and expiratory wheezing. The child may have crackles on auscultation of the chest. Diffuse hyperinflation of the lungs is classic on chest radiograph; look for flattened diaphragms. Treat supportively (e.g., oxygen, mist tent, bronchodilators, IV fluids).

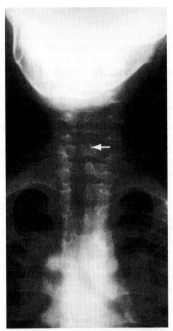

Fig. 20.7 Anteroposterior radiograph of the neck region of child with croup. Note the steeple sign *(white arrow)*. (From Wetmore RF. *Pediatric Otolaryngology: Requisites.* 1st ed. Philadelphia, PA: Mosby; 2007 [fig. 11-1].)

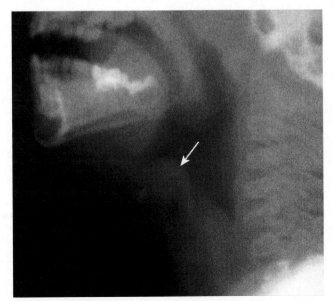

Fig. 20.8 Lateral neck radiograph demonstrating epiglottis with the "thumb sign." (From Zaoutis LB, Chiang VW. *Comprehensive Pediatric Hospital Medicine.* 1st ed. Philadelphia, PA: Elsevier; 2007 [fig. 66-3].)

51. **What "old-school" pediatric infection causes pseudomembranes and myocarditis? What about whooping cough?**

    Diphtheria (*Corynebacterium diphtheriae*) and pertussis (*Bordetella pertussis*), respectively. Diphtheria is quite uncommon in the United States because of mandatory vaccination. Pertussis was uncommon, but the incidence has been increasing significantly over the past 20 years. If a child is unimmunized, don't forget these two entities. Diphtheria causes grayish pseudomembranes (necrotic epithelium and inflammatory exudate) on the pharynx, tonsils, and uvula as well as myocarditis. Pertussis is associated with severe paroxysmal coughing and a high-pitched whooping inspiratory noise (traditionally called "whooping cough"), particularly in children and especially those under 1 year of age. Treat diphtheria with antitoxin and either penicillin or erythromycin. Treat pertussis with azithromycin or erythromycin.

52. **In what clinical scenario does rabies occur in the United States? Describe the classic physical findings.**

    Rabies in the United States is due to bites from bats, skunks, raccoons, or foxes; rabies due to bites from dogs is rare due to vaccination. The incubation period is usually around 1 to 2 months. The classic findings are hydrophobia (fear of water due to painful swallowing) and central nervous system (CNS) signs (e.g., paralysis).

53. **What should you do after a patient is bitten by an animal?**

    1. Treat the local wound. Cleanse thoroughly with soap. Do *not* cauterize or suture the wound. Amoxicillin-clavulanate is often given for cellulitis prophylaxis.
    2. Observe the animal. If possible, capture and observe the dog or cat to see if it develops rabies. If a wild animal is caught, it should be killed and the brain tissue examined for rabies.
    3. If the wild animal escapes or has rabies, give rabies immunoglobulin and vaccinate the patient. In cases of a dog or cat bite, do *not* give prophylaxis or vaccine unless the animal acted strangely or bit the patient without provocation and rabies is prevalent in the area (rare). Do not give prophylaxis or vaccine for rabbit or small rodent bites (e.g., rats, mice, squirrels, chipmunks).

54. **What are the two main infections caused by *S. pyogenes* (group A streptococci)? What are the common sequelae?**

    S. pyogenes causes pharyngitis and skin infections. Sequelae include rheumatic fever, scarlet fever, and postinfectious glomerulonephritis.

55. **How does streptococcal pharyngitis present? How do you diagnosis and treat it?**

    Look for sore throat with fever, tonsillar exudate, enlarged tender cervical nodes, and leukocytosis. A positive streptococcal throat culture confirms the diagnosis. Elevated titers of antistreptolysin O (ASO) and anti-DNase antibody can be used for a retrospective diagnosis in patients with rheumatic fever or postinfectious glomerulonephritis. Treat streptococcal pharyngitis with penicillin, amoxicillin, cephalosporin, macrolide, or clindamycin to avoid rheumatic fever and scarlet fever.

56. **What are the major and minor Jones criteria for rheumatic fever? Why is rheumatic fever less common today?**

    The five major Jones criteria include migratory polyarthritis, carditis, CNS involvement (chorea), erythema marginatum, and subcutaneous nodules. The minor Jones criteria include fever, arthralgia, elevation in erythrocyte sedimentation rate or C-reactive protein (CRP), and prolonged PR interval on electrocardiogram (ECG). The diagnosis of rheumatic fever requires a history of streptococcal infection and the presence of two of the major criteria or one major criterion plus two minor criteria. Treatment of streptococcal pharyngitis with antibiotics markedly reduces the incidence of rheumatic fever, thus it is less common today. Give all patients affected by rheumatic fever endocarditis prophylaxis before surgical procedures.

57. **How do you recognize postinfectious glomerulonephritis? How is it treated?**

    Postinfectious glomerulonephritis occurs most commonly after a streptococcal skin infection, but it also may occur after pharyngitis. Patients are usually children and generally present with a history of infection with a nephritogenic strain of *Streptococcus* species 1 to 3 weeks earlier and abrupt onset of hematuria, proteinuria (mild, not in nephrotic range), red blood cell casts, hypertension, edema (especially periorbital), and elevated blood urea nitrogen and creatinine. Treat supportively. Control blood pressure and use diuretics for severe edema. Treatment of streptococcal infections does not reduce the incidence of poststreptococcal glomerulonephritis.

58. **Distinguish between impetigo and erysipelas.**

    Both are superficial skin infections due to streptococci or *S. aureus* and often occur after a break in the skin (e.g., trauma, scabies, insect bite). **Impetigo** (Fig. 20.6) classically changes first from maculopapules to vesicopustules and bullae and then to honey-colored, crusted lesions. Staphylococci are a more frequent cause than streptococci. Definitely think of staphylococci if a furuncle or carbuncle is present; think of streptococci if glomerulonephritis develops. Impetigo is contagious; watch for sick contacts. If there are a limited number of lesions without bullae, topical mupirocin may be used. If there are bullous or many lesions, treat with dicloxacillin, cephalexin, or clindamycin. **Erysipelas** (Fig. 20.9) is a superficial cellulitis (it involves the upper dermis and superficial lymphatics) that appears red, shiny, and swollen; it is tender and may be associated with vesicles and bullae, fever, and lymphadenopathy. Erysipelas typically has well-demarcated and raised borders. Treat with penicillin or amoxicillin, though erysipelas may require parenteral therapy with a cephalosporin (ceftriaxone or cefazolin) if systemic symptoms such as fever and chills are present.

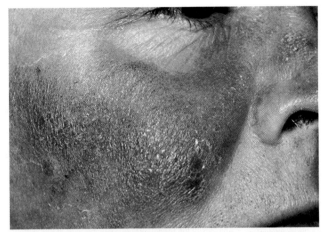

Fig. 20.9 Sharply defined erythema and edema, characteristic of erysipelas. (From Zaoutis LB, Chiang VW. *Comprehensive Pediatric Hospital Medicine.* 1st ed. Philadelphia, PA: Elsevier; 2007 [fig. 156-2].)

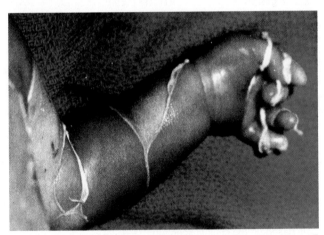

Fig. 20.10 Scalded appearance from widespread desquamation seen in staphylococcal scalded skin syndrome. (From Baren JM, Rothrock SG, Brennan J, et al. *Pediatric Emergency Medicine.* 1st ed. Philadelphia, PA: Saunders; 2007 [fig. 126-4].)

59. **What organisms typically cause cellulitis? What special circumstances should make you think of atypical causes?**
Streptococci and staphylococci cause most cases. Think of *Pseudomonas* species with burns or severe trauma, of *Pasteurella multocida* after dog or cat bites (treat with ampicillin), of *Vibrio vulnificus* in fishermen or other patients exposed to saltwater (treat with tetracycline). Diabetic patients with foot ulcers tend to have polymicrobial infections and need powerful broad-spectrum antibiotic coverage.

60. **Describe the physical findings of cellulitis.**
In patients with cellulitis, the involved overlying skin is red, hot, and frequently tender. It looks like erysipelas but involves deeper dermis and subcutaneous fat. Antibiotic selection depends on whether the cellulitis is purulent or nonpurulent. These are newer terms and are designations within the 2011 Infectious Diseases Society of America clinical practice guidelines for methicillin-resistant *Staphylococcus aureus* (MRSA). The idea is that a purulent infection may be caused by *S. aureus.* Oral treatment options for purulent cellulitis are trimethoprim-sulfamethoxazole, doxycycline, clindamycin, and linezolid. Oral treatment options for nonpurulent cellulitis are dicloxacillin, cephalexin, and clindamycin.

61. **Define necrotizing fasciitis. How is it treated?**
Necrotizing fasciitis is defined as the progression of cellulitis to necrosis and gangrene, which can quickly become limb and life threatening. Watch for crepitus and signs of systemic toxicity (e.g., tachycardia, fever, and hypotension). Often

multiple organisms are involved (aerobes and anaerobes). Treat with IV fluids, aggressive surgical debridement, and broad-spectrum antibiotics. This includes a carbapenem (imipenem or meropenem) plus clindamycin plus vancomycin.

62. What is the most common cause of endometritis (puerperal fever)? How do you recognize and treat it?
Consider endometritis, an infection of the endometrial lining, in any postpartum woman with a fever. The hallmarks are uterine tenderness and purulent lochia, and the most common cause is *Streptococcus* species, though it is often polymicrobial. Treat with clindamycin plus gentamicin after getting local cultures.

63. What infection in neonates is caused by *Streptococcus agalactiae* (group B streptococci)?
Streptococcus agalactiae is the most common cause of neonatal meningitis or sepsis. The organism is often part of normal vaginal flora and may be acquired from the birth canal. Group B streptococci are penicillin sensitive. Expectant mothers are cultured for group B strep, and if it is present around the time of delivery, then prophylactic IV penicillin (preferred) or IV ampicillin is given to the mother to prevent meningitis in the newborn.

64. Other than pneumonia, what infections does *S. pneumoniae* commonly cause?
Otitis media, meningitis, sinusitis, and spontaneous bacterial peritonitis.

65. What are the main infections caused by *S. aureus*?
The list is long. *S. aureus* is a common cause of the following infections:
- Skin and soft tissue abscesses (especially in the breast after breastfeeding or in the skin after a furuncle)
- Endocarditis (especially in drug users)
- Osteomyelitis (the most common cause unless sickle cell disease is present)
- Septic arthritis
- Infection of prosthetic material (e.g., grafts, shunts, orthopedic devices)
- Food poisoning (via a preformed toxin)
- Toxic shock syndrome (via a preformed toxin)
- Scalded skin syndrome (via a preformed toxin; affects younger children who often present with impetigo, then desquamate) (Fig. 20.10)
- Impetigo
- Cellulitis
- Wound infections
- Pneumonia (often forms lung abscess or empyema)
- Furuncles and carbuncles

66. What is the treatment of choice for staphylococcal infections on the USMLE?
An antistaphylococcal penicillin (e.g., methicillin, dicloxacillin). Use vancomycin, clindamycin, doxycycline, trimethoprim-sulfamethoxazole, daptomycin, or linezolid if the staphylococcal species is known to be methicillin resistant or if MRSA is suspected. MRSA is a rapidly growing problem. Most abscesses (regardless of the causative organism) must be treated first with surgical incision and drainage because antibiotics cannot penetrate through the walls of an abscess cavity.

67. Cover up the right-hand column in the following table, then describe the preferred treatment for tuberculosis based on the clinical scenario.

Clinical Setting/Findings	Treatment
Exposed adult with negative PPD skin test	None
Exposed child <5 years old with negative PPD	Isoniazid (INH) for 3 mo, then repeat PPD
Treatment for PPD conversion (negative to positive), no active disease	INH for 9 mo
Active pulmonary disease/positive culture	INH/rifampin/pyrazinamide/ethambutol for 2 mo, then INH/rifampin for 4 mo in most patients

PPD, Purified protein derivative.

68. Name some other important tuberculosis treatment issues.
- Multidrug-resistant strains are an increasing problem and require four-drug therapy (pyrazinamide, isoniazid, ethambutol, and rifampin) in most circumstances.
- If the patient is nonadherent, directly observed therapy (someone watches the patient take medications every day) is recommended.
- Consider supplementation with vitamin B_6 (pyridoxine) for patients on isoniazid (INH), or watch for signs of deficiency, such as neuropathy, confusion, angular cheilitis, or a seborrheic dermatitis-like rash.
- Watch for liver dysfunction in patients on therapy. Patients should be advised to abstain from alcohol while on treatment and should have their transaminase levels monitored.

CHAPTER 21

LABORATORY MEDICINE

1. In the table are the standard reference ranges for common laboratory values used on the USMLE Step 2 exam. These values (and more) will be provided for you on test day, but knowing the acceptable ranges for common labs will save you precious time during your exam

Study Ordered	Blood, Plasma, Serum	Reference Range
Basic metabolic panel (BMP)	Sodium (Na$^+$)	136–145 mEq/L
	Chloride (Cl$^-$)	95–105 mEq/L
	Potassium (K$^+$)	3.5–5 mEq/L
	Bicarbonate (HCO$_3^-$)	22–28 mEq/L
	Blood urea nitrogen (BUN)	7–18 mg/dL
	Creatinine (Cr)	0.6–1.2 mg/dL
	Glucose	70–110 mg/dL (fasting)
Liver function tests (LFTs)	Alanine aminotransferase (ALT)	8–20 U/L
	Aspartate aminotransferase (AST)	8–20 U/L
	Bilirubin (total)	0.1–1 mg/dL
	Bilirubin (direct/conjugated)	0–0.3 mg/dL
	Alkaline phosphatase (ALP)	20–70 U/L
	Albumin	3.5–5.5 g/dL
	Total protein	6–7.8 g/dL
Arterial blood gas (ABG)	pH	7.35–7.45
	PaCO$_2$	33–45 mmHg
	Bicarbonate (HCO$_3^-$)	22–28 mEq/L
	PaO$_2$	75–105 mmHg
Complete blood count (CBC)	Leukocyte count (WBCs)	4500–11,000/mm^3
	Platelet count	150,000–400,000/mm^3
	Hemoglobin (Hb)	Male: 13.5–17.5 g/dL Female: 12–16 g/dL
	Hematocrit (Hct)	Male: 41%–53% Female: 36%–46%
Coagulation panel	Bleeding time	2–7 min
	Activated partial thromboplastin time (aPTT)	25–40 sec
	Prothrombin time (PT)	11–15 sec
	International normalized ratio (INR)	2–3 target therapeutic range when on anticoagulants

2. **What may cause a false lab report of hyperkalemia?**
Hemolysis of the blood sample. Remember that potassium is mainly intracellular, so if a blood sample sits out for too long before being processed, cell lysis will occur and cause a falsely elevated value. Repeat the test if a high value doesn't make sense (e.g., hyperkalemia reported by the lab with no peaked T waves, lengthened PR interval, or QRS widening seen on electrocardiogram).

3. **Which electrolyte abnormality may mimic the ascending muscle weakness typically associated with Guillain-Barré syndrome?**
Hyperkalemia. Sphincter tone and cranial nerve function will remain intact, which may be useful to distinguish these patients from patients with Guillain-Barré syndrome experiencing acute diarrhea and oculomotor or facial nerve palsies. Unlike patients with Guillain-Barré syndrome, patients with hyperkalemia are **not** at risk of respiratory muscle weakness. Resolve the hyperkalemia and you will resolve the weakness.

4. **What conditions may cause a "false" hyponatremia (pseudohyponatremia)?**
Pseudohyponatremia may be caused by hyperglycemia, hyperproteinemia (e.g., multiple myeloma), or hyperlipidemia. The apparent hyponatremia will resolve with correction of the abnormal glucose, protein, or lipid levels. You can determine if the hyponatremia is true (hypotonic hyponatremia) or pseudo (isotonic hyponatremia) by measuring the plasma osmolality. Causes of true hyponatremia may be investigated by assessing extracellular volume status.

5. **What adverse event may result from rapid correction of hyponatremia?**
Osmotic demyelination syndrome (formerly called central pontine myelinolysis), which can present with dysarthria, paresis, behavioral disturbances, lethargy, confusion, coma, and death. These symptoms are typically irreversible. There is greater risk for this complication when attempting to correct chronic hyponatremia. In general, you should not give hypertonic saline (3% NaCl) to correct hyponatremia except in severe or symptomatic cases, and then it should be given only in limited quantities.

6. **What adverse events may result from rapid correction of hypernatremia?**
Cerebral edema and potentially life-threatening herniation, as the aggressive administration of relatively hypotonic fluids may cause free water to shift out of the vasculature, across the blood-brain barrier, and into the surrounding tissue. When considering the potentially harmful effects of rapidly correcting abnormally high or abnormally low serum sodium levels, remember the mnemonic "**from low to high the pons will die** (ODS); **from high to low the brain will blow** (cerebral edema and herniation)."

7. **Which electrolyte abnormality is associated with the Chvostek sign and Trousseau sign? Describe the maneuvers that elicit each sign**
Hypocalcemia is associated with Chvostek and Trousseau signs, due to latent tetany and neuromuscular irritability. The **Ch**vostek sign is elicited by tapping the patient's **ch**eek, causing contraction of ipsilateral facial muscles due to facial nerve stimulation. The Trousseau sign is elicited by overinflating a sphygmomanometer for at least 3 minutes to induce relative ischemia, increasing local nerve excitability and causing carpal spasm of the wrist and digits. Trousseau sign is considered to be more sensitive for hypocalcemia than the Chvostek sign.

8. **How is the serum anion gap calculated? In what clinical scenario should a serum anion gap be calculated?**
The serum anion gap is calculated by subtracting the two main anionic electrolytes (Cl^- and HCO_3^-) from the main cationic electrolyte, sodium (Na^+). While exact thresholds vary between clinical sites, a **serum anion gap greater than 12 mEq/L** is considered abnormal for USMLE purposes. Calculate the serum anion gap when investigating the etiology of metabolic acidosis. Use the mnemonic **MUDPILES** to remember the commonly tested etiologies of anion gap metabolic acidosis:

M—methanol (commonly also presents with vision problems)
U—uric acid
D—diabetic ketoacidosis
P—polyethylene glycol
I—iron toxicity, isoniazid
L—lactate (e.g., seizures, ischemic bowel, metformin toxicity)
E—ethylene glycol (commonly also presents with acute renal dysfunction)
S—salicylates

9. **What effect does serum acid-base status have on potassium and calcium levels?**
In the setting of serum alkalosis, patients may experience hypokalemia and symptoms of hypocalcemia (perioral numbness, tetany), whereas serum acidosis may cause hyperkalemia. Correction of acid-base status will correct the potassium and calcium derangements. If you find it difficult to remember the effects of acidosis vs. alkalosis, remember that serum levels of potassium and calcium will mimic the change in H^+ ions. Low serum levels of H^+ ions (alkalosis) will lead to low serum levels of potassium and calcium, while high serum levels of H^+ ions (acidosis) will lead to elevated potassium levels due to cellular shift.

10. Besides pancreatic disease, what other pathologies may cause elevated levels of amylase and/or lipase?

Damage to the salivary glands or bowel, renal failure, and ruptured tubal pregnancy may cause elevations in amylase and/or lipase. Elevation of both amylase and lipase in the same patient, however, is usually due to pancreatitis. Your exam may try to trick you with an isolated elevation of amylase; be sure to confirm the presence of elevated lipase as well before jumping to a pancreatic-related diagnosis.

11. Which diseases can cause elevated levels of alkaline phosphatase? What additional lab tests may be used to distinguish among these diseases?

Alkaline phosphatase may be elevated in biliary disease, bone disease, or pregnancy (the placenta produces alkaline phosphatase). If the elevation is due to biliary disease, gamma-glutamyltranspeptidase (GGT; also called gamma-glutamyltransferase) and/or 5'-nucleotidase (5'-NT) will also be elevated. In bone disease and pregnancy, however, GGT and 5'-NT will be within normal limits.

12. True or False: Hypothyroidism can cause elevated cholesterol

True. This is primarily due to reduced LDL-receptor activity, as T3 naturally plays a role in regulating HMG-CoA reductase activity. Thyroid hormone replacement will correct the elevated cholesterol.

13. Injury to what organ (other than the heart) causes elevated levels of creatine kinase (CK)?

Skeletal muscle. Watch for trauma, burns, and rhabdomyolysis. HMG-CoA reductase inhibitors (statins) may cause muscle damage, especially if combined with fibrate medications such as gemfibrozil or CYP3A4 inhibitors such as cyclosporine, macrolide antibiotics, systemic azole antifungals, or protease inhibitors. Neuroleptic malignant syndrome (NMS) caused by antipsychotic medications may also present with elevated CK levels.

14. Explain the relationship between low serum levels of potassium and calcium with low serum levels of magnesium?

If a patient has refractory hypokalemia or idiopathic hypocalcemia, check the serum magnesium level. These deficiencies may be due to hypomagnesemia, as magnesium has been shown to prevent renal potassium wasting and indirectly maintains serum calcium levels by regulating parathyroid hormone receptor responsiveness. If hypomagnesemia is present, it is often impossible to correct the hypokalemia or hypocalcemia until you correct the hypomagnesemia.

15. Which two electrolytes are classically depleted in the setting of diabetic ketoacidosis and hyperosmolar hyperglycemic state?

Potassium and phosphorus.

16. What does a BUN-to-creatinine ratio greater than 15 or 20 generally imply?

Prerenal acute kidney injury (AKI) caused by dehydration.

17. What measurements are included in an "iron study"?

Serum ferritin, serum iron, and total iron-binding capacity (TIBC; also referred to as the transferrin level) are directly measured in an iron study. Transferrin saturation (TSAT) is calculated by dividing serum iron by TIBC and converting the result into a percentage (i.e., multiplying by 100%). Be careful not to mistake transferrin level (TIBC – a measured value) with transferrin saturation (TSAT – a calculated percentage).

18. What disease classically causes a false-positive result on the rapid plasma reagin (RPR) or Venereal Disease Research Laboratory (VDRL) syphilis test?

Systemic lupus erythematosus (SLE). A false-positive result on the RPR or VDRL test is actually one of the diagnostic criteria for SLE.

19. What does an elevated erythrocyte sedimentation rate mean in pregnancy?

Nothing of clinical significance. This is a normal finding in pregnancy (i.e., it is not a useful test to order in an otherwise healthy pregnant patient).

20. True or False: Renal disease should be suspected in a pregnant patient despite normal serum levels of BUN or creatinine

True. BUN and creatinine are decreased significantly in pregnancy after the first trimester in women with normal renal function. Serum levels within normal limits during pregnancy may indicate relatively impaired kidney function.

21. Why do pregnant patients often develop anemia as their pregnancy progresses?

During pregnancy the mother's erythrocyte cell mass increases, but her plasma volume increases to a greater degree. This gives a relative dilutional anemia (also called physiologic anemia), which will present as a reduced hemoglobin concentration despite the increased red blood cell (RBC) production.

22. How can iron-deficiency anemia be distinguished from physiologic anemia during pregnancy?

The single best lab test to distinguish these two anemias during pregnancy is serum ferritin. Consider calculating the transferrin saturation (TSAT) if serum ferritin is within normal limits but there is high clinical suspicion for iron-deficiency anemia. However, remember that iron supplements may falsely elevate TSAT (i.e., falsely appearing to be normal when in fact TSAT is low). Although iron-deficiency anemia is considered a microcytic anemia, microcytosis is typically a later-stage finding, meaning your pregnant patient with low-normal mean corpuscular volume (MCV) may actually be experiencing iron deficiency. Order a serum ferritin to confirm one way or the other.

23. What serum screening tests are performed during the first trimester of pregnancy?
Serum levels of beta-hCG and PAPP-A (pregnancy-associated plasma protein A) are measured during the first trimester.

24. When are the triple and quadruple screening tests performed during pregnancy? What do these tests measure?
The triple and quadruple screening tests are performed during the second trimester. The triple screen measures serum levels of hCG, alpha-fetoprotein (AFP), and estriol. The quadruple screen measures the same three as the triple screen, plus inhibin A (see Chapter 25 for further details).

25. Which three antibodies are typically tested for when suspecting antiphospholipid syndrome during pregnancy?
Anticardiolipin, anti-beta$_2$ glycoprotein I, and lupus anticoagulant.

26. Define isosthenuria. What condition does it suggest?
Isosthenuria is the inability to concentrate or dilute the urine. The specific gravity of urine and serum is the same—classically 1.010. Isosthenuria is often associated with sickle cell trait or disease.

27. How is the anion gap calculated for urinalysis? What is the clinical value of calculating a urine anion gap?
Urine anion gap is calculated by adding urine sodium levels to urine potassium levels, then subtracting urine chloride levels (urine $Na^+ + K^+ - Cl^-$). Calculating the urine anion gap is useful when investigating ammonium (NH_4^+) excretion in a patient with metabolic acidosis. A negative urine anion gap (more Cl^- in the urine than Na^+ and K^+ combined) suggests increased NH_4^+ excretion. In metabolic acidosis, this suggests chronic or large-volume diarrhea. A positive urine anion gap suggests low or normal NH_4^+ excretion; in metabolic acidosis, this would be expected in distal renal tubular acidosis (RTA).

28. How are hemoglobinuria and myoglobinuria distinguished from each other on urinalysis?
Both hemoglobinuria and myoglobinuria may present as a red urine sample with a positive urine dipstick test. Hemoglobinuria will have a significant number of RBCs in the urine while myoglobinuria will not. CK levels may also be increased in a setting of myoglobinuria but will be within normal limits for hemoglobinuria.

29. On the USMLE exams there are five classes of illicit substances commonly measured on a urine drug screen (UDS). Cover the table to see how many you can name, along with the various substances that may cause a false-positive result for each

Illicit Substance Measured on Urine Drug Screen	Substances Potentially Causing False-Positive Results
Amphetamines	Bupropion, selegiline, levodopa/carbidopa, atenolol, propranolol, pseudoephedrine, phenylephrine
Cannabis (THC)	Dronabinol, hemp-containing products
Cocaine	None—UDS is highly specific
Opioids	Poppy seeds
PCP (phencyclidine)	Tramadol, ketamine, dextromethorphan, diphenhydramine, venlafaxine, lamotrigine

30. Which substances of abuse (illicit or prescription) are not measured on a standard UDS?
Benzodiazepines, barbiturates, and LSD (lysergic acid diethylamide) are not typically included on a standard UDS. Synthetic or semisynthetic substances are also not typically captured on a standard UDS, meaning patients with signs and symptoms of acute intoxication but negative UDS may have used one of these substances instead.

31. In the table, cover the substances/presentation and identify the substances that may mimic the substance/presentation

Clinical Presentation or Suspected Intoxication	Substances That May Mimic the Intoxication
Amphetamine- or stimulant-like	MDMA (ecstasy), bath salts
Cannabis (THC)–like	Synthetic cannabinoids
Cocaine-like	None—UDS is highly sensitive
Opioid-like	Hydrocodone, oxycodone, hydromorphone, fentanyl, methadone, meperidine
PCP-like	None—UDS is highly sensitive

32. True or False: A positive urine drug screen indicates active substance intoxication
    False. This is an important concept that is often misunderstood by patients and clinicians alike. A positive screen indicates the presence of a substance or metabolite that reaches the lab's established threshold but does **not** necessarily reflect a state of intoxication or level of physiologic significance. For example, a patient exposed to an illicit substance may experience intoxication for a few hours but test positive on UDS for 3 to 7 days after the effects wear off. It just happens to still be in the patient's system at levels high enough to trigger a "positive" assay result. This is important to remember for your psychotic patient with UDS positive for cocaine or PCP. Be very, very careful that your first instinct does not cause you to miss a true case of encephalitis in a patient who happened to use cocaine or PCP earlier that week.

CHAPTER 22

NEPHROLOGY

1. **What are the signs and symptoms of acute kidney injury (AKI)?**

   Signs: increased blood urea nitrogen (BUN) and creatinine levels, metabolic acidosis, hyperkalemia, tachypnea (caused by acidosis and hypervolemia), and hypervolemia (bilateral rales on lung examination, elevated jugular venous pressure, dilutional hyponatremia)

   Symptoms: fatigue, nausea and vomiting, anorexia, shortness of breath, mental status changes, oliguria

2. **What are the three broad categories of AKI?**

   Prerenal, renal/intrarenal, and postrenal

3. **Define prerenal AKI. What are the causes? How do you recognize it?**

   In prerenal AKI, the kidney is not adequately perfused. The most common cause is hypovolemia (dehydration, hemorrhage). Look for a BUN-to-creatinine ratio greater than 20 and signs of hypovolemia (e.g., tachycardia, weak pulse, depressed fontanelle). Fractional excretion of sodium (FeNa) will be less than 1% (as the body tries to retain sodium). Give intravenous (IV) fluids and/or blood. Other common prerenal causes are sepsis (treat the sepsis and give IV fluids), heart failure (give inotropes and diuretics), liver failure (hepatorenal syndrome; trial an albumin challenge followed by octreotide/midodrine to maintain renal perfusion), and renal artery stenosis.

4. **Define postrenal AKI. What causes it?**

   In postrenal AKI, urine is blocked from being excreted at some point beyond the kidneys (ureters, prostate, urethra). The most common cause is benign prostatic hyperplasia (BPH). Patients are men over age 50 with BPH symptoms (e.g., hesitancy, dribbling, weak stream, nocturia); ultrasound demonstrates bilateral hydronephrosis. Additional scenarios may include females with complicated gynecologic history (e.g., recent cesarean section with ureter transection). Treat with catheterization (suprapubic, if necessary) or urologic intervention (e.g., nephrostomy tube) to relieve the obstruction and prevent further renal damage. Alpha-blockers (e.g., terazosin) or a 5-alpha-reductase inhibitor (e.g., finasteride) can improve the symptoms, and surgery should be considered (transurethral resection of the prostate). Other causes are nephrolithiasis (but remember that stones generally have to be bilateral to cause renal failure), retroperitoneal fibrosis (watch for a history of radiation therapy or methysergide, bromocriptine, methyldopa, or hydralazine use), and pelvic/intraabdominal malignancies.

5. **What is the most common cause of intrarenal AKI?**

   Intrarenal AKI, which results from a problem within the kidney itself, is most commonly due to **acute tubular necrosis** from various causes.

6. **What do you need to know about intravenous contrast and acute kidney injury?**

   IV contrast can precipitate AKI, usually in diabetic patients and patients with preexisting renal disease. Avoid contrast in such patients, if possible. If you must give IV contrast, administer IV hydration before and after the contrast is given, and avoid the use of nonsteroidal antiinflammatory drugs (NSAIDs) to decrease the chance of AKI. The data on the use of acetylcysteine are conflicting.

7. **True or False: Muscle breakdown can cause acute kidney injury**

   True. Myoglobinuria or rhabdomyolysis due to strenuous exercise (e.g., running marathons), alcohol, burns, muscle trauma, muscle compression (e.g., prolonged immobilization after a fall), seizure activity, heat stroke, and neuroleptic malignant syndrome may cause AKI. The cellular debris that results from muscle breakdown plugs the renal filtration system, and myoglobin breakdown products are directly nephrotoxic. Look for very high levels of creatine phosphokinase (CPK). Urinalysis may reveal red urine that is positive for blood on dipstick (caused by the heme contained in myoglobin) but has no red blood cells. Treat with aggressive hydration. Alkalinization of the urine (with bicarbonate) may be helpful in severe cases. Diuretics may be helpful if the patient develops volume overload but have not been shown to be useful in preventing AKI. Monitor calcium and potassium levels carefully during treatment of rhabdomyolysis.

8. **What medications commonly cause AKI renal failure?**

   Chronic use of NSAIDs may cause acute tubular necrosis, acute interstitial nephritis, or papillary necrosis; additionally, consider cyclosporine, aminoglycosides, and methicillin.

9. **Define nephritic syndrome. What is the classic cause? How is it treated?**
Nephritic syndrome is generally defined as oliguria, azotemia (rising BUN/creatinine), hypertension, and hematuria. The patient may have some degree of proteinuria but not in the nephrotic range. The classic cause is poststreptococcal glomerulonephritis (PSGN). Treatment is supportive and includes control of hypertension and maintenance of urine output with IV fluids and diuretics.

10. **Define Goodpasture syndrome. How does it present?**
Goodpasture syndrome (a cause of rapidly progressive glomerulonephritis [RPGN]) is due to the presence of measurable antiglomerular basement membrane antibodies, which cause a linear immunofluorescence pattern on renal biopsy. These antibodies react with and damage both the kidneys and the lungs. Look for a young man with hemoptysis, dyspnea, and renal failure. Treat with steroids and cyclophosphamide.

11. **Define granulomatosis with polyangiitis. How does it present?**
Granulomatosis with polyangiitis is a vasculitis that also affects the lungs and kidneys. Look for nasal involvement (bloody nose, nasal perforation, saddle nose deformity) or hemoptysis and pleurisy as presenting symptoms, along with renal disease. Patients test positive for **antineutrophil cytoplasmic antibody (ANCA)** titers (specifically, c-ANCA/PR3-ANCA). Treat with cyclophosphamide and glucocorticoids. Methotrexate is an alternative.

12. **How do you recognize PSGN? How is it treated?**
PSGN occurs most commonly after a streptococcal skin infection but may also occur after pharyngitis. Patients are usually children (although older age is a predictor of poorer outcomes) and generally have a history of infection with a nephritogenic strain of *Streptococcus* species 1 to 3 weeks previously and abrupt onset of edema (especially periorbital), hypertension, proteinuria (mild, not in the nephrotic range), hematuria (red blood cell casts), and elevated BUN and creatinine. Red blood cell casts on urinalysis confirm the diagnosis of nephritic syndrome. Laboratory tests that support a PSGN diagnosis include proof of recent streptococcal infection (e.g., antistreptolysin O and antiDNAse B titers) and evidence of complement-mediated glomerular inflammation (low C3 and C4 levels).
Treat supportively. Control blood pressure and use diuretics for severe edema. Unlike rheumatic fever, treatment of the initial streptococcal infection does not reduce the incidence of PSGN. Nonetheless, any residual infection should be treated with antibiotics. Another nephritic condition, IgA nephropathy (Berger syndrome), can occur within 1 to 2 days of an upper respiratory tract infection or viral pharyngitis and is hence termed *synpharyngitic*. The differentiation on the USMLE would be the delay of only a few days from pharyngitis to nephritic syndrome in IgA nephropathy versus the delay of a few weeks for PSGN.

13. **What are the indications for dialysis in patients with renal failure?**
When renal failure is present, first try to determine the cause and fix it, if possible, to correct the renal failure. Indications for acute dialysis are remembered by the mnemonic **AEIOU**: **a**cidosis (severe metabolic, roughly a pH <7.2), **e**lectrolytes (hyperkalemia, typically >6.5 mEq/L or rapidly rising potassium levels), **i**ngestion of a dialyzable drug or toxin, **o**verload, and **u**remia (includes uremic pericarditis or encephalopathy).

14. **Define nephrotic syndrome. What causes it? How is it diagnosed?**
Nephrotic syndrome is defined by proteinuria (>3.5 g/day), hypoalbuminemia, edema (the classic pattern is morning periorbital edema), and hyperlipidemia with lipiduria. In children it is usually due to minimal change disease (podocytes with missing "feet" on electron microscopy), which is most commonly idiopathic but also follows infections or is associated with underlying malignancy. Measure 24-hour urine protein or spot urine protein-to-creatinine ratio to confirm the diagnosis. Treat with steroids. Causes in adults include membranous nephropathy, diabetes, hepatitis B and C, HIV, amyloidosis, lupus erythematosus, and drugs (e.g., penicillamine, captopril).

15. **What causes chronic kidney disease (CKD)?**
Any of the causes of acute renal failure can cause CKD if the insult is severe or prolonged. Most cases of CKD are due to diabetes mellitus (leading cause) or hypertension (second most common cause). A popular cause on the Step 2 exam is polycystic kidney disease (PKD). Watch for multiple cysts in the kidney, and look for a positive family history (usually autosomal dominant; the autosomal recessive form presents in children), hypertension, hematuria, palpable renal masses, berry aneurysms in the circle of Willis, and cysts in liver (Fig. 22.1).

16. **What metabolic derangements are seen in end-stage renal disease (ESRD)?**
   - Azotemia (high levels of BUN and creatinine)
   - Metabolic acidosis
   - Hyperkalemia
   - Fluid retention (may cause hypertension, edema, congestive heart failure, and pulmonary edema)
   - Hypocalcemia and hyperphosphatemia (impaired vitamin D production with secondary hyperparathyroidism; bone loss leads to renal osteodystrophy). Treat with phosphorus binders (sevelamer), vitamin D repletion (calcitriol), and parathyroid hormone–lowering therapy (cinacalcet).
   - Anemia (due to lack of erythropoietin; give synthetic erythropoietin to correct)
   - Anorexia, nausea, vomiting (from buildup of toxins)

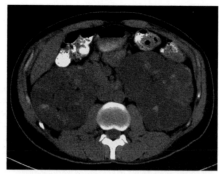

Fig. 22.1 This noncontrast computed tomography image demonstrates autosomal dominant polycystic kidney disease. The kidneys are markedly enlarged bilaterally with multiple low-density cysts throughout both kidneys. The little remaining renal parenchyma is noted by the sparse higher density material squeezed by the cysts. (From Brenner B. *Brenner and Rector's The Kidney.* 8th ed. Philadelphia: Saunders; 2008 [fig. 27.30].)

- Central nervous system disturbances (mental status changes and even convulsions or coma from toxin buildup; dialysis disequilibrium syndrome with seizures can occur from rapid correction of BUN during hemodialysis)
- Bleeding (due to uremic platelet dysfunction)
- Uremic pericarditis (friction rub may be heard)
- Skin pigmentation and pruritus (skin turns yellowish-brown and itches because of metabolic by-products)
- Increased susceptibility to infection (due to decreased cellular immunity)

17. **How is ESRD treated?**
    Treat renal failure with regular hemodialysis (usually three times/week), water-soluble vitamins (which are removed during dialysis), phosphate restriction and binders (calcium carbonate, calcium acetate, or sevelamer), erythropoietin as needed, and hypertension control. The only cure is renal transplant.

18. **What are the signs and symptoms of urinary tract infection (UTI)? What are the most likely organisms?**
    Signs and symptoms include urgency, dysuria, suprapubic and/or low back pain, and low-grade fever. UTIs are usually caused by *Escherichia coli* (75%–85% of cases) but may also be caused by *Staphylococcus saprophyticus* or *Proteus, Pseudomonas, Klebsiella, Enterobacter,* and/or *Enterococcus* species (or other enteric organisms). Patients who acquire UTIs in the hospital or from a chronic indwelling Foley catheter are more likely to have organisms other than *E. coli.* While rare, if urinary cultures grow *S. aureus,* the patient should receive repeat urinary cultures as well as assessment for bacteremia/endocarditis with blood cultures and transthoracic echocardiography.

19. **What factors increase the likelihood of UTIs?**
    Female gender and conditions that promote urinary stasis (BPH, pregnancy, stones, neurogenic bladder, vesicoureteral reflux) or bacterial colonization (indwelling catheter, fecal incontinence, surgical instrumentation) predispose to UTI.

20. **How do you diagnose and treat UTIs?**
    The gold standard for diagnosis is a positive urine culture with at least 100,000 colony-forming units (measure of bacterial load) of specific bacteria. At the least, get a midstream sample; the best method is a catheterized sample or suprapubic tap. Urinalysis shows white blood cells, bacteria (on Gram stain of the urine), positive leukocyte esterase, and/or positive nitrite.
    Empiric treatment is usually based on symptoms and urinalysis while awaiting culture results. Commonly used antibiotics include trimethoprim-sulfamethoxazole, amoxicillin, nitrofurantoin, ciprofloxacin, or a first-generation cephalosporin for about 5 days.

21. **Why are UTIs in children and males of special concern?**
    In children, a UTI is cause for concern because it may be the presenting symptom of a genitourinary malformation. The most common examples are vesicoureteral reflux and posterior urethral valves. Urine culture should be obtained. Order an ultrasound and either a voiding cystourethrogram (VCUG) or radionuclide cystogram (RNC) to evaluate the urinary tract in any child 2 months to 2 years with a first UTI. Recommendations for imaging in older children are less clear cut.
    If a male has symptoms and a urinalysis suggestive of a UTI, consider the possibility of prostatitis (the prostate may be tender and boggy on exam). Bacterial prostatitis requires 6 weeks of antibiotics to ensure eradication.

22. **True or False:** You should treat asymptomatic bacteriuria in most patients
    False. The exception is the pregnant patient, in whom asymptomatic bacteriuria is treated because of the high risk of progression to pyelonephritis. Use antibiotics that are safe in pregnancy, such as penicillins. Patients undergoing urologic procedures should also be treated to avoid translocation of bacteria from mucosal damage.

23. **How does pyelonephritis usually occur? What are the signs and symptoms? How is it treated?**
    Pyelonephritis is most often due to an ascending UTI caused by *E. coli* (>80% of cases). Patients present with high fever, shaking chills, costovertebral angle tenderness, flank pain, and/or UTI symptoms. Order urinalysis and urine and blood cultures to establish the diagnosis. If the patient cannot tolerate oral antibiotics, the patient should be admitted for IV antibiotics, typically IV ceftriaxone or fluoroquinolones. Outpatient management in uncomplicated pyelonephritis typically consists of an oral fluoroquinolone. Always choose an antibiotic regimen with good *E. coli* coverage. If the patient continues to have fevers, leukocytosis, or hemodynamic instability while being treated over 48 to 72 hours, consider imaging evaluation for a perinephric abscess.

24. **How do you differentiate among the common pediatric hematologic disorders that affect the kidney?**

	HUS	*HSP*	*TTP*	*ITP*
Most common age	Children	Children	Young adults	Children or adults
Previous infection	Diarrhea (*E. coli*)	URI	None	Viral (especially in children)
Red blood cell count	Low	Normal	Low	Normal
Platelet count	Low	Normal	Low	Low
Peripheral smear	Hemolysis	Normal	Hemolysis	Normal
Kidney effects	ARF, hematuria	Hematuria	ARF, proteinuria	None
Treatment	Supportive*	Supportive*	Plasmapheresis, NSAIDs; no platelets‡	Steroids,† splenectomy if drugs fail
Key differential points	Age, diarrhea	Rash, abdominal pain, arthritis, melena (Fig. 22.2)	CNS changes, age	Antiplatelet antibodies

ARF, Acute renal failure; *CNS,* central nervous system; *HSP,* Henoch-Schönlein purpura; *HUS,* hemolytic uremic syndrome; *ITP,* idiopathic thrombocytopenia; *NSAIDs,* nonsteroidal antiinflammatory drugs; *TTP,* thrombotic thrombocytopenic purpura; *URI,* upper respiratory infection.
*In HUS and HSP, patients may need dialysis and transfusions.
†Give steroids only if the patient is bleeding or platelet counts are very low (<20,000–30,000/μL).
‡Do not give platelet transfusions to patients with TTP; clots may form.

25. **Which is more likely to be seen on a plain abdominal radiograph: kidney stones or gallbladder stones?**
    Kidney stones (85%), which more commonly calcify (Fig. 22.3), are more likely to be seen than gallstones (15%).

26. **What are the signs and symptoms of renal stones? How are they diagnosed and treated?**
    Kidney stones (nephrolithiasis) generally present with severe, intermittent, unilateral flank and/or groin pain when the stone dislodges and gets stuck in the ureter (ureterolithiasis). Most stones can be seen on abdominal radiographs and are composed of calcium. Renal ultrasound or computed tomography (CT) scan can be used to detect a stone if clinical suspicion is high but plain abdominal radiographs are negative. Symptomatic urolithiasis should be treated with lots of hydration and pain control (to see if the stone will pass). Most stones less than 5 mm will pass on their own. If the stone does not pass, it needs to be removed surgically (preferably endoscopically) or by lithotripsy.

27. **What causes kidney stones?**
    Nephrolithiasis is often idiopathic, but on the Step 2 exam watch for one of the following underlying disorders that predispose to the development of kidney stones:
    Hypercalcemia: due to hyperparathyroidism or malignancy (calcium stones).
    Infection: from ammonia-producing bugs (*Proteus* spp., staphylococci). Look for **staghorn calculi** (large stones composed of magnesium, ammonia, and phosphate [struvite] that fill the renal calyceal system) (Fig. 22.4).

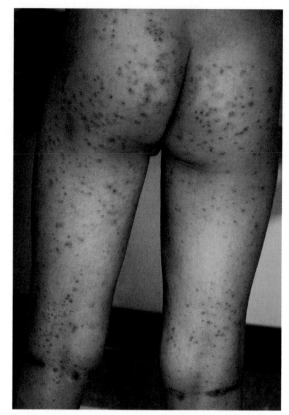

Fig. 22.2 Henoch-Schönlein purpura. Nonblanchable macules and papules on the buttocks and lower extremities. (From Taal M. *Brenner and Rector's The Kidney.* 9th ed. Philadelphia: Saunders; 2011 [fig. 59-20].)

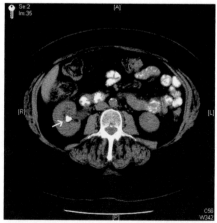

Fig. 22.3 Computed tomography image of a urinary calculus in the right kidney. All stones (with the exception of some medication calculi) appear as dense, white objects within the urinary collecting system. (From Wein AJ, Kavoussi LR, Novick AC, et al. *Campbell-Walsh Urology.* 9th ed. Philadelphia: Saunders; 2007 [fig. 43.2].)

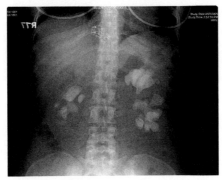

Fig. 22.4 Plain film of a patient with bilateral staghorn calculi composed entirely of struvite. This patient had a 15-year history of recurrent urinary tract infections. (From Wein AJ, Kavoussi LR, Novick AC, et al. *Campbell-Walsh Urology*. 9th ed. Philadelphia: Saunders; 2007 [fig. 43.9].)

Hyperuricemia: uric acid stones due to gout or leukemia treatment (allopurinol and IV hydration are given before leukemia chemotherapy to prevent this complication).

Cystinuria/aminoaciduria: should be suspected if the stone is made of cystine or you are presented with a repetitive stone-forming patient.

Note: Send any recovered stones to the lab for stone analysis to determine the type of stone.

CHAPTER 23

NEUROLOGY

1. In what common situation is a lumbar puncture contraindicated?

   With acute head trauma, intracranial hypertension (signs include papilledema), coagulopathy, suspicion for intracranial hemorrhage, or suspicion for a spinal epidural abscess. You should do a lumbar tap only after you have a negative computed tomography (CT) scan or magnetic resonance imaging (MRI) of the head in these settings. Otherwise you may cause uncal herniation and death.

2. Cover all but the left-hand column and describe the classic findings of cerebrospinal fluid (CSF) analysis in the following conditions

Condition	Appearance	Cells (mm)[a]	Glucose (mg/dL)	Protein (mg/dL)	Pressure (mm Hg)
Normal CSF	Clear	0–3 (L)	50–100	20–45	100–200
Bacterial meningitis	Clear, cloudy, or purulent	>1000 (PMN)	<50	Around 100	>200
Viral/aseptic meningitis	Clear	>100 (L)	Normal	Normal/ slightly increased	Normal/slightly increased
Pseudotumor cerebri	Clear	Normal	Normal	Normal	>200
Guillain-Barré syndrome[b]	Clear	0–100 (L)	Normal	>100	Normal
Cerebral hemorrhage[c]	Xanthochromia, bloody, or clear	Bloody (RBC)	Normal	>45	>200
Multiple sclerosis[d]	Clear	Normal/ slightly increased (L)	Normal	Normal/ slightly increased	Normal

Note: Tuberculous and fungal meningitis have low glucose (<50) with increased cells (>100), which are predominantly lymphocytes. In patients with fungal meningitis, a positive India ink preparation equals *Cryptococcus neoformans*.

[a]Main cell type is in parentheses after number (*L*, lymphocytes; *PMN*, neutrophils; *RBC*, red blood cells).

[b]Guillain-Barré syndrome is also known as albuminocytologic dissociation.

[c]Think of subarachnoid hemorrhage, but this pattern also may occur after an intracerebral bleed.

[d]On electrophoresis of CSF look for oligoclonal bands due to increased IgG production and an increased level of myelin basic protein in the CSF during active demyelination.

3. Give a classic case description of multiple sclerosis

   Multiple sclerosis classically presents with an insidious onset of neurologic symptoms in white women aged 20 to 40 years with exacerbations and remissions. Common presentations include paresthesias and numbness, weakness and clumsiness, visual disturbances (decreased vision and pain due to optic neuritis, diplopia due to cranial nerve involvement), gait disturbances, incontinence and urgency, and vertigo. Also look for emotional lability, other mental status changes, scanning speech (spoken words are broken into syllables separated by a noticeable pause with stress occasionally on the wrong syllable), and worsening of symptoms with hot showers. The patient may have a positive Babinski sign. The patient's symptoms do not follow a single neurologic lesion. Classic initial symptoms to recognize include:

   1. **Internuclear ophthalmoplegia:** a disorder of conjugate gaze in which the affected eye shows impairment of adduction.
   2. **Transverse myelitis:** a disorder in which one or more continuous segments of the spinal cord (most commonly thoracic) becomes inflamed, leading to a motor and sensory loss below the level of the lesion, autonomic dysfunction (bowel and bladder dysfunction), and eventual spastic paralysis and hyperreflexia.
   3. **Optic neuritis:** a disorder characterized by unilateral vision loss, eye pain with movement, afferent pupillary defect, and red color desaturation.

4. **What is the most sensitive test for diagnosis of multiple sclerosis? How is it treated?**
MRI is the most sensitive diagnostic tool and shows demyelination plaques in the periventricular white matter. Also look for increased IgG/oligoclonal bands and possibly myelin basic protein in the CSF. Treatment is not highly effective but includes interferon, glatiramer, mitoxantrone, natalizumab, cyclophosphamide, and methotrexate. Acute exacerbations are treated with glucocorticoids.

5. **Define Guillain-Barré syndrome (GBS)**
GBS is a postinfectious autoimmune polyneuropathy. Look for a history of mild infection, especially upper respiratory infection (*Campylobacter* infection is the most commonly identified precipitant of GBS), or immunization roughly 1 week before onset of symmetric, distal weakness or paralysis with mild paresthesias beginning in the feet and legs with loss of deep tendon reflexes in affected areas. The hallmark of the disease is that motor function is often affected with intact or only minimally impaired sensation. As the ascending paralysis or weakness progresses, respiratory paralysis may occur. Watch carefully; usually spirometry is done to follow inspiratory ability. Intubation may be required. Diagnosis is by clinical presentation. CSF shows markedly increased protein with normal white blood cell count (albuminocytologic dissociation). Nerve conduction velocities are slowed. The disease usually resolves spontaneously. Plasmapheresis (for adults) and intravenous (IV) immune globulin (for children) reduce the severity and length of disease. Do *not* use steroids; they no longer have a role in the treatment of GBS.

6. **What causes nerve conduction velocity to be slowed?**
Demyelination. Watch for GBS and multiple sclerosis as causes.

7. **What causes an electromyography (EMG) study to show fasciculations or fibrillations at rest?**
A lower motor neuron lesion (i.e., a peripheral nerve problem).

8. **What causes an EMG study with no muscle activity at rest and decreased amplitude of muscle contraction upon stimulation?**
Intrinsic muscle disease, such as the muscular dystrophies or inflammatory myopathies (e.g., polymyositis). You now know enough about EMG for the USMLE.

9. **What is the most common cause of syncope? What other conditions should you consider?**
Vasovagal syncope is the most common cause and is classically seen after stress or fear. Arrhythmias and orthostatic hypotension are also common. Always remember to consider hypoglycemia as a cause. The other main categories to worry about include:
    1. **Cardiac problems** (arrhythmias, hypertrophic cardiomyopathy, valvular disease, tamponade). Always check an electrocardiogram. Further testing with echocardiography or treadmill stress testing can be performed based upon the electrocardiogram findings and degree of suspicion for cardiac etiology for syncope.
    2. **Neurologic disorders** (e.g., seizures, migraine headache, brain tumor, stroke). Consider an electroencephalogram or CT/MRI if history suggests seizures or intracranial lesion.
    3. **Vascular disease** (consider transient ischemic attacks or carotid stenosis, which can be ruled out with carotid artery ultrasound/duplex scanning, though this is not a common cause of syncope).
    4. **Medication effects** (e.g., anticholinergic agents, beta-blockers, narcotics, vasodilators, alpha-agonists, antipsychotics).
    5. **Sleep disturbances** (e.g., narcolepsy and cataplexy).
       As many as half of patients have syncope of unknown cause after a standard diagnostic evaluation.

10. **Cover the right-hand column, and localize the neurologic lesion for each of the following signs and symptoms**

Symptom/Sign	Area
Decreased or no reflexes, fasciculations, atrophy	Lower motor neuron disease (or possibly muscle problem)
Hyperreflexia, clonus, increased muscle tone	Upper motor neuron lesion (cord or brain)
Apathy, inattention, disinhibition, labile affect	Frontal lobes
Broca (motor) aphasia	Dominant frontal lobe[a]
Wernicke (sensory) aphasia	Dominant temporal lobe[a]
Memory impairment, hyperaggression, hypersexuality	Temporal lobes
Inability to read, write, name, or do math	Dominant parietal lobe[a]

Symptom/Sign	Area
Ignoring one side of body, trouble with dressing	Nondominant parietal lobe[a]
Visual hallucinations/illusions	Occipital lobes
Cranial nerves 3 and 4	Midbrain
Cranial nerves 5, 6, 7, and 8	Pons
Cranial nerves 9, 10, 11, and 12	Medulla
Ataxia, dysarthria, nystagmus, intention, tremor, dysmetria, scanning speech, dysdiadochokinesia	Cerebellum

[a]The left side is dominant in more than 95% of population (99% of right-handed people and 60%–70% of left-handed people).

11. When evaluating a delirious or unconscious patient with no history of trauma, for what three common conditions should you think about giving empiric treatment?
    1. **Hypoglycemia** (give glucose)
    2. **Opioid overdose** (give naloxone)
    3. **Thiamine deficiency** (give thiamine before giving glucose in a suspected alcoholic)
       Other common causes are alcohol, illicit drugs, prescription drugs, diabetic ketoacidosis, stroke, and epilepsy or postictal state.

12. What are the classic differences between delirium and dementia?

	Delirium	Dementia
Onset	Acute and dramatic	Chronic and insidious
Common causes	Illness, toxin, withdrawal	Alzheimer disease, multiinfarct dementia, HIV/AIDS
Reversible	Usually	Usually not
Attention	Poor	Usually unaffected
Orientation	Impaired and fluctuating	Often normal but may be impaired
Arousal level	Fluctuates	Normal

13. What signs and symptoms do delirium and dementia have in common?
    Both may have hallucinations, illusions, delusions, memory impairment (usually global in delirium, whereas remote memory is spared in early dementia) and "sundowning" (worse at night). However, a new pattern of "sundowning" should be presumed to be delirium.

14. What is a differential diagnosis for dementia? What findings can help you distinguish between them?

Disease	Clinical Finding
Alzheimer dementia	Memory affected first and then personality and executive function (e.g., patient will get lost on the way to the grocery store)
Vascular dementia	Stepwise decrease in function; also usually has risk factors similar to stroke, such as smoking
Dementia with Lewy bodies	Parkinson symptoms plus dementia[1]
Frontotemporal dementia (Pick disease)	Personality and behavior first, then memory
Creutzfeldt-Jakob disease	Rapidly progressive dementia with myoclonus
Huntington disease	Chorea first and then dementia

Disease	Clinical Finding
Normal pressure hydrocephalus	"Wet, weird, and wobbly" (urinary incontinence, dementia, and ataxia)
Normal aging	Decreased executive function and decreased memory; however, preserved procedural memory and able to perform daily tasks

[1]In classic Parkinson disease, dementia symptoms do not occur until much later.

15. Define pseudodementia

    Depression can cause some clinical signs and symptoms of dementia, classically in the elderly. This type of "dementia" is reversible with treatment. Step 2 questions will give you other signs and symptoms of depression (e.g., sadness, loss of loved one, weight or appetite loss, suicidal ideation, poor sleep, feelings of worthlessness).

16. What treatable causes of dementia must always be ruled out?

    Vitamin B_{12} deficiency and hypothyroidism, for which the American Academy of Neurology recommends screening. Other treatable causes of dementia for which you might consider screening in some patients with specific risk factors include hyperhomocysteinemia, endocrine disorders (thyroid and parathyroid), uremia, liver disease, hypercalcemia, syphilis, Lyme disease, brain tumors, and normal-pressure hydrocephalus. Treatment of Parkinson disease may reverse dementia if it is present.

17. Define Wernicke encephalopathy and Korsakoff syndrome. What causes them?

    Thiamine deficiency, classically in alcoholics, causes the acute delirium of **Wernicke encephalopathy**, which results in ataxia, ophthalmoplegia, nystagmus, and confusion. If untreated, this acute encephalopathy may progress to **Korsakoff syndrome**, which is characterized by memory loss with confabulation; because patients cannot remember, they make things up. Korsakoff syndrome is usually irreversible. Always give thiamine before glucose in an alcoholic to prevent precipitating Wernicke encephalopathy.

18. Differentiate among tension, cluster, and migraine headaches. How is each treated?

    Tension headaches are the most common; look for a long history of headaches and stress, plus a feeling of tightness or stiffness, usually frontal or occipital and bilateral. Treat with stress reduction and acetaminophen/nonsteroidal antiinflammatory drugs (NSAIDs).

    Cluster headaches are unilateral, severe, and tender; they occur in clusters (e.g., three in 1 week, then none for 2 months) and are usually accompanied by autonomic symptoms such as ptosis, lacrimation, rhinorrhea, and nasal congestion. Supplemental oxygen and subcutaneous sumatriptan are first-line therapy for acute attacks.

    Migraine headaches are classically associated with an aura (a peculiar sensation, such as a noise or a flash of light, that lets the patient know that an attack is about to start). Remember the mnemonic **POUND**: **p**ulsatile quality, **o**nset/duration of 4 to 72 hours, **u**nilateral, **n**ausea/vomiting, and **d**isabling. Often, signs and symptoms also include photophobia, phonophobia, and a positive family history. Occasionally neurologic symptoms are seen during attacks. Migraines usually begin between the ages of 10 and 30 years. Medications used for the acute treatment of migraines include NSAIDs, triptans, ergotamine, and antiemetics. Prophylaxis can be achieved with beta-blockers, tricyclic antidepressants, topiramate, valproic acid, and calcium channel blockers.

19. How do you recognize a headache secondary to brain tumor or intracranial mass?

    By the presence of associated neurologic signs and symptoms of intracranial hypertension (papilledema; nausea/vomiting, which may be projectile; and mental status changes or ataxia). The classic headache occurs every day and is worse in the morning. Watch for a headache that wakes the patient from sleep. Headaches from an intracranial mass get worse with a Valsalva maneuver, exertion, or sex. Get a CT or MRI scan of the head.

20. Define idiopathic intracranial hypertension (IIH; formerly pseudotumor cerebri). How is it diagnosed and treated?

    Idiopathic intracranial hypertension is a fairly benign condition that can mimic a tumor because both cause intracranial hypertension with papilledema and daily headaches that are classically worse in the morning and may be accompanied by nausea and vomiting. The difference, however, is that IIH is usually found in young, obese females who are unlikely to have a brain tumor. Negative CT and MRI scans rule out a tumor or mass. The main worrisome sequela is vision loss. Treatment is supportive; weight loss usually helps, and repeated lumbar punctures or a CSF shunt may be needed. Large doses of vitamin A, tetracyclines, and withdrawal from corticosteroids are possible causes of IIH.

21. How do you recognize a headache due to meningitis?

    The adult patient has a fever, **Brudzinski** or **Kernig sign**, altered mental status, focal neurologic signs, seizures, vomiting, and positive CSF findings (the classic findings in bacterial meningitis are significantly elevated white

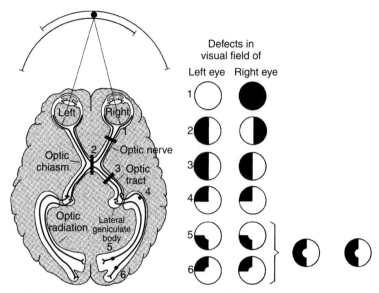

Fig. 23.1 Visual field defects produced by lesions at various levels of the visual pathway. *1,* Right optic nerve; *2,* optic chiasm; *3,* optic tract; *4,* Meyer loop; *5,* cuneus; *6,* lingual gyrus; *bracket,* occipital lobe (with macular sparing). (From Berne R. *Physiology.* 5th ed. Philadelphia: Mosby; 2003 [fig. 8.10].)

blood cells, decreased glucose, protein ~100 mg/dL, and increased opening pressure) if a lumbar tap is done. Photophobia is also common.

22. **What causes the "worst headache" of a patient's life?**
This is a classic description for a subarachnoid hemorrhage. The most common causes are ruptured congenital berry aneurysm or trauma. Look for blood around the brain, within sulci, or within basal cisterns (star sign) on a CT/MRI scan or xanthochromic (pink-yellow coloration due to breakdown of hemoglobin >6 hours after onset) grossly bloody CSF on lumbar puncture. Treatment is supportive. Aneurysms require surgical treatment to prevent rebleeding and death.

23. **What are the common extracranial causes of headache?**
    - Eye pain (optic neuritis, eyestrain from refractive errors, iritis, glaucoma)
    - Middle ear pain (otitis media, mastoiditis)
    - Sinus pain (sinusitis)
    - Oral cavity pain (toothache)
    - Herpes zoster infection with cranial nerve involvement
    - Toxins (e.g., carbon monoxide poisoning)
    - Nonspecific headache (e.g., malaise from any illness, studying for Step 2)

24. **What does a lesion of the first cranial nerve (CN I) cause? What exotic syndrome should you watch for clinically?**
CN I lesions cause anosmia (inability to smell). Watch for **Kallmann syndrome**, which is anosmia plus hypogonadism due to gonadotropin-releasing hormone deficiency.

25. **True or False: Brain lesions can be localized based on the visual field defect**
True. Remember this stuff from basic science? Review it again for at least one easy point on the USMLE Step 2 (Fig. 23.1). If you really hate this stuff, at least remember bitemporal hemianopsia due to an optic chiasm lesion, usually caused by a pituitary tumor.

Visual Field Defect	Location of Lesion
Right anopsia (monocular blindness)	Right optic nerve
Bitemporal hemianopsia	Optic chiasm (classically due to pituitary tumor)
Left homonymous hemianopsia	Right optic tract

Visual Field Defect	Location of Lesion
Left upper quadrant anopsia	Right optic radiations in the right temporal lobe
Left lower quadrant anopsia	Right optic radiations in the right parietal lobe
Left homonymous hemianopsia with macular sparing	Right occipital lobe (from posterior cerebral artery occlusion)

26. **How do you distinguish between a benign and serious cause of CN III deficit?**
    With benign causes (i.e., hypertension and diabetes) of a CN III palsy, the pupil is normal in size and reactive; no treatment is needed. With serious causes (i.e., aneurysm, tumor, or uncal herniation), the pupil is dilated and nonreactive ("blown"). Urgent diagnosis and treatment are required. Additional neurologic symptoms also indicate a serious cause.
    The first step in serious cases is to get a CT/MRI scan of the head. Careful observation is preferred in benign cases, but if the patient does not improve within a few months or does not have hypertension or diabetes, you should order a CT/MRI scan of the head just in case.

27. **What does CN V (trigeminal nerve) innervate? What classic peripheral nerve disorder affects its function?**
    CN V innervates the muscles of mastication and facial sensation, including the afferent limb of the corneal reflex. Watch for **trigeminal neuralgia** (tic douloureux), which is classically described as unilateral shooting pains in the face in older adults and often triggered by activity (e.g., brushing the teeth). This condition is best treated with antiepilepsy medications (e.g., carbamazepine). If the patient is younger and female, or the symptoms are bilateral, consider multiple sclerosis, and rule out other causes, such as tumor or stroke.

28. **What structures does CN VII innervate? What is the difference between an upper and lower motor neuron lesion of the facial nerve?**
    CN VII (facial nerve) innervates the muscles of facial expression, taste in the anterior two-thirds of the tongue, skin of the external ear, lacrimal and salivary glands (except the parotid gland), and stapedius muscle. With an upper motor neuron lesion of CN VII, the forehead is spared on the affected side, and the cause is usually a stroke or tumor. With a lower motor neuron lesion, the forehead is involved on the affected side, and the cause is usually Bell palsy or tumor.

29. **What problems (other than facial droop) affect patients with a CN VII lesion?**
    Patients may be unable to close their eyes. Give artificial tears to prevent corneal ulceration. Also watch for **hyperacusis** (quiet noises sound extremely loud) in Bell palsy due to stapedius muscle paralysis.

30. **What rare tumor is a classic cause of lower motor neuron lesions of CN VII and CN VIII?**
    Cerebellopontine angle tumors (e.g., acoustic neuroma, classically seen in patients with neurofibromatosis).

31. **Describe the function of CN VIII. What symptoms do lesions cause?**
    CN VIII (the vestibulocochlear nerve) is needed for hearing and balance. Lesions can cause deafness, tinnitus, and/or vertigo. In children, think of meningitis as a cause. In adults, symptoms may be due to a toxin or medication (e.g., aspirin, aminoglycosides, loop diuretics, cisplatin), infection (labyrinthitis), tumor, or stroke.

32. **What does CN IX innervate? What physical findings are associated with a lesion?**
    CN IX (the glossopharyngeal nerve) innervates the pharyngeal muscles and mucous membranes (afferent limb of gag reflex), parotid gland, taste in the posterior third of the tongue, skin of the external ear, and the carotid body/sinus. With lesions (due to stroke or tumor), look for loss of gag reflex and loss of taste in the posterior third of the tongue.

33. **Describe the function of CN X. Specify the physical findings and causes of lesions.**
    CN X innervates muscles of the palate, pharynx, and larynx (efferent limb of gag reflex); taste buds in the base of the tongue; abdominal viscera; and skin of the external ear. Look for hoarseness, dysphagia, and loss of gag or cough reflex. Lesions are commonly due to stroke, but do not forget aortic aneurysms or tumors (especially apical/Pancoast lung tumors), or recent nearby surgery (classically thyroidectomy) as a cause of recurrent laryngeal nerve palsy and hoarseness.

34. **What muscles does CN XI innervate? How do you know on which side the lesion is located?**
    CN XI (the spinal accessory nerve) innervates the sternocleidomastoid and trapezius muscles. Patients with CN XI lesions have trouble turning their head to the side opposite the lesion and have ipsilateral shoulder droop.

35. **What does a lesion of CN XII cause?**
    CN XII (the hypoglossal nerve) innervates the muscles of the tongue. A protruded tongue deviates to the same side as the lesion. A helpful mnemonic for remembering the direction of deviation is, "Patients with CN XII lesions lick their wounds."

36. Which vitamin deficiencies may present with neurologic signs or symptoms?

Vitamin B_{12}: dementia, peripheral neuropathy, loss of vibration sense in lower extremities, loss of position sense, ataxia, spasticity, hyperactive reflexes, paresthesia, and positive Babinski sign

Thiamine: peripheral neuropathy, confusion, ophthalmoplegia, nystagmus, ataxia, confusion, delirium, dementia, psychosis

Vitamin E: loss of proprioception/vibratory sensation, areflexia, ataxia, and gaze palsy

Vitamin A: vision loss

Vitamin B_6: peripheral sensory neuropathy (watch for isoniazid as a cause, and give prophylactic B_6 to patients taking isoniazid, if given the choice)

37. What are the two overarching types of seizures and their subtypes that you should be able to recognize?

1. Partial (focal) seizure
   a. Simple partial seizure
   b. Complex partial seizure
2. Generalized seizure
   a. Absence (petit mal)
   b. Myoclonic
   c. Tonic-clonic
   d. Tonic
   e. Atonic

38. Describe simple partial seizures. How are they treated?

Simple partial (local or focal) seizures may be motor (e.g., Jacksonian march), sensory (e.g., hallucinations), or psychic (cognitive or affective symptoms). The key point is that consciousness is *not* impaired. The first-line agents for treatment are carbamazepine, lamotrigine, oxcarbazepine, and levetiracetam.

39. Describe complex partial seizures. How are they treated?

Complex partial (psychomotor) seizures are any simple partial seizure followed by impairment of consciousness. Patients perform purposeless movements and may become aggressive if restraint is attempted (however, people who get in fights or kill other people are not having a seizure). The first-line agents for treatment are valproate, lamotrigine, and levetiracetam.

40. Give the classic description of an absence seizure

Absence (petit mal) seizures are brief (10–30 seconds in duration) generalized seizures in which the main manifestation is loss of consciousness, often with eye or muscle fluttering. They do not begin after the age of 20 years. The classic description is a child in a classroom who stares into space in the middle of a sentence and then 20 seconds later resumes the sentence as if nothing happened. The child is *not* daydreaming but is having a seizure. There is no postictal state (an important difference between absence and complex seizures). The first-line treatment agents are ethosuximide and valproate.

41. How do you recognize a tonic-clonic seizure?

Tonic-clonic (grand mal) seizures are the classic seizures that we knew about before we went to medical school. They may be associated with an aura. Tonic muscle contraction is followed by clonic contractions, usually lasting 2 to 5 minutes. Associated symptoms may include incontinence and tongue lacerations. The postictal state is characterized by drowsiness, confusion, headache, and muscle soreness. The first-line agents for treatment are valproate, lamotrigine, or levetiracetam.

42. Define febrile seizure and distinguish between a simple and complex febrile seizure

Children between the ages of 6 months and 5 years may have a seizure caused by fever. Always assume another cause outside this age range. Simple febrile seizures are of the tonic-clonic, generalized type, are less than 15 minutes in duration, and occur only once in a 24-hour period. A febrile seizure that is more than 15 minutes is associated with focal neurologic signs or recurs within 24 hours is considered complex. For simple febrile seizures, no specific seizure treatment is required, but you should treat the underlying cause of the fever, if possible, and give acetaminophen to reduce fever. Such children do *not* have epilepsy, and the chances of their developing it are slightly higher than in the general population. For all febrile seizures, but especially for those classified as complex, make sure that the child does not have meningitis, tumor, or another serious cause of the seizure. The Step 2 question will give clues in the case description if you should pursue workup for a serious condition.

43. What are the common causes of secondary seizures? How are they treated?

- Mass effect (tumor, hemorrhage)
- Metabolic disorder (hypoglycemia, hypoxia, phenylketonuria, hyponatremia)
- Toxins (lead, cocaine, carbon monoxide poisoning)
- Drug withdrawal (alcohol, barbiturates, benzodiazepines, withdrawing anticonvulsants too rapidly)

- Cerebral edema (severe or malignant hypertension; also watch for pheochromocytoma and eclampsia)
- Central nervous system infections (meningitis, encephalitis, toxoplasmosis, cysticercosis)
- Trauma
- Stroke

Treat the underlying disorder and use a benzodiazepine (lorazepam or diazepam) and/or phenytoin or fosphenytoin acutely to control seizures. For all seizures (primary or secondary), secure the airway and, if possible, side-roll the patient to prevent aspiration.

44. **Define status epilepticus. How is it treated?**
Status epilepticus is defined as a seizure that lasts for a sufficient length of time (usually ≥30 minutes, though considering the need for rapid evaluation and intervention to avoid cardiovascular morbidity and refractory status, an accepted operation definition is ≥5 minutes of continuous seizures) or is repeated frequently enough that the individual does not regain consciousness between seizures. Status epilepticus may occur spontaneously or result from withdrawing anticonvulsants too rapidly. Treat with IV lorazepam. Give fosphenytoin if the seizures persist. As with all seizures, remember your ABCs (airway, breathing, circulation). Protect the airway. Intubate if necessary, and side-roll the patient to prevent aspiration.

45. **True or False: Hypertension can cause seizures**
True. Always remember hypertension as a cause of seizures or convulsions, headache, confusion, stupor, and mental status changes.

46. **What do you need to remember when giving anticonvulsants to women?**
All anticonvulsants are teratogenic, and women of reproductive age need counseling about the risks of pregnancy. Do a pregnancy test before starting an anticonvulsant and offer birth control. Polypharmacy increases the risk of teratogenicity. Valproic acid is well known for its association with an increased incidence of neural tube defects. There is limited human information on the risks to the fetus with the newer antiepileptic medications.

47. **What causes strokes? How common are they?**
Cerebrovascular disease (stroke) is the most common cause of neurologic disability in the United States—and the third leading cause of death. Ischemia due to atherosclerosis (atherothrombotic ischemia) is by far the most common type of stroke (>85% of cases). Hypertension is another cause of stroke and typically causes hemorrhagic stroke, most commonly in the basal ganglia, thalamus, or cerebellum. Having said this, be aware of more exotic causes of stroke, such as atrial fibrillation with resultant clot formation and emboli to the brain, septic emboli from endocarditis, paradoxic emboli through a patent foramen ovale, and sickle cell disease.

48. **How is an acute stroke treated?**
Treatment for an acute ischemic stroke in evolution is supportive (e.g., airway, oxygen, IV fluids). The first step is to get a CT scan of the head without contrast to evaluate for bleeding or mass (Fig. 23.2). If no blood is seen on CT scan, aspirin is usually the medication of choice. Heparin is not recommended for the treatment of acute ischemic stroke and should be avoided on the USMLE. Chapter 39 discusses the role of carotid endarterectomy, which is not done emergently. Thrombolysis with t-PA (tissue plasminogen activator) can be attempted if patients present within 3 hours (up to 4.5 hours in certain circumstances) and meet strict criteria for its use.

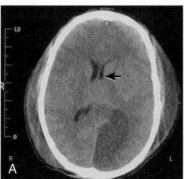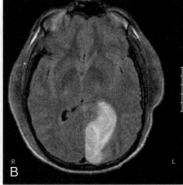

Fig. 23.2 Stroke on computed tomography (CT) and magnetic resonance imaging (MRI) scans. The CT scan (A) done 3 days after a stroke shows a low-density area posteriorly on the left with mass effect and clear midline shift *(arrow)*. The MRI scan (B) done on the same day shows the infarcted area much more clearly. (From Mettler F. *Essentials of Radiology*. 2nd ed. Philadelphia: Saunders; 2004 [fig. 2.17].)

49. Define transient ischemic attack (TIA). How is it managed?
    TIA is a brief episode of neurologic dysfunction resulting from temporary cerebral ischemia not associated with cerebral infarction. This newer definition is tissue based rather than time based. TIA is often a precursor to stroke and is due to ischemia. The classic presentation is ipsilateral blindness (amaurosis fugax) and/or unilateral hemiplegia, hemiparesis, weakness, or clumsiness that lasts less than 5 minutes.
    Order a carotid duplex scan to look for carotid stenosis. The correct choice for long-term therapy is aspirin and antiplatelet medications. Choose carotid endarterectomy over aspirin if the degree of carotid stenosis is 70% to 99%.

50. Describe the signs and symptoms of Huntington disease. How is it acquired? What is the classic CT finding?
    Huntington disease is an autosomal dominant condition that usually presents between the ages of 35 and 50 years. Look for choreiform movements (irregular, spasmodic, involuntary movements of the limbs or facial muscles) and progressive intellectual deterioration, dementia, or psychiatric disturbances (suicidal ideation is common). **Atrophy of the caudate nuclei** may be seen on CT or MRI. Treatment is supportive; tetrabenazine or atypical neuroleptics (olanzapine, risperidone, or aripiprazole) may help with the chorea and agitation/psychosis.

51. Define Parkinson disease. How do you recognize it on the Step 2 exam?
    Parkinson disease has a classic tetrad of (1) slowness or poverty of movement, (2) muscular ("lead pipe" and "cog-wheel") rigidity, (3) "pill-rolling" tremor at rest (which disappears with movement and sleep), and (4) postural instability (manifested by the classic shuffling gait and festination). Patients may also have dementia and depression. The mean age of onset is around 60 years.

52. Describe the pathophysiology of Parkinson disease. How is it treated pharmacologically?
    The cause is thought to be a loss of dopaminergic neurons, especially in the **substantia nigra**, which project to the basal ganglia. The result is decreased dopamine in the basal ganglia. Drug therapy, which aims to increase dopamine, includes dopamine precursors (levodopa with carbidopa), dopamine agonists (bromocriptine, apomorphine, pergolide, pramipexole, and ropinirole), monoamine oxidase-B inhibitors (selegiline), COMT inhibitors (entacapone and tolcapone), anticholinergics (trihexyphenidyl and benztropine), and amantadine.

53. What is the classic iatrogenic cause of parkinsonian signs and symptoms?
    Antipsychotics may cause parkinsonian symptoms in schizophrenics. This is a favorite Step 2 question. Treat this side effect of antipsychotic medication with anticholinergics (benztropine, trihexyphenidyl) or antihistamines (diphenhydramine).

54. What brain lesions cause a resting tremor and an intention tremor? What about hemiballismus?
    A resting tremor, if due to a brain lesion, is generally a sign of basal ganglia disease, as is chorea. An intention tremor is usually due to cerebellar disease. Hemiballismus (random, violent, unilateral flailing of the limbs) is classically due to a lesion in the **subthalamic nucleus**.

55. What other common conditions other than Parkinson disease cause a resting tremor?
    A resting tremor may be due to hyperthyroidism, anxiety, or drug withdrawal or intoxication. A common action tremor is called benign (essential) hereditary tremor. Benign hereditary tremor is usually autosomal dominant; look for a positive family history or improvement with consumption of alcohol, and use beta-blockers to reduce the tremor. Also watch for Wilson disease (hepatolenticular degeneration), which can cause chorea-like movements; asterixis (slow, involuntary flapping of outstretched hands) may be seen in patients with liver failure.

56. What diseases should come to mind in children with cerebellar findings?
    • Brain tumor (cerebellar astrocytoma, medulloblastomas)
    • Hydrocephalus (enlarging head in an infant age <6 months, Arnold-Chiari or Dandy-Walker malformations)
    • Friedreich ataxia (starts between ages 5 and 15 years; autosomal recessive; look for areflexia, loss of vibration/position sense, and cardiomyopathy)
    • Ataxia-telangiectasia (progressive cerebellar ataxia, oculocutaneous telangiectasias, and immune deficiency)

57. What diseases should come to mind in adults with cerebellar findings?
    Alcoholism, brain tumor, ischemia or hemorrhage, and multiple sclerosis.

58. How do you recognize amyotrophic lateral sclerosis (ALS) on the Step 2 exam?
    ALS (Lou Gehrig disease) is the only condition that you are likely to be asked about that causes both upper and lower motor neuron lesion signs and symptoms. This idiopathic neurodegenerative disease is more common in men, and the mean age at onset is 55. The key is to notice a combination of upper motor neuron lesion signs (spasticity, hyperreflexia, positive Babinski sign) and lower motor neuron lesion signs (fasciculations, atrophy, flaccidity) present at the same time. Treatment is generally supportive, and riluzole may have survival benefit and increase time to tracheostomy. Fifty percent of patients die within 3 years of disease onset.

59. What are the two classic causes of a "floppy" (flaccid) baby? How do you differentiate the two?

Genetic disorders, the most common of which is Werdnig-Hoffmann disease (WHD), and infant botulism. History easily differentiates the two. WHD is an autosomal recessive degeneration of anterior horn cells in the spinal cord and brainstem (lower motor neuron disease). Most infants are hypotonic at birth, and all are affected by 6 months. Look for a positive family history and a long, slowly progressive disease course. Treatment is supportive only.

Infant botulism is caused by a *Clostridium botulinum* toxin. Look for sudden onset and a history of ingesting honey or other home-canned foods. Diagnosis is made by finding *C. botulinum* toxin or organisms in the feces. Treatment involves inpatient monitoring and support with a close watch of respiratory status. The child may need intubation for respiratory muscle paralysis. Spontaneous recovery usually occurs within 1 week, and supportive care is all that is needed.

60. List the causative categories of peripheral neuropathy and give examples of each
    1. Metabolic/endocrine: diabetes mellitus (autonomic and sensory neuropathy), uremia, hypothyroidism.
    2. Nutritional: deficiencies of vitamin B_{12}, vitamin B_6 (look for history of isoniazid), thiamine ("dry" beriberi), and vitamin E.
    3. Toxins/medications: lead (the classic symptom is wristdrop or footdrop; look for coexisting central nervous system or abdominal symptoms) or other heavy metals, isoniazid, vincristine, ethambutol (optic neuritis), aminoglycosides (especially CN VIII).
    4. Immunization and autoimmune disorders: Guillain-Barré syndrome, lupus erythematosus, polyarteritis nodosa, scleroderma, sarcoidosis, amyloidosis.
    5. Trauma: carpal tunnel syndrome (entrapment of the median nerve at the wrist; usually due to repetitive physical activity but may be a presentation of acromegaly or hypothyroidism; look for positive Tinel and Phalen signs), pressure paralysis (radial nerve palsy in alcoholics), fractures (causing nerve compression).
    6. Infectious: Lyme disease, diphtheria, HIV, leprosy.

61. What test can be used to prove the presence of a peripheral neuropathy, regardless of etiology?

Nerve conduction velocity is slowed with a peripheral neuropathy.

62. Describe the pathophysiology of myasthenia gravis (MG). Who is affected? What are the classic physical findings?

MG is an autoimmune disease that destroys acetylcholine receptors. Most patients have antibodies to acetylcholine receptors in their serum. The disease usually presents in women between the ages of 20 and 40 years. Look for ptosis, diplopia, and general muscle fatigability, especially toward the end of the day or with repetitive use.

63. How is MG diagnosed? What tumor is associated with it?

Diagnosis is made with the Tensilon test. After injection of edrophonium (Tensilon), a short-acting anticholinesterase inhibitor, muscle weakness improves. Nerve stimulation studies can also be used. Watch for associated **thymomas** (a tumor of the thymus). Thymectomy is generally recommended for patients under age 60 years without thymoma. Chronic medical treatment consists of long-acting anticholinesterase inhibitors (pyridostigmine) and immunotherapy (glucocorticoids, mycophenolate, azathioprine, and cyclosporine).

64. What three conditions may cause an MG-like clinical picture?
    1. **Eaton-Lambert syndrome** is a paraneoplastic syndrome (classically seen with small cell lung cancer) associated with muscle weakness. The extraocular muscles are spared, whereas MG is almost always characterized by prominent involvement of extraocular muscles. Eaton-Lambert syndrome has a different mechanism of action (impaired release of acetylcholine from nerves) and a differential response to repetitive nerve stimulation. The weakness in MG worsens with repetitive use or stimulation, whereas the weakness in Eaton-Lambert syndrome improves.
    2. **Organophosphate poisoning** also causes MG-like muscle weakness. Poisoning is usually due to agricultural exposure. Look for symptoms of parasympathetic excess (e.g., miosis, excessive bronchial secretions, urinary urgency, and diarrhea). Edrophonium causes worsening of the muscular weakness. Treat with atropine and pralidoxime.
    3. **Aminoglycosides in high doses** may cause MG-like muscular weakness and/or prolong the effects of muscular blockade after anesthesia.

65. What is the most common type of muscular dystrophy? How is it inherited? What are the classic findings?

The most common type is Duchenne muscular dystrophy, an X-linked recessive disorder of dystrophin that usually presents in boys between the ages of 3 and 7 years. Look for muscle weakness, markedly elevated levels of creatine phosphokinase, pseudohypertrophy of the calves (due to fatty and fibrous infiltration of the degenerating muscle), and often a lower-than-normal IQ. Gower sign is also classic: The patient "walks" his hands and feet toward each other to rise from a prone position (Fig. 23.3). Muscle biopsy establishes the diagnosis. Treatment is supportive. Most patients die by age 20.

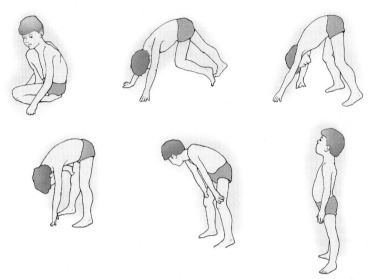

Fig. 23.3 Gower sign. Child must use hands to rise from sitting position. (From Canale ST, Beaty JH. *Campbell's Operative Orthopaedics.* 11th ed. Philadelphia: Mosby; 2011 [fig. 32.5]. Redrawn from Siegel IM. *Clinical Management of Muscle Disease.* London: William Heinemann; 1977.)

66. **List the five less common types of muscular dystrophies**
    1. Becker muscular dystrophy: also, an X-linked recessive dystrophin disorder but milder.
    2. Facioscapulohumeral dystrophy: an autosomal dominant disorder that affects the areas in the name (face, shoulder girdle). Symptoms begin between the age of 7 and 20 years. Life expectancy is normal.
    3. Limb-girdle dystrophy: affects pelvic and shoulder muscles; begins in adulthood.
    4. Mitochondrial myopathies: of interest because they are inherited mitochondrial defects (passed only from mother to offspring; cannot be transmitted by men). The key phrase is "ragged red fibers" on biopsy specimen. Ophthalmoplegia is usually present.
    5. Myotonic dystrophy: an autosomal dominant disorder that presents between the ages of 20 and 30 years. Myotonia (inability to relax muscles) classically presents as an **inability to relax the grip or release a handshake.** Look for coexisting mental retardation, baldness, and testicular or ovarian atrophy. Treatment is supportive, including genetic counseling. The diagnosis is clinical.

67. **What class of inherited metabolic disorders affects muscle and may resemble muscular dystrophy?**
    The rare glycogen storage diseases (autosomal recessive inheritance) can cause muscular weakness, especially **McArdle disease**, a deficiency in glycogen phosphorylase that is relatively mild and presents with weakness and cramping after exercise due to lactic acid buildup.

CHAPTER 24

NEUROSURGERY

1. List the four major types of intracranial hemorrhages.
   1. Subdural hematoma
   2. Epidural hematoma
   3. Subarachnoid hemorrhage
   4. Intracerebral hemorrhage

2. What causes a subdural hematoma? How do you recognize and treat it?
   Subdural hematomas are due to bleeding from veins that bridge the cortex and dural sinuses. On computed tomography (CT) scan the hematoma is crescent shaped (Fig. 24.1). The blood does not cross the falx cerebri (midline), because the dura is attached to the skull. Subdural hematomas are common in alcoholics and victims of head trauma. They may present immediately after trauma or as long as 1 to 2 months later. The bleeding is relatively slow because it is venous blood. If the patient has a history of head trauma, always consider the diagnosis of subdural hematoma. If large, expanding, or accompanied by neurologic deficits, treat with surgical evacuation.

3. What causes an epidural hematoma? How do you recognize and treat it?
   Epidural hematomas are due to bleeding from meningeal arteries (classically, the middle meningeal artery). Bleeding tends to occur quickly because it is higher-pressure arterial blood, and the hematoma pushes away the dura as it expands. On CT scan, the hematoma is lenticular in shape (Fig. 24.2). At least 85% of epidural hematomas are associated with a skull fracture (classically, a temporal bone fracture), and many patients have an ipsilateral "blown" pupil (dilated, fixed, nonreactive pupil on the side of the hematoma). The classic history includes head trauma with loss of consciousness, followed by a lucid interval of minutes to hours, and then neurologic deterioration. Treatment usually includes surgical evacuation.

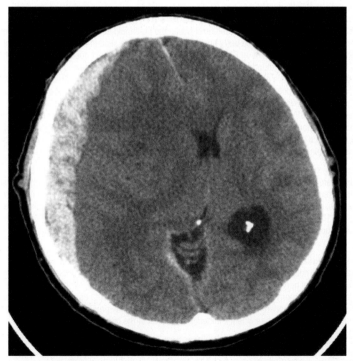

Fig. 24.1 Subdural hematoma. The crescent-shaped blood clot is causing a severe midline shift and brain herniation. (From Standring S. *Gray's Anatomy.* Elsevier; 2016:429-441.)

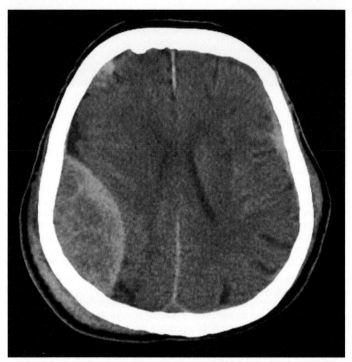

Fig. 24.2 A head computed tomography scan showing a right-sided epidural hematoma. The blood clot is biconvex. (From Standring S. *Gray's Anatomy.* Elsevier; 2016:429-441.)

4. **Define subarachnoid hemorrhage. What causes it? How is it treated?**
   A subarachnoid hemorrhage describes bleeding between the arachnoid and pia mater. The most common cause is trauma, followed by ruptured berry aneurysms. Blood can be seen in the cerebral ventricles and surrounding the brain or brainstem on CT scan (Fig. 24.3). The classic patient describes the "worst headache of my life," also known as a "thunderclap" headache, although many die or are unconscious before they reach the hospital. Patients who are awake have signs of meningitis (positive Kernig and Brudzinski signs). Remember the association between polycystic kidney disease and berry aneurysms. CT is the test of choice and should be performed before performing lumbar puncture (see question 12). A lumbar puncture shows grossly bloody cerebrospinal fluid (CSF) or xanthochromia (yellowish color of the CSF due to breakdown of heme into bilirubin).
   Treat with support of vital functions, anticonvulsants, and observation. Once the patient is stable, do a CT or magnetic resonance angiogram to look for aneurysms or arteriovenous malformations, which may be treatable with surgical clipping or catheter-directed angiographic procedures.

5. **What causes an intracerebral hemorrhage? How do you recognize and treat it?**
   Intracerebral hemorrhage describes bleeding into the brain parenchyma (Fig. 24.4). The most common cause is hypertension, but it also may be due to other forms of stroke, trauma, arteriovenous malformations, coagulopathies, or tumors. Two-thirds of intracerebral hemorrhages occur in the basal ganglia (especially with hypertension). The patient may present with coma or, if awake, contralateral hemiplegia and hemisensory deficits. Blood (which appears white on CT scan) can be seen in the brain parenchyma and may extend into the ventricles. Surgery is reserved for large, accessible hemorrhages, although usually it is not helpful.

6. **What does a unilateral, dilated, nonreactive pupil after head trauma suggest?**
   A unilateral, dilated, nonreactive pupil in the setting of head trauma most likely represents impingement of the ipsilateral third cranial nerve and impending uncal herniation due to increased intracranial pressure. Of the different intracranial hemorrhages, this scenario is seen most commonly with epidural hemorrhages. Do *not* do a lumbar puncture in any patient with a "blown" pupil because you may precipitate uncal herniation and death. Instead, order a CT or magnetic resonance imaging (MRI) scan of the head.

7. **List four classic signs of a basilar skull fracture**
   1. Periorbital ecchymosis ("raccoon eyes")
   2. Postauricular ecchymosis (Battle sign)
   3. Hemotympanum (blood behind the eardrum)
   4. CSF otorrhea or rhinorrhea (leakage of CSF, which is clear in appearance, from the ears or nose)

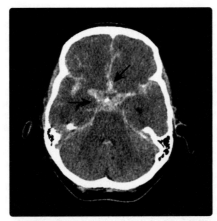

Fig. 24.3 Computed tomography scan showing a subarachnoid hemorrhage. The subarachnoid appears white and fills the space around the brain that would normally contain cerebrospinal fluid and would appear dark. (From Fuller G, Manform M. *Neurology.* Churchill Livingstone; 2010:72-73.)

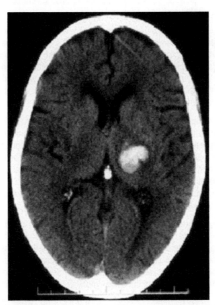

Fig. 24.4 Intracerebral hemorrhage. A computed tomography scan shows a parenchymal hemorrhage involving the left thalamus and posterior internal capsule. (From Goldman L. *Goldman's Cecil Medicine.* 24th ed. Philadelphia: Saunders; 2011 [fig. 415.4]. Courtesy Gregory W. Albers, Stanford University, Stanford, CA.)

8. **What is the imaging test of choice for skull fractures of the calvarium? How are they managed?**

   Skull fractures of the calvarium (roof of the skull) are best seen on CT scan (preferred over plain x-rays). Surgical indications include contamination (surgical cleaning and debridement), depression with impingement on brain parenchyma, or open fracture with CSF leak. Otherwise, such fractures can be observed and generally heal on their own.

9. **True or False: Severe, permanent neurologic deficits may occur after head trauma, even with a negative CT or MRI scan of the head.**

   True. Head trauma can cause cerebral contusion or shear injury of the brain parenchyma (diffuse axonal injury), both of which may not show up on a CT or MRI scan but may cause temporary or permanent neurologic deficits.

10. **What finding suggests increased intracranial pressure?**
Increased intracranial pressure (intracranial hypertension) is highly suggested in the setting of bilaterally dilated and fixed pupils. Normal intracranial pressure is between 5 and 15 mm Hg. Less specific symptoms include headache, papilledema, nausea and vomiting, and mental status changes. Look also for the classic Cushing triad, which consists of increasing blood pressure, bradycardia, and respiratory irregularity.

11. **How should increased intracranial pressure be managed?**
The first step is to elevate the head of the bed and intubate the patient. Once intubated, the patient should be hyperventilated for rapid lowering of intracranial pressure through decreased intracranial blood volume (due to cerebral vasoconstriction). **Mannitol** diuresis or boluses of hypertonic saline (3% normal saline) can be tried to lessen cerebral edema. Furosemide is also used but is less effective. Ventriculostomy should be performed if hydrocephalus is identified. Therapeutic hypothermia can be used to protect the brain from secondary injury. Barbiturate coma and decompressive craniotomy (burr holes) are last-ditch measures. Anticonvulsant therapy should be started if seizures are suspected; prophylactic anticonvulsants are controversial but may be warranted in some cases.
  Remember that cerebral perfusion pressure equals blood pressure minus intracranial pressure. In other words, do *not* treat hypertension initially in a patient with increased intracranial pressure, because hypertension is the body's way of trying to increase cerebral perfusion. Lowering blood pressure in this setting may worsen symptoms or even cause a stroke.

12. **True or False: Lumbar puncture is the first test that should be performed in a patient with increased intracranial pressure.**
False. *Never* do a lumbar puncture in any patient with signs of increased intracranial pressure until a CT scan is done first. If the CT is totally negative, you can proceed to a lumbar puncture, if needed. If you do a lumbar puncture first, you may precipitate uncal herniation and death.

13. **How do patients with spinal cord trauma present? How are they managed?**
Patients with spinal cord trauma often present with "spinal shock" (loss of reflexes and motor function, hypotension). Order standard trauma radiographs (cervical spine, chest, pelvis) as well as additional spine radiographs or CT scans based on physical exam. Also give corticosteroids (proven to improve outcome). Moderate hypothermia is increasingly being utilized in the management of patients with spinal cord trauma. Surgery is done for incomplete neurologic injury (some residual function maintained) with external compression (e.g., subluxation, bone chip). MRI can visualize cord injury noninvasively.

14. **What causes spinal cord compression? How do patients present?**
Spinal cord compression is usually defined as acute or subacute. Most cases of acute cord compression result from trauma. Look for the appropriate history. Subacute compression is often due to metastatic cancer but may also result from a primary neoplasm, subdural or epidural abscess (classically seen in diabetics and due to *Staphylococcus aureus*), or hematoma (especially after a lumbar tap or epidural/spinal anesthesia in a patient with a bleeding disorder or a patient taking anticoagulation).
  Patients present with local spinal pain (especially with bone metastases) and neurologic deficits below the lesion (e.g., hyperreflexia, positive Babinski sign, weakness, sensory loss).

15. **How should patients with subacute spinal cord compression be diagnosed and treated?**
The first step in the emergency department is to give high-dose corticosteroids and order an MRI scan (preferred over CT) (Fig. 24.5). If the cause is cancer or tumor, give local radiation if the metastases are from a known primary tumor that is radiosensitive. Surgical decompression can be used if the tumor is not radiosensitive. For a hematoma or subdural/epidural abscess, surgery is indicated for decompression and drainage. Prognosis is related most closely to pretreatment function; the longer you wait to treat, the worse the prognosis.

16. **Define syringomyelia. What causes it? How does it usually present?**
Syringomyelia is a central pathologic cavitation of the spinal cord, usually in the cervical or upper thoracic region. Most cases are idiopathic, but syringomyelia may also follow trauma or be related to congenital cranial base malformations (e.g., Arnold-Chiari malformation). The classic presentation, due to involvement of the lateral spinothalamic tracts, is bilateral loss of pain and temperature sensation below the lesion in the distribution of a "cape." The cavitation in the cord gradually widens to involve other tracts, causing motor and sensory deficits. MRI scan is the diagnostic imaging study of choice. The primary treatment available is surgical creation of a shunt.

17. **Define spina bifida. How can it be prevented?**
Spina bifida is a congenital abnormality in which lack of fusion of the spinal column, specifically the posterior vertebral arches, allows protrusion of spinal membranes, with or without spinal cord. Spina bifida occulta, the mildest form of the disease (bone deficiency without dural membrane or cord protrusion), is often asymptomatic and should be suspected in patients with a triangular patch of hair over the lumbar spine. More serious defects are usually obvious and occur most often in the lumbosacral region. A **meningocele** is protrusion of the meninges outside the spinal canal, whereas a **myelomeningocele** is protrusion of meninges plus central nervous system

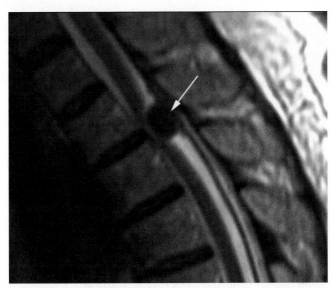

Fig. 24.5 Meningioma. Sagittal T2-weighted image demonstrates a hypointense extramedullary dural-based mass lesion that causes marked spinal cord compression *(arrow)*. (From Daroff RB. *Bradley's Neurology in Clinical Practice.* 6th ed. Philadelphia: Saunders; 2012 [fig. 33A.88].)

tissue outside the spinal canal. Patients with a myelomeningocele almost always have an associated Arnold-Chiari malformation. Giving folate supplementation to potential mothers reduces the incidence of spina bifida and other neural tube defects.

18. **Define hydrocephalus. How is it recognized in children?**
    Hydrocephalus is excessive accumulation of CSF in the cerebral ventricles. In children, look for increasing head circumference, increased intracranial pressure, bulging fontanelle, scalp vein engorgement, and paralysis of upward gaze. The most common causes include congenital malformations, tumors, and inflammation (e.g., hemorrhage, meningitis). Treat the underlying cause, if possible; otherwise, a surgical shunt is created to decompress the ventricles.

19. **In what setting does dural venous sinus thrombosis occur? How is it diagnosed and treated?**
    The risk factors are similar to those for deep venous thrombosis in other areas, including hypercoagulable state, trauma, dehydration, pregnancy, oral contraceptive use, infections (e.g., extension of sinusitis or mastoiditis intracranially), nephrotic syndrome, and local tumor invasion. The diagnostic test of choice is MRI. Though hemorrhagic infarcts are common with dural venous thrombosis, treatment with anticoagulation improves outcomes.

CHAPTER 25

OBSTETRICS

1. A patient of reproductive age who is taking birth control pills presents with amenorrhea. What is the most likely cause?

   Pregnancy. No form of contraception is 100% effective (including tubal ligation), especially when patient compliance is required. Always order a urine pregnancy test for reproductive-age female patients presenting with amenorrhea, no matter what distractors may be included in the patient's history.

2. List the signs and symptoms of pregnancy

   Symptoms of pregnancy:
   - Amenorrhea
   - Nausea or morning sickness
   - Breast enlargement or tenderness; possible darkening of the areola
   - Fatigue
   - Weight gain

   Signs of pregnancy:
   - Hegar sign (softening and compressibility of the lower uterine segment)
   - Chadwick sign (color change of the vulva, cervix, and vaginal walls; often darkening or becoming bluish)
   - Suprapubic palpation/ballottement of uterine fundus
   - Linea nigra (linear stripes of hyperpigmented skin across the abdomen)
   - Melasma (also known as chloasma or the "mask of pregnancy")

3. Explain how to determine a patient's gestational age and how it differs from embryonic age. Which method is most commonly used in a clinical setting? Why?

   Gestational age is measured in weeks since the first day of the patient's last menstrual period (LMP). Embryonic age (also called postconception age) is defined as the number of weeks since the ovulated egg was fertilized. Embryonic age is therefore approximately 2 weeks behind that patient's gestational age. Due to the varied length of each patient's follicular phase, it is difficult to identify an exact ovulation or fertilization date; the first day of most menstrual periods is fairly unambiguous, therefore gestational age is typically used to date pregnancies in most clinical settings. When a clinician says, "The patient is at X weeks," you can bet the clinician is talking about gestational age.

4. How is pregnancy diagnosed? At what gestational age will each method show a positive result?

   There are four ways that pregnancy can be definitively diagnosed:
   - Detection of elevated beta-hCG (e.g., the beta subunit of human chorionic gonadotropin) in the patient's blood or serum
   - Detection of elevated beta-hCG in the patient's urine
   - Detection of a gestational sac, yolk sac, or fetal pole by transvaginal ultrasound (TVUS)
   - Detection of fetal cardiac activity on Doppler ultrasound

     While there is variability when measuring beta-hCG in real-life patients, for the purpose of your licensing exams, elevated beta-hCG may be detected in blood and serum samples as early as 3 weeks of gestation (i.e., 1 week after fertilization), while elevated beta-hCG is not detectable in urine until at least 4 weeks of gestation (i.e., at least 2 weeks after fertilization). TVUS can typically identify a gestational sac at 4.5 weeks, yolk sac at 5 weeks, and fetal pole with cardiac activity around 5.5 weeks. Due to the reduced image resolution of transabdominal ultrasound compared to the transvaginal approach, TVUS is preferred. Doppler ultrasound can first detect fetal cardiac activity between weeks 10 and 12.

5. Visualization of a gestational sac via *transvaginal* ultrasound typically correlates with what serum levels of beta-hCG?

   Levels are 1000 to 2000 mIU/mL.

6. Visualization of a gestational sac via *transabdominal* ultrasound typically correlates with what serum levels of beta-hCG?

   Levels are 5000 to 6000 mIU/mL.

7. Describe Naegele's rule used to determine a patient's estimated due date (EDD)

A patient's EDD is the day she reaches a gestational age of exactly 40 weeks (i.e., 280 days since LMP). Naegele's rule can be used to quickly estimate EDD by taking the date of the patient's LMP, subtracting 3 months, and adding 7 days. For example, a patient with LMP of April 15 would have an EDD of January 22 the following year, since January is 3 months before April and January 22 is 7 days after January 15.

8. Which vitamin should be recommended to all women of reproductive age? Why?

All women of reproductive age should take vitamin B_9 (folate), dosed at 400 µg/day, to prevent neural tube defects. Folate is essential to prevent neural tube defects, with its most critical window occurring early in the first trimester before many women may know they are pregnant. If an expectant mother waits to start folate until after pregnancy is confirmed, she still runs the risk of fetal neural tube defects.

9. What lab tests should be performed on all pregnant patients during the first prenatal visit?

According to the American College of Obstetrics and Gynecology (ACOG), there are 11 lab tests that every pregnant patient should get on their first prenatal visit. These include:

- **Hemoglobin, hematocrit, and platelet count:** to establish baseline values as you monitor for anemia or thrombocytopenia during future visits.
- **Blood type, rhesus (Rh) type, and Rh antibody screen:** to investigate possible isoimmunization.
- **VDRL/RPR test:** to assess for syphilis.
- **Hepatitis B surface antigen (HBsAg) screen:** to prevent perinatal HBV transmission.
- **Human immunodeficiency virus (HIV) test:** current ACOG guidelines recommend an opt-out approach rather than an opt-in approach to increase screening rates.
- **Rubella antibody titer:** if the patient if found to be nonimmune, counsel her to get postpartum immunization. **No live vaccines** should be given during pregnancy.
- **Urinalysis and culture:** to establish baseline protein content and screen for bacteriuria.
  There are additional supplemental lab tests that may be performed during the initial prenatal visit, but only if indicated. These include:
- **Pap smear:** if the patient is due; pregnancy does not change the frequency of screening.
- **Human papilloma virus (HPV) screen:** if indicated.
- **Chlamydia and gonorrhea screening:** typically in teenage patients or if clinical suspicion is high.
- **Varicella antibody titer:** as with rubella, vaccination can be offered postpartum for nonimmune patients, but a live vaccine should **not** be given during pregnancy.
- **Hemoglobin electrophoresis:** if high risk for sickle cell disease or thalassemia.
- **Tuberculosis test:** typically by PPD if the patient is considered high risk.
- **Thyroid function:** maternal hypothyroidism may affect fetal neurologic development. Maternal hyperthyroidism can lead to fetal and maternal complications.
- **Down syndrome screening:** should be offered to all pregnant patients. There are multiple ways to screen.

10. How often should a pregnant patient attend antenatal visits?

Antenatal appointments should be scheduled every 4 weeks until week 28, then every 2 weeks until week 36, then weekly until week 40. If the patient has not delivered by week 40, schedule twice-weekly visits until week 42.

11. On every prenatal visit, listen to fetal heart tones and measure fundal height. When can these two features first be noticed?

As mentioned previously, **fetal heart tones** can be heard with Doppler ultrasound at 10 to 12 weeks and can be auscultated with a normal stethoscope around 16 to 20 weeks. **Fundal height** is measured as the distance in centimeters from the symphysis pubis to the top of the uterine fundus. The uterine fundus becomes palpable above the symphysis pubis around week 12 and reaches the umbilicus around week 20. In a patient with normal body habitus and uncomplicated singleton pregnancy, the fundal height should roughly equal the gestational age between weeks 16 and 36. After week 36, the fundal height may appear to decrease as the fetus begins to descend and engage with the lower pelvis in anticipation of labor.

12. How is a size/date discrepancy identified? What is the next step?

A discrepancy of more than 2 to 3 cm between the measured fundal height and the gestational age is considered a **size/date discrepancy**. This may have a benign explanation such as multiple gestations or an incorrectly estimated date of conception, or it may represent complications such as intrauterine growth restriction (IUGR), molar pregnancy, or fetal demise. An ultrasound exam should be performed for further evaluation.

13. When in pregnancy is ultrasound most accurate at estimating the fetal age? Which parameters are used to estimate gestational age during the first, second, and third trimesters?

Dating by ultrasound is more accurate when done early in the pregnancy. The most accurate first-trimester estimation of gestational age is achieved by measuring the crown-rump length (CRL), which can be done as soon as a fetal pole can be identified (around 5.5 weeks) and continues to be the primary dating method until week 13+6 (i.e., the end of the first trimester). Starting week 14 and continuing into the third trimester, dating is usually done by a composite measurement of four fetal biometric characteristics: the fetal head circumference, biparietal diameter, abdominal circumference, and femur length. Of these, the biparietal diameter is generally considered the most reliable.

14. **How is fetal biparietal diameter (BPD) measured? Which two landmarks must be visible to ensure an accurate measurement?**
Fetal biparietal diameter is measured as the distance between the outer edge of the proximal skull to the inner edge of the distal skull. The third ventricle and thalami must be visible to ensure an accurate BPD is measured.

15. **How is intrauterine growth retardation defined? List the possible etiologies of symmetric and asymmetric IUGR**
IUGR is defined as fetal size below the 10th percentile for gestational age. Symmetric IUGR (e.g., proportional decrease in all four biometric measurements) is typically caused by intrinsic maternal or fetal factors. Maternal factors may include TORCH infections, underlying medical conditions (e.g., hypertension, diabetes, chronic renal disease), or exposure to growth-restricting substances (e.g., alcohol, tobacco, cocaine, heroin and methadone, warfarin, antiepileptic medications, or antineoplastic medications), while fetal factors may include aneuploidy (e.g., trisomy 13 or 18) or structural anomalies (e.g., gastroschisis, cardiac malformation, renal agenesis).

Asymmetric IUGR (typically seen as normal head measurements with abnormally low limb and abdomen measurements) is most often caused by extrinsic factors during the third trimester, such as uteroplacental dysfunction, causing inadequate nutrient delivery or inadequate waste and carbon dioxide removal. Other placental factors include preeclampsia, placental abruption, and twin-twin transfusion.

16. **How is fetal well-being evaluated?**
A **nonstress** test (NST) is the easiest initial screen for fetal well-being. A fetal heart rate tracing is obtained over the course of 20 minutes. A normal NST has at least two accelerations of heart rate during those 20 minutes. For gestational age 32 or more weeks, each acceleration must be 15 beats per minute above baseline and last at least 15 seconds. For gestational age less than 32 weeks, each acceleration must be 10 beats per minute above baseline and last for 10 seconds each.

A **biophysical profile** (BPP) is composed of a **nonstress test** plus an **ultrasound** evaluation, scoring fetal (i) breathing, (ii) movement, (iii) muscle tone, (iv) heart rate, and (v) amniotic fluid index.

If the fetus scores poorly on the biophysical profile, the next test is the **contraction stress test**, which looks for uteroplacental dysfunction. Oxytocin is given, and a fetal heart strip is monitored. If late decelerations are seen on the fetal heart strip with each contraction, the test is positive. In most cases of a positive contraction stress test, delivery is performed by cesarean section.

17. **True or False: A biophysical profile is often used in high-risk pregnancies despite the absence of obvious problems**
True. For patients referred for antenatal testing, a nonstress test or biophysical profile may be done once or twice a week from the start of the third trimester until delivery to monitor for potential problems.

18. **What is quickening? When does it typically occur?**
Quickening refers to when the first fetal movements are felt. It may occur as early as week 16, but it may not occur until as late as week 20 in primigravid patients.

19. **True or False: Aspirin should be avoided during pregnancy**
False. Low-dose aspirin reduces the frequency of preeclampsia and related adverse pregnancy outcomes such as preterm birth and growth restriction when given to women at moderate to high risk of the disease. There is no consensus on the exact criteria that confer high risk, though the following are generally accepted:
• Previous pregnancy with preeclampsia
• Multifetal gestation
• Chronic hypertension
• Type 1 or type 2 diabetes mellitus
• Chronic kidney disease
• Autoimmune disease with potential vascular complications
Further, it is reasonable to offer low-dose aspirin for preeclampsia prevention with two or more of the following moderate risk factors:
• Nulliparity
• Obesity
• Family history of preeclampsia in mother or sister
• Age ≥35 years
• Low socioeconomic status

20. **Define postterm pregnancy. Why is it a major concern? How is postterm pregnancy treated?**
Posterm pregnancy is defined as more than 42 weeks of gestation. Both prematurity and postmaturity increase perinatal morbidity and mortality rates. With postmaturity, **dystocia** (or difficult delivery) becomes more common

because of the increased size of the infant. Placental insufficiency or meconium aspiration may also occur in postterm pregnancies.

In general, if the gestational age is known to be accurate and the cervix is favorable, labor is induced (e.g., with oxytocin). If the cervix is not favorable or the dates are uncertain, twice-weekly biophysical profiles are done. At 41 weeks, most obstetricians advise induction of labor. A 2012 meta-analysis demonstrated that routine labor induction at greater than 41 weeks compared with expectant management resulted in **lower perinatal mortality** and a lower rate of meconium aspiration syndrome.

21. What two rare disorders are associated with prolonged gestation?
Anencephaly and placental sulfatase deficiency

22. What lab test is used to screen for neural tube defects, and at what time during pregnancy is it measured? Explain the significance of low or high levels in maternal serum
Maternal alpha-fetoprotein (AFP) is most accurate when measured between 15 and 20 weeks of gestation. A low AFP may represent **Down syndrome**, fetal demise, or inaccurate dates. A high AFP may represent **neural tube defects** (e.g., anencephaly, spina bifida), **ventral wall defects** (e.g., omphalocele, gastroschisis), multiple gestation, or inaccurate dates.

23. What should be done if the AFP is elevated?
Repeat the test. As many as 30% of elevated maternal serum AFP test results may be elevated but are normal upon repeat testing. The initial elevation is not associated with an increased risk of neural tube defects.

24. What further testing should a patient undergo if the AFP remains elevated?
If the AFP remains elevated, the patient is advised first to undergo ultrasound to determine whether a neural tube defect or abdominal anomaly is present. The ultrasound is also used to confirm gestational age, number of fetuses, and fetal viability. Further evaluation with amniocentesis may be required if the ultrasound findings are uncertain or there is a concern for nonvisualized neural tube defects (via elevated AFP level in amniotic fluid or detection of acetylcholinesterase in amniotic fluid). There is a small risk of miscarriage after amniocentesis.

25. What is the first trimester combined test? When is it performed?
The first trimester combined test is performed at 11 to 13 weeks of gestation. The test involves determination of nuchal translucency (NT) by ultrasound, combined with serum pregnancy-associated plasma protein-A (PAPP-A) and serum hCG. If positive, chorionic villus sampling (CVS) is used to confirm the diagnosis. The combined test is most appropriate for women who place a higher value on identifying Down syndrome during the first trimester than on the risk of pregnancy loss from invasive diagnostic testing such as CVS.

26. Describe the full-integrated and serum-integrated screening tests
The full-integrated test includes an ultrasound measurement of nuchal translucency at 10 to 13 weeks of gestation, serum PAPP-A at 10 to 13 weeks of gestation, and serum levels of AFP, unconjugated estradiol (uE3), hCG, and inhibin A measured at 15 to 18 weeks of gestation. No matter which results come back first, all results of the full-integrated test are withheld until the second trimester. The full-integrated test is most appropriate for women who place a higher value on minimizing the risk of pregnancy loss from invasive diagnostic testing than on first-trimester identification of Down syndrome.

The serum-integrated screening test measures the same lab markers as the full-integrated test, but it excludes the ultrasound evaluation of NT. This test is used in areas where expertise in the ultrasound measurement of NT is not available. Results of the serum-integrated test are not available until the second trimester.

Stepwise sequential testing has been developed to provide a risk estimate during the first trimester. The first-trimester portion of the integrated screen is performed. If the tests indicate a very high risk of having an affected fetus, CVS is offered. Those women whose results do not place them at very high risk of having an affected fetus go on to have the second-trimester portion of the screening.

Contingent testing has not yet been proven efficacious in a prospective clinical trial.

27. What is the quadruple test? For whom is it typically used? When is it performed?
The quadruple test includes the serum markers AFP, uE3, hCG, and inhibin A. The quadruple test is the best available test for women who present for prenatal care in the second trimester but can be used for women who receive earlier prenatal care. It is typically performed around 15 to 18 weeks of gestation.

28. What is a maternal plasma–based test?
This is the newest option that is just becoming widely available to screen for genetic aneuploidies such as trisomy 21 (Down syndrome), trisomy 18, and trisomy 13. This test, also called cell-free fetal DNA (cfDNA) testing, detects fetal DNA in the maternal circulation. It has a detection rate greater than 98%, false-positive rate of 1%, and false-negative rate of 1.4% for Down syndrome (the detection rates are lower and the false-negative rate higher for trisomy 18 and trisomy 13). cfDNA testing is not yet validated in low-risk women and is not commonly used as a primary screening test in the United States. However, it can be used in higher-risk women (i.e., women who

will be age >35 years at the time of delivery or those with sonographic findings associated with fetal aneuploidy, history of previous pregnancy with fetal trisomy, positive screening results on tests such as the first trimester combined test, the integrated test, or the quadruple test). As such, it is commonly used as a secondary screening test.

29. **What is the next step if a woman has a positive screening test for Down syndrome?**
Offer fetal karyotype determination. This is done by CVS in the first trimester and by amniocentesis in the second trimester.

30. **Why is CVS done instead of amniocentesis in some cases?**
CVS can be done at 9 to 12 weeks of gestation (earlier than amniocentesis) and is generally reserved for women with previously affected offspring or known genetic disease. It offers the advantage of a first-trimester abortion if the fetus is affected. CVS is associated with a slightly higher miscarriage rate than amniocentesis.

31. **True or False: CVS can detect neural tube defects but not genetic disorders**
False. CVS can detect genetic or chromosomal disorders but not neural tube defects.

32. **What is a hydatidiform mole? What are the clues to its presence?**
A hydatidiform mole is one form of gestational trophoblastic neoplasia, in which the products of conception essentially become a tumor. Look for the following clues:
- Hyperemesis gravidarum
- Very high hCG levels during pregnancy and levels that do not return to zero after delivery (or abortion/miscarriage)
- First- or second-trimester bleeding with possible expulsion of "grapes" from the vagina (grossly, the tumor looks like a "bunch of grapes") and excessive nausea/hyperemesis
- Uterine size/date discrepancy, with the uterus larger than expected for dates
- "Snowstorm" pattern on ultrasound

33. **Distinguish between complete and partial hydatidiform moles. How are hydatidiform moles treated?**
Complete moles have a karyotype of 46 XX or 46 XY (with all chromosomes from the father) and no fetal tissue. **Incomplete (partial) moles** usually have a karyotype of 69 XXY with fetal tissue in the tumor.
    Treat hydatidiform moles with uterine dilation and curettage and follow with serial measurements of hCG levels until they fall to zero. If the hCG level does not fall to zero or begins to rise, the patient either has an invasive mole or a choriocarcinoma. If a choriocarcinoma occurs, these increasingly aggressive forms of gestational trophoblastic neoplasia require chemotherapy—methotrexate or dactinomycin are most effective.

34. **Cover the right-hand column, then specify the effects of the following classic teratogens on an exposed fetus**

Agent	Defect(s) Caused
Thalidomide	Phocomelia (absence of long bones, with flipperlike appearance of hands)
Antineoplastics	Many
Tetracycline	Yellow or brown teeth
Aminoglycosides	Deafness
Valproic acid	Spina bifida, hypospadias
Progesterone	Masculinization of female fetus
Cigarettes	IUGR, low birth weight, prematurity
Lithium	Cardiac (Ebstein) anomalies
Radiation	IUGR, central nervous system defects, eye defects, malignancy (e.g., leukemia)
Alcohol	Fetal alcohol syndrome
Phenytoin	Craniofacial, limb, and cerebrovascular defects; intellectual disability; fetal hydantoin syndrome
Warfarin	Craniofacial defects, IUGR, central nervous system malformation, stillbirth
Carbamazepine	Fingernail hypoplasia, craniofacial defects, fetal hydantoin syndrome

Agent	Defect(s) Caused
Isotretinoin*	Central nervous system, craniofacial, ear, and cardiovascular defects
Iodine	Goiter, neonatal hypothyroidism
Cocaine	Cerebral infarcts, intellectual disability
Diazepam	Cleft lip and/or palate
Diethylstilbestrol (DES)	Clear cell vaginal cancer, adenosis, cervical incompetence

IUGR, Intrauterine growth restriction.
*Vitamin A in general is considered teratogenic when recommended intake levels are exceeded.

35. Define macrosomia. What is the likely cause?
Macrosomia is defined as a fetus or newborn who weighs more than 4000 g (~9 lb). The cause is maternal diabetes mellitus until proven otherwise.

36. List the teratogenic effects of maternal diabetes mellitus. What is the best way to reduce these complications?
Maternal diabetes may cause any of the following fetal defects:
- Cardiovascular malformations
- Cleft lip and/or palate
- Caudal regression (lower half of the body is incompletely formed)
- Neural tube defects
- Left colon hypoplasia or immaturity
- Macrosomia (most common and classic effect)
- Microsomia (can occur if the mother has long-standing diabetes)
    Tight control of glucose during pregnancy, typically by a strict insulin regimen, dramatically reduces these complications.

37. What other problems does maternal diabetes cause in pregnancy?
In the mother, diabetes can result in polyhydramnios and preeclampsia (as well as the complications of diabetes). Problems in infants born to a diabetic mother (other than birth defects) include an increased risk of respiratory distress syndrome, transposition of the great arteries, and postdelivery **hypoglycemia**. After birth, the infant is cut off from the mother's glucose and the hyperglycemia resolves, but the infant's islet cells still overproduce insulin and may cause hypoglycemia. The risk can be decreased before delivery with strict glucose control. After delivery, treat infant hypoglycemia with IV glucose.

38. True or False: Oral hypoglycemic agents should not be used during pregnancy
Historically, this has been true, though some obstetricians are now using oral agents. Use insulin to treat diabetes if diet and exercise cannot control glucose levels. Oral hypoglycemics, unlike insulin, may cross the placenta and cause fetal hypoglycemia.

39. What commonly used drugs are generally considered safe in pregnancy?
A short list of drugs that are generally safe in pregnancy includes acetaminophen, penicillins, cephalosporins, erythromycin, nitrofurantoin, histamine-2 receptor blockers, antacids, heparin, hydralazine, methyldopa, labetalol, insulin, and docusate.

40. What are the TORCH syndromes? What do they cause?
TORCH is an acronym for several maternal infections that can cross the placenta and cause devastating intrauterine fetal complications. Most TORCH infections can cause mental retardation, microcephaly, hydrocephalus, hepatosplenomegaly, jaundice, anemia, low birth weight, and IUGR.

T = *Toxoplasma gondii:* look for exposure to cats. Specific defects include intracranial calcifications and chorioretinitis.
O = **O**ther: varicella-zoster causes limb hypoplasia and scarring of the skin. Syphilis causes rhinitis, saber shins, Hutchinson teeth, interstitial keratitis, and skin lesions.
R = **R**ubella: worst in the first trimester (some recommend abortion if the mother has rubella in the first trimester). Always check antibody status on the first visit in patients with a poor immunization history. Look for cardiovascular defects (e.g., patent ductus arteriosus), deafness, cataracts, and microphthalmia.
C = **C**ytomegalovirus: most common infection of the TORCH group. Look for deafness, intracerebral calcifications, and microphthalmia.
H = **H**erpes: look for vesicular skin lesions (with positive Tzanck smears) and history of maternal herpes lesions.

41. **True or False: With most in utero infections that can cause birth defects, obvious clues are present in the mother and/or fetus at birth**
False. Although the USMLE probably will give clues, the mother may be asymptomatic (i.e., she may have a subclinical infection), and the infant may be asymptomatic at birth, only developing symptoms later in life, such as learning disability, intellectual disability, or autism.

42. **What do you need to know about HIV testing and transmission in mother and child?**
In untreated HIV-positive patients, HIV is transmitted to the fetus in roughly 25% of cases. Roughly one-third of transmissions occur antenatally, one-third in the peripartum period, and one-third postpartum, most commonly via breastfeeding. Transmission rates are much higher in the setting of acute HIV infection, in which a woman seroconverts during pregnancy.

When multidrug antiretroviral therapy is given to the mother prenatally and zidovudine is given to the infant for 6 weeks after birth, HIV transmission is reduced to less than 2%. A noninfected infant may still have a positive HIV antibody test at birth because maternal antibodies can cross the placenta. Within 6 to 18 months, however, the test reverts to negative. This is why infants of HIV-positive mothers are tested using a direct HIV DNA polymerase chain reaction (PCR) test at birth, at 4 to 6 weeks of age, and 4 months of age. Babies who have these three negative tests should have an HIV antibody test at 12 and 18 months of age. Cesarean section is recommended for viremic women with a viral load greater than 1000 copies at the time of delivery to prevent HIV transmission to the child. Mothers with HIV should avoid breastfeeding, since the virus crosses into breast milk (the World Health Organization recommends that in developing countries mothers continue breastfeeding while the mother or infant takes antiretroviral drugs).

43. **What should you do if a pregnant woman has genital herpes?**
A decision is generally made when the mother goes into labor, not beforehand. If, at the time of true labor, the mother has active, visible genital herpes lesions, do a cesarean section to prevent transmission to the fetus. If, at the time of true labor, the mother has no visible genital herpes lesions, the child may be delivered vaginally. Women with a history of genital herpes should be offered suppressive therapy with acyclovir to maximize their chance at a vaginal delivery.

44. **What should you do for the child if the mother has chronic hepatitis B or chickenpox?**
If the mother has chronic hepatitis B confirmed by HBsAg measurement, give the infant the first hepatitis B vaccine shot plus hepatitis B immunoglobulin at birth and a bath as soon as possible. If the mother contracts chickenpox in the last 5 days of pregnancy or the first 2 days after delivery, give the infant varicella-zoster immunoglobulin.

45. **How do you treat gonorrheal and chlamydial genital infections during pregnancy?**
The treatment for gonorrhea remains unchanged because ceftriaxone is safe during pregnancy. For chlamydial infection, give azithromycin, amoxicillin, or erythromycin base instead of doxycycline or erythromycin estolate.

46. **How is tuberculosis treated in pregnancy?**
Use isoniazid, rifampin, and ethambutol to treat tuberculosis in pregnancy if the risk of a drug-resistant organism is low. Pyrazinamide should be used with caution because of a lack of data on the risk of teratogenicity. However, pyrazinamide should be added if a drug-resistant organism is suspected. Streptomycin, which is a rarely used second-line agent, should be avoided. Give vitamin B_6 to pregnant patients treated with isoniazid to avoid a deficiency.

47. **What are the signs of placental separation during the third stage of labor?**
There are three primary signs of placental separation: a fresh show or "gush" of blood from the vagina; lengthening of the umbilical cord; and a rising fundus that becomes firm and globular. If placental separation does not occur within 30 minutes of delivery, retained placenta may be diagnosed.

48. **True or False: After cesarean section, a patient may have a vaginal delivery in the future**
It depends on the type of cesarean. After a classic (vertical) uterine incision, patients must have cesarean sections for all future deliveries because of the increased rate of uterine rupture with vaginal delivery. After a low transverse (horizontal) uterine incision, a patient may deliver future pregnancies vaginally with only a slightly increased (i.e., acceptable) risk of uterine rupture.

49. **Define lochia. When is it a problem?**
For the first several days after delivery, some vaginal discharge (known as lochia) is normal. It is red for the first few days and gradually turns white or yellowish-white by day 10. If the lochia is foul smelling, suspect endometritis.

50. **What treatment may be given to a woman who does not want to breastfeed?**
Because the breasts can be become engorged with milk and thus quite painful, you may prescribe tight-fitting bras, ice packs, and analgesia to reduce symptoms. Medications for the suppression of lactation (e.g., bromocriptine and estrogens or oral contraceptive pills) are generally no longer recommended due to risks of thromboembolism and stroke.

51. **List the common contraindications for breastfeeding**
    - Use of alcohol or illicit drugs (with a few caveats that won't be tested on the USMLE)
    - HIV infection (though the World Health Organization recommends breastfeeding in developing countries because of the risks of unsafe drinking water)
    - Some medications, including antineoplastic agents, antimetabolic agents (cyclophosphamide, mercaptopurine), some anticonvulsants (topiramate), amiodarone.
      Note that hepatitis C is **not** a breastfeeding contraindication—this fact happens to be a board exam favorite.

52. **What are the options for anesthesia in obstetric patients? Why?**
    Many women elect to manage the pain of labor with breathing and other relaxation techniques. Epidural anesthesia is the most common method in obstetric patients and is generally safe and effective. Spinal anesthesia can interfere with the mother's ability to push and is associated with a higher incidence of hypotension than epidural anesthesia but is commonly used for anesthesia during cesarean section deliveries. General anesthesia is the method of choice for emergent cesarean sections when time is of the essence, but it involves a higher risk of aspiration and resulting pneumonia because the gastroesophageal sphincter is relaxed in pregnancy, and patients usually have not refrained from eating before going into labor. There is also concern about the effect of general anesthetic agents on the fetus.

53. **True or False: Asymptomatic bacteriuria, detected on routine urinalysis, should be treated during pregnancy**
    True. Up to 20% of patients develop cystitis or pyelonephritis if untreated. This rate is much higher than in nonpregnant patients, who should not be treated for asymptomatic bacteriuria. In pregnancy, the gravid uterus can compress the ureters, and increased progesterone can decrease the tone of the ureters, increasing urinary stasis and the risk of urinary tract infection. Treat with nitrofurantoin, cephalexin, or amoxicillin-clavulanate.

54. **What do you need to know about vaginal group B streptococcal (GBS) colonization during pregnancy?**
    Pregnant women should be tested for vaginal GBS at 35 to 37 weeks of gestation. Women who are carriers should be treated during labor with intrapartum penicillin G or ampicillin. Earlier testing and treatment (e.g., second trimester) is ineffective because GBS frequently returns. The exception is for women with GBS bacteriuria (often detected on first trimester screening urine culture)—these women are not retested later but are instead treated empirically during labor, as they are assumed to be chronically colonized with GBS. The reason for treating asymptomatic carriers is to prevent neonatal sepsis and endometritis, both of which are commonly caused by GBS.

55. **When does mastitis occur? How do you recognize and treat it?**
    Mastitis (inflammation of the breast) usually develops in the first 2 months postpartum. Breasts are red, indurated, and painful, and nipple cracks or fissuring may be seen. The patient with mastitis will be febrile but there will be no fluctuance; if fluctuance is present, it is an abscess. *Staphylococcus aureus* is the usual cause. Treat mastitis with analgesics (e.g., acetaminophen, ibuprofen), warm and/or cold compresses, and continued breastfeeding with the affected breast(s) even though it is painful. Advise the patient to use a breast pump to empty breast, if needed. Despite the pain, continued breastfeeding is important to prevent further milk duct blockage and abscess formation. An antistaphylococcal antibiotic (e.g., cephalexin, dicloxacillin) is usually given.

56. **What are the diagnostic signs and symptoms of preeclampsia? When does it occur?**
    Preeclampsia is new-onset **hypertension** after week 20, defined as two blood pressure readings greater than 140/90 mm Hg, separated by at least 4 hours, in a woman with previously normal blood pressure, or a greater than 30-point increase in systolic or a greater than 15-point increase in diastolic blood pressure over baseline in a woman with underlying hypertension. Other signs and symptoms include **proteinuria** ($\geq$2+ protein on urinalysis, >0.3 on a spot urine protein/creatinine ratio, or >300 mg on a 24-hour urine collection), end-organ damage such as oliguria, edema of the hands or face, headache, visual disturbances, or the HELLP syndrome (**h**emolysis, **e**levated **l**iver enzymes, **l**ow **p**latelets, and right upper quadrant or epigastric **p**ain).

57. **What are the main risk factors for preeclampsia? How is it treated?**
    The risk factors (in decreasing order of importance) include preeclampsia in a prior pregnancy, chronic renal disease, chronic hypertension, family history of preeclampsia, multiple gestations, nulliparity, extremes of reproductive age, diabetes, and black race. The definitive treatment is delivery. This is the treatment of choice if the patient is at term ($\geq$37 weeks). In a preterm patient with mild disease, the hypertension can be treated with hydralazine, labetalol, or methyldopa. Advise bed rest and observe. If the patient has severe disease (defined as oliguria, mental status changes, headache, blurred vision, pulmonary edema, cyanosis, HELLP syndrome, blood pressure >160/110 mm Hg, or progression to eclampsia [seizures]), deliver the infant once the mother is stabilized.

58. **Define the different types of hypertension in pregnancy**
    Chronic hypertension (cHTN): hypertension diagnosed before pregnancy, or elevated blood pressure of at least 140/90 mm Hg measured on two occasions, taken at least 4 hours apart, either before 20 weeks of gestation or persisting beyond 12 weeks postpartum.

Gestational hypertension (gHTN): new-onset hypertension after 20 weeks of gestation with *no proteinuria*. If a patient presents for care after 20 weeks of pregnancy, you may not be able to differentiate chronic hypertension from gestational hypertension.

Preeclampsia: hypertension that begins after week 20, plus new-onset proteinuria. Proteinuria is considered positive if at least 300 mg of protein is collected in a 24-hour urine sample, or a urinary protein/creatinine ratio of 0.3 or greater is measured. A single severe feature representing end-organ damage in combination with hypertension is also sufficient for the diagnosis. The following are severe features of preeclampsia:

- Elevated blood pressure (systolic ≥160 mm Hg, diastolic ≥110 mm Hg)
- Elevated creatinine level (>1.1 mg/dL or ≥2 times baseline)
- Hepatic dysfunction (transaminase levels ≥2 times upper limit of normal) or right upper quadrant or epigastric pain
- New-onset headache or visual disturbances
- Platelet count <100,000
- Pulmonary edema

59. What are the recommended gestational ages for delivery for cHTN? gHTN? Preeclampsia?
cHTN: consider delivery at 38 weeks of gestation (depending on blood pressure control throughout pregnancy)
gHTN: delivery at 37 weeks of gestation
Preeclampsia with no severe features: delivery at 37 weeks of gestation
Preeclampsia with severe features: timing is based on maternal factors and fetal considerations, with delivery ideally occurring at 34 weeks of gestation. However, urgent delivery may be required earlier, with the use of betamethasone to accelerate fetal lung maturity indicated between 24 and 34 weeks of gestation.

60. What are the potential complications of chronic maternal hypertension in pregnancy?
Preexisting hypertension (present before conception) increases the risk for IUGR and preeclampsia.

61. When is edema normal during pregnancy? When is it not?
Mild ankle edema is normal in pregnancy, but severe edema of the lower extremities or edema of the hands or face is likely to indicate preeclampsia.

62. What should you consider if preeclampsia develops before the third trimester?
The possibility of gestational trophoblastic disease (i.e., the presence of hydatidiform mole or choriocarcinoma).

63. Distinguish between preeclampsia and eclampsia. How can eclampsia be prevented?
Preeclampsia plus seizures equals eclampsia. Eclampsia can be prevented by regular prenatal care so that you catch the disease in the preeclamptic stage and treat appropriately.

64. What should you use to treat seizures in eclampsia? What are the toxic effects?
Use **magnesium sulfate** for eclamptic seizures; it also lowers blood pressure. Toxic effects include hyporeflexia (first sign of toxicity), respiratory depression, central nervous system depression, coma, and death. If toxicity occurs, the first step is to stop the magnesium infusion. Consider giving calcium gluconate to reverse magnesium toxicity.

65. True or False: When eclampsia occurs, you must deliver the infant immediately, regardless of maternal status
False. Do *not* try to deliver the infant until the mother is stable (e.g., do not perform a cesarean section while the mother is actively seizing).

66. What are the major complications associated with preeclampsia and eclampsia?
Preeclampsia and eclampsia cause uteroplacental insufficiency, IUGR, fetal demise, and increased maternal morbidity and mortality rates.

67. True or False: Preeclampsia and eclampsia are risk factors for development of hypertension in the future
False, but they are risk factors for later cardiovascular disease.

68. What are the major causes of maternal mortality associated with childbirth?
In decreasing order: pulmonary embolism, pregnancy-induced hypertension (preeclampsia/ eclampsia), and hemorrhage.

69. How do you recognize an amniotic fluid embolism?
Look for a recently postpartum mother who develops sudden shortness of breath, tachypnea, and chest pain within minutes of delivery. Hypotension and disseminated intravascular coagulation may soon follow. Treatment is supportive.

70. **Define oligohydramnios. What causes it? Why is it worrisome?**
Oligohydramnios means a deficiency amount of amniotic fluid is present (<500 mL or an amniotic fluid index <5). Causes include IUGR, premature rupture of the membranes (PROM), postmaturity, and renal agenesis (Potter disease). Oligohydramnios is worrisome because it may cause fetal problems, including pulmonary hypoplasia, cutaneous or skeletal abnormalities due to compression (Potter sequence), and hypoxia due to cord compression.

71. **Define polyhydramnios. What causes it? Why is it worrisome?**
Polyhydramnios means an overabundance of amniotic fluid is present (>2 L or an amniotic fluid index >25). Causes include maternal diabetes, multiple gestation, neural tube defects (e.g., anencephaly, spina bifida), gastrointestinal anomalies (e.g., omphalocele, esophageal atresia), chromosomal abnormalities (e.g., trisomies 18 and 21), and hydrops fetalis. Polyhydramnios is worrisome because it may cause maternal problems, including postpartum uterine atony (with resultant postpartum hemorrhage) and maternal dyspnea (an overdistended uterus compromises pulmonary function).

72. **When does a standard home pregnancy test become positive?**
Roughly 2 weeks after conception, which is about 4 weeks after the patient's LMP. This is also roughly the time when the woman realizes that her period is late.

73. **Define the characteristics and duration of the normal stages of labor**

Stage	Characteristics	Nulligravida	Multigravida
First stage (latent + active phase)	Onset of true labor (contractions + cervical dilation) to full cervical dilation (10 cm)	Highly variable	Highly variable
Latent phase	From 0–6 cm cervical dilation (slow, irregular)	<20 hr	<14 hr
Active phase	From 6–10 cm dilation (rapid, regular)	>1.2 cm/hr dilation	>1.5 cm/hr dilation
Second stage	From full dilation to birth of baby	30 min–3 hr	5 min–2 hr
Third stage	Delivery of baby to delivery of placenta	0–30 min	0–30 min
Fourth stage	Placental delivery to maternal stabilization	Up to 48 hr	Up to 48 hr

74. **Distinguish between true labor and false labor**
In true labor, normal contractions occur at least every 3 minutes, are fairly regular, and are associated with cervical changes (effacement and dilation). In false labor, known as Braxton-Hicks contractions, the patient experiences contractions that are irregular with no cervical changes.

75. **Distinguish between protracted labor and arrest of labor. How do you manage these conditions?**
Protracted labor occurs if labor is progressing (noted by cervical dilation or fetal descent), but this progress is occurring slower than it should be. Most practitioners are becoming more relaxed about following "normal labor curves," as labor course can be highly variable. Manage protracted labor with labor augmentation (e.g., oxytocin, prostaglandins).

   Arrest of labor is the failure to progress and is diagnosed once true labor has begun if no cervical dilation has occurred after 4 hours of adequate contractions (e.g., 200 Montevideo units over 10 minutes measured with an intrauterine pressure catheter) or no cervical dilation has occurred after 6 hours of inadequate contractions. Labor augmentation will not resolve arrest of labor—the next step in management is delivery by cesarean section.

76. **What is the most common cause of protracted labor or arrest of labor?**
Cephalopelvic disproportion, defined as a disparity between the size of the infant's head and the mother's pelvis. Labor augmentation is contraindicated in this setting—the infant must be delivered by cesarean section.

77. **What problems may be encountered when oxytocin is used to augment labor?**
On the USMLE Step 2 exam, watch for uterine hyperstimulation (painful, overly frequent, and poorly coordinated uterine contractions), uterine rupture, fetal heart rate decelerations, and water intoxication/hyponatremia (due to the antidiuretic hormone effect of oxytocin). The first step to manage all these complications is to discontinue the oxytocin infusion. The effects of oxytocin will wear off quickly, as its half-life is less than 10 minutes.

78. **What problems are associated with the use of intravaginal prostaglandin and amniotomy?**
    Prostaglandin E2 (dinoprostone) or misoprostol may be used locally to induce the cervix (a process sometimes called "ripening") and is highly effective in combination with (or before) oxytocin. However, these uterotonics may also cause uterine hyperstimulation. **Amniotomy** (manual rupture of the amniotic membrane) also hastens labor but exposes the fetus and uterine cavity to possible infection if labor does not progress promptly.

79. **What are the contraindications to labor induction or augmentation?**
    The list is almost the same as the list of contraindications to vaginal delivery: placenta or vasa previa, umbilical cord prolapse, prior classical (vertical) cesarean section, transverse fetal lie, active genital herpes, cephalopelvic disproportion, and cervical cancer.

80. **Define abortion**
    Abortion is the termination (intentional or not) of a pregnancy at less than 20 weeks of gestation or when the fetus weighs less than 500 g. *Miscarriage* is the term used to describe a spontaneous abortion. After week 20, the term *fetal demise* is used.

81. **What are the different categories of spontaneous abortion?**
    Threatened abortion: uterine bleeding *without* cervical dilation and no expulsion of tissue. Treat with pelvic rest.
    Inevitable abortion: uterine bleeding *with* cervical dilation but no tissue expulsion.
    Incomplete abortion: passage of some products of conception through the cervix.
    Complete abortion: expulsion of *all* products of conception through the cervix, often without cervical dilation. Manage with serial testing of hCG level to ensure it returns to zero.
    Missed abortion: fetal death with no expulsion of tissue (in some cases not for several weeks). Treat with misoprostol or dilation and curettage, or consider induction termination if the pregnancy is a more advanced gestation.
       All of the abovementioned terms apply only to patients who have not yet reached 20 weeks of gestation. If the mother has an Rh-negative blood type with a negative Rh-antibody screen, be sure to give her RhoGAM as well to avoid possible alloimmunization.

82. **Define induced and recurrent abortions. What do recurrent abortions suggest?**
    Induced or therapeutic abortion: an elective termination of pregnancy at less than 20 weeks of gestation. Methotrexate is the most commonly used medication for this purpose.
    Recurrent abortion: two or more sequential, unplanned abortions. History and physical exam may suggest the cause:
    - Infection (*Listeria, Mycoplasma,* or *Toxoplasma* species, syphilis)
    - Inherited thrombophilia (factor V Leiden, G20210A gene mutation, antithrombin deficiency, deficiency of protein C or protein S)
    - Substance use (alcohol, tobacco, drugs)
    - Diabetes mellitus
    - Hypothyroidism
    - Systemic lupus erythematosus (especially with positive antiphospholipid/lupus anticoagulant antibodies, sometimes an isolated syndrome without coexisting lupus)
    - Cervical insufficiency (watch for a history of cervical procedures [e.g., LEEP or cold-knife cone procedure] or exposure to diethylstilbestrol [DES] in the patient's mother during pregnancy and/or a patient with recurrent painless second trimester abortions; treat future pregnancies with intramuscular or vaginal progesterone and cervical cerclage)
    - Congenital female tract abnormalities (if possible, correct to restore fertility)
    - Fibroids (remove them by performing a myomectomy)
    - Chromosomal abnormalities (e.g., maternal or paternal translocations)

83. **True or False: hCG roughly doubles every 2 days in the first trimester**
    True

84. **What are two possible reasons the patient's hCG levels would *not* double every 2 days during the first weeks of pregnancy?**
    An hCG level that stays the same or increases only slowly with serial testing suggests that the fetus is in trouble. In cases like this, the two conditions you should be most concerned for are threatened abortion or ectopic pregnancy.

85. **What are the risk factors for developing an ectopic pregnancy?**
    The major risk factor for ectopic pregnancy is scarring of the fallopian tube. You might see this in a patient with previous history of pelvic inflammatory disease (PID), which increases the ectopic pregnancy rate 10-fold. Other risk factors include a previous ectopic pregnancy, history of tubal ligation or tuboplasty, and pregnancy that occurs with an intrauterine device in place.

86. **What are the classic signs and symptoms of a ruptured ectopic pregnancy?**
A recent history of amenorrhea with current signs of peritonitis and acute, severe abdominal pain. Patients also have a positive hCG pregnancy test.

87. **What should you do if you suspect an ectopic pregnancy?**
Order a transvaginal ultrasound to look for a gestational sac or fetus. When the diagnosis is in doubt and the patient is hemodynamically unstable (e.g., hypovolemia, shock, severe abdominal pain, rebound tenderness), perform laparoscopic exploration for definitive diagnosis and treatment.

88. **How is unruptured ectopic pregnancy managed?**
An unruptured ectopic pregnancy is also definitively managed with surgery, but a different procedure is performed than in the case of a ruptured ectopic. An unruptured tubal pregnancy, if stable and less than 3 cm in diameter, can be treated with salpingostomy and removal of the products of conception. The tube is left open to heal on its own; this strategy retains normal tubal function and fertility. Methotrexate is an alternative medical treatment for small (<3 cm), unruptured tubal pregnancies. If the patient is unstable, the ectopic pregnancy has ruptured, or the fallopian tube has dilated to greater than 3 cm in diameter, a salpingectomy must be performed. In Rh-negative patients, give RhoGAM after treatment to prevent possible alloimmunization.

89. **In fetal heart monitoring, what is the difference between early decelerations, variable deceleration, and late decelerations?**
In **early decelerations** (Fig. 25.1), the peaks are aligned (nadir of fetal heart deceleration and peak of uterine contraction). This pattern signifies **head compression** (probably a vagal response) and is not a concerning heart tracing.
  Variable decelerations (Fig. 25.2) are so called because the fetal heart rate deceleration does not appear to be related to uterine contractions—the timing of the decelerations is *variable*. Note that in variable decelerations, each deceleration lasts no more than 30 seconds. This is the most commonly encountered type of deceleration pattern and signifies **cord compression**. If variable decelerations are seen, place the mother in the lateral decubitus position, administer oxygen by face mask, stop any oxytocin infusion, and consider giving an intravenous fluid bolus to increase intravascular volume.
  Late decelerations (Fig. 25.3) occur when fetal heart rate deceleration begins after uterine contraction, with the nadir of each deceleration occurring after the peak of contraction and at regular intervals. This pattern signifies **uteroplacental insufficiency** and is the most worrisome fetal heart tracing. If it is seen, first place the mother in the lateral decubitus position; then give oxygen by face mask and stop oxytocin, if applicable. Next, give a tocolytic (often a beta$_2$-agonist such as ritodrine or magnesium sulfate) if the mother is not in active labor and intravenous fluids (if the mother is hypotensive). If the late decelerations persist, measure the fetal oxygen saturation or scalp pH and prepare for operative delivery.

90. **What other patterns of fetal distress may be seen on a fetal heart tracing? What is a normal fetal heart rate?**
Loss of variability may signify fetal acidemia. This may present as loss of short-term (beat-to-beat) or long-term (baseline changes in heart rate >1 minute) variability. Prolonged fetal tachycardia (>160 beats/min) can be an early sign of infection such as chorioamnionitis. The normal fetal heart rate is 110 to 160 beats/minute.

91. **What if the question gives you a value for fetal oxygen saturation or scalp pH?**
Any fetal scalp pH less than 7.2 or significantly decreased oxygen saturation is an indication for immediate cesarean delivery. If the pH is greater than 7.2 or oxygenation is normal, immediate surgical intervention is not warranted.

92. **What should you do if shoulder dystocia or impaction occurs during vaginal delivery?**
The first step is to try the McRoberts maneuver. Have the mother sharply flex her thighs against her abdomen, which may free the impacted shoulder. Other maneuvers include applying suprapubic pressure, performing the Woods screw maneuver (applying pressure to the anterior aspect of the fetus's posterior shoulder), the Rubin maneuver (applying pressure to the posterior aspect of the anterior shoulder), and delivery of the posterior arm. Some clinicians may intentionally fracture the clavicle by pulling the anterior clavicle outward, though this comes with its own set of complications and is not a universally practiced method of management. If these maneuvers fail, options are limited. Delivery by cesarean section is usually the procedure of choice and must be performed after performing the Zavanelli maneuver (pushing the infant's head back into the birth canal).

93. **What causes third trimester bleeding? How do you distinguish the four major causes from one another?**
The four most notable causes of third trimester bleeding include:
  • Placenta previa (painless bleeding with no fetal bradycardia)
  • Vas previa (painless bleeding with fetal bradycardia)

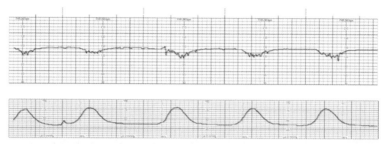

Fig. 25.1 *Early deceleration* of the fetal heart rate (FHR) is defined as a gradual decrease (onset to nadir <30 seconds) in FHR from the baseline and a subsequent return to baseline associated with a uterine contraction. In most cases the onset, nadir, and recovery of the deceleration occur at the same time as the beginning, peak, and end of the contraction, respectively. Early decelerations are considered to represent a fetal autonomic response to changes in intracranial pressure and/or cerebral blood flow caused by intrapartum compression of the fetal head during uterine contractions. Early decelerations are not associated with interruption of fetal oxygenation or adverse neonatal outcome and are considered clinically benign. (From Miller DA. Intrapartum fetal evaluation. In: Gabbe SG, Niebyl JR, Simpson, et al., eds. *Obstetrics: Normal and Problem Pregnancies.* Philadelphia: Elsevier; 2017.)

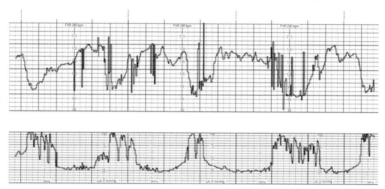

Fig. 25.2 *Variable deceleration* of the fetal heart rate (FHR) is defined as an abrupt decrease (onset to nadir <30 seconds) in FHR below the baseline. The decrease is at least 15 beats/minute below the baseline, the deceleration lasts at least 15 seconds, and fewer than 2 minutes pass from onset to return to baseline. Variable decelerations can occur with or without uterine contractions. A variable deceleration represents a fetal autonomic reflex response to transient mechanical compression or stretch of the umbilical cord. (Miller DA. Intrapartum fetal evaluation. In: Gabbe SG, Niebyl JR, Simpson, et al., eds. *Obstetrics: Normal and Problem Pregnancies.* Philadelphia: Elsevier; 2017.)

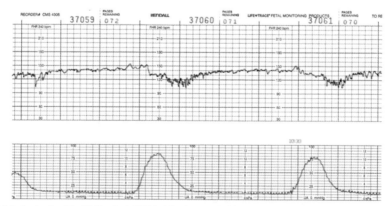

Fig. 25.3 *Late deceleration* of the fetal heart rate (FHR) is defined as a gradual decrease (onset to nadir ≥30 seconds) of the FHR from the baseline and subsequent return to the baseline associated with a uterine contraction. Late decelerations are associated with uteroplacental insufficiency and are considered an emergency of fetal distress that requires immediate delivery. (Miller DA. Intrapartum fetal evaluation. In: Gabbe SG, Niebyl JR, Simpson, et al., eds. *Obstetrics: Normal and Problem Pregnancies.* Philadelphia: Elsevier; 2017.)

- Abruptio placentae (painful bleeding)
- Uterine rupture

Other causes to consider include:

- Cervical or vaginal infections (e.g., herpes simplex virus, gonorrhea, chlamydial or candidal infection)
- Cervical or vaginal trauma (usually from sexual intercourse)
- Bleeding disorders (rare before delivery; more common after delivery)
- Cervical cancer (which may occur in pregnant patients)
- "Bloody show"

94. **True or False: Ultrasound must be performed before performing a pelvic exam when investigating the cause of third-trimester bleeding**
True. You may perform a history and partial physical exam before performing the ultrasound, but *always* do an ultrasound before you do a pelvic exam to better understand the patient's uterine anatomy and placental placement. In the case of placenta previa, for example, disturbing the placenta by performing a pelvic exam may make the bleeding worse and turn a worrisome case into an emergency.

95. **Define placenta previa. How does it present? How is it diagnosed and treated?**
True placenta previa occurs when the placenta implants and grows to cover the cervical opening (os). Predisposing factors include multiparity, increasing maternal age, multiple gestation, and a history of prior placenta previa. Placenta previa typically presents as painless third trimester bleeding, and the bleeding may be profuse. Because of this condition, you *always* do an ultrasound before a pelvic exam for third trimester bleeding. Ultrasound is 95% to 100% accurate in diagnosis. The only delivery option for placenta previa is by cesarean section.

96. **Define placental abruption. How does it present? How is it managed?**
Placental abruption (or abruptio placentae) is premature detachment of a normally situated placenta. Predisposing factors include hypertension (with or without preeclampsia), trauma, polyhydramnios with rapid decompression after membrane rupture, cocaine or tobacco use, and preterm PROM. Patients can have this condition without visible vaginal bleeding; the blood may be contained behind the placenta. Usual symptoms include pain (which may be described as abdominal, pelvic, or back pain), uterine tenderness, increased uterine tone with a hyperactive contraction pattern, and fetal distress. Placental abruption may also cause disseminated intravascular coagulation if fetal products enter the maternal circulation. Ultrasound detects only a small percentage of cases. Treat with intravenous fluids (and blood if needed) and rapid delivery (vaginal preferred).

97. **What factors predispose to uterine rupture? How does it present? How is it managed?**
Predisposing factors include previous uterine surgery (especially prior classic cesarean section with vertical incision), trauma, oxytocin, grand multiparity (several previous deliveries), excessive uterine distention (e.g., multiple gestation, polyhydramnios), abnormal fetal lie, cephalopelvic disproportion, and shoulder dystocia. Uterine rupture is very painful, has a sudden and dramatic onset with loss of fetal station, and often is accompanied by maternal hypotension or shock. Other classic signs are the ability to feel fetal body parts on abdominal exam and a sudden change in the abdominal contour. Maternal distress usually is more pronounced than fetal distress (unlike abruptio placentae, in which fetal distress is greater). Treat with immediate laparotomy and delivery. Hysterectomy is usually required after delivery.

98. **What causes fetal bleeding to present as third-trimester vaginal bleeding?**
Visible fetal bleeding usually is due to vasa previa or velamentous insertion of the cord, which occurs when umbilical vessels present in advance of the fetal head, usually traversing the membranes and crossing the cervical os. The biggest predisposing risk factor is multiple gestation (the higher the number of fetuses, the higher the risk). Bleeding is painless, and the mother is typically stable, whereas the fetus shows worsening distress (tachycardia initially, then bradycardia as the fetus decompensates). An Apt test may be performed on vaginal blood, which will be positive for fetal blood if fetal bleeding is occurring. Treat with immediate cesarean section delivery.

99. **Explain the term *bloody show*. How is it diagnosed?**
With cervical effacement, a blood-tinged mucous plug may be released from the cervical canal and mark the onset of labor. This normal occurrence is a diagnosis of exclusion when investigating third trimester bleeding.

100. **For Rh-negative, antibody-negative patients, how is the dose of RhoGAM determined?**
A Kleihauer-Betke test is used to quantify fetal blood in the maternal circulation and calculate the necessary dose of RhoGAM.

101. **Define preterm labor. How is it managed?**
Preterm labor is true labor that begins between 20 and 37 weeks of gestation. Put the mother in the lateral decubitus position, order bed and pelvic rest, and give oral or IV fluids and oxygen. In some cases, these maneuvers stop the contractions. If they fail, you can give a tocolytic if no contraindications are present (e.g., heart disease, hypertension, diabetes, hemorrhage, ruptured membranes, cervix dilated >4 cm).

208 OBSTETRICS

102. **What are tocolytics? When is it not appropriate to give them?**
Tocolytics are medications that slow or stop uterine contractions. Common examples are beta$_2$-agonists (terbutaline, ritodrine), indomethacin, and magnesium sulfate. Do not give tocolytics to the mother in the presence of preeclampsia, severe hemorrhage, chorioamnionitis, IUGR, fetal demise, or fetal anomalies incompatible with survival. Indomethacin cannot be used after 32 weeks of gestation, as it risks premature closure of the ductus arteriosus.

103. **What is fetal fibronectin? When is a test for this substance useful? Is the test more helpful when positive or negative?**
Fetal fibronectin is an extracellular matrix protein that helps attach the amniotic membranes to the uterine lining. It can be detected in the vaginal secretions of some women presenting with signs and symptoms of preterm labor. The test is most helpful when negative between 22 and 34 weeks of gestation because it indicates a very low likelihood of impending delivery over the next 2 weeks. Thus a more conservative, observational approach can be used. When fetal fibronectin is positive in this setting, the woman is at a higher risk for delivery within the next 2 weeks, and a more aggressive approach to tocolysis and fetal lung maturity hastening is typically taken. In other words, fetal fibronectin has a high negative predictive value.

104. **When should fetal lung maturity be evaluated?**
Evaluation of fetal lung maturity is indicated before elective deliveries that are, or may be, less than 39 weeks of gestation. Testing is not necessary for well-documented pregnancies that are 39 or more weeks of gestation, pregnancies that are less than 32 weeks of gestation (because fetal lung maturity is unlikely), or when delaying delivery will place the mother or fetus at significant risk.

105. **What tests can be used to assess fetal lung maturity?**
   • Lamellar body count
   • Lecithin/sphingomyelin ratio
   • Phosphatidylglycerol
   • Surfactant/albumin ratio
   • Optical density at 650 nm
   • Foam stability index
      For the purposes of the USMLE exam, it is not necessary to know the details of these tests. No test performs better than another. All of these tests are better at predicting the absence, rather than the presence, of respiratory distress.

106. **What is the role of steroids in preterm labor?**
Steroids (e.g., betamethasone) typically are given in the setting of preterm labor between 24 and 37 weeks of gestation to hasten fetal lung maturity and thus decrease the risk of respiratory distress syndrome in the neonatal period.

107. **Define quickening. When does it occur?**
Quickening is the term used to describe when the mother first detects fetal movements, usually between 18 and 20 weeks of gestation in a primigravida and 16 and 18 weeks of gestation in a multigravida.

108. **List the order of fetal positions that occur during normal labor and delivery**
   1. Descent
   2. Flexion
   3. Internal rotation
   4. Extension
   5. External rotation
   6. Expulsion

109. **What subtype of maternal antibody can cross the placenta?**
IgG is a monomer and is therefore the only type of maternal antibody that crosses the placenta. IgM antibodies are pentamers and are too large to cross the placenta. This is an important diagnostic point: An elevated neonatal IgM concentration is never normal, whereas an elevated neonatal IgG often represents maternal antibodies.

110. **Explain Rh incompatibility. In what situations does it occur?**
Rh blood-type incompatibility is of concern because it can lead to hemolytic disease of the newborn. Rh incompatibility occurs when the mother is Rh negative and her infant is Rh positive. This is only possible if the father is Rh positive. If both the mother and the father are Rh negative, there is no possibility of producing an Rh-positive infant; if the mother is Rh positive, there is no possibility of her producing Rh antibodies.

111. **How do you detect and manage potential hemolytic disease of the newborn?**
If Rh incompatibility is a concern based on maternal and paternal blood type, check maternal titers of Rh antibody every month, starting in the seventh month of gestation. Give RhoGAM automatically at 28 weeks and again within 72 hours after delivery, as well as after any procedures that may cause mixing of maternal and fetal blood.

112. **True or False: The first child is usually the most severely affected by Rh incompatibility**

False. Previous maternal sensitization is required for disease to occur. In other words, if a nulliparous Rh-negative mother has never received blood products, her first Rh-positive infant will not be affected by hemolytic disease because the antibodies generated will be IgM that cannot cross the placenta. The second Rh-positive infant, however, will be affected because IgG antibodies that can cross the placenta will be generated. This is why, in Rh-negative mothers, you must administer RhoGAM at 28 weeks and within 72 hours after delivery during the first pregnancy to prevent the generation of anti-Rh antibodies that will affect the next Rh-positive fetus.

113. **How do you recognize, monitor, and treat hemolytic disease of the newborn?**

Hemolytic disease of the newborn in its most severe form causes hydrops fetalis (edema, ascites, pleural and/or pericardial effusions) and death. Amniotic fluid spectrophotometry and ultrasound can help gauge the severity of fetal hemolysis. Treatment of hemolytic disease involves (1) delivery, if the fetus is mature (check lung maturity with a lecithin-to-sphingomyelin ratio); (2) intrauterine transfusion; and (3) phenobarbital, which helps the fetal liver break down bilirubin.

114. **True or False: ABO blood group incompatibility can cause hemolytic disease of the newborn**

True. ABO blood group incompatibility can cause hemolytic disease of the newborn when the mother is type O and the infant is type A, B, or AB. *This condition does not require previous sensitization* because IgG antibodies with transplacental potential occur naturally in mothers with blood type O—but not in mothers with other blood types. The hemolytic disease is usually less severe than with Rh incompatibility, but treatment is the same.

115. **When should RhoGAM be given?**

RhoGAM should only be given when the mother is Rh negative and antibody negative, and the father is Rh positive or his blood type is unknown. During routine prenatal care, check for Rh antibodies at the first visit. If the test is positive, do not give RhoGAM—you are too late and the mother has already generated anti-Rh antibodies. Giving RhoGAM will not change this. Otherwise, give RhoGAM routinely in these patients at 28 weeks and immediately after delivery. Also give RhoGAM after an abortion, stillbirth, ectopic pregnancy, amniocentesis, chorionic villus sampling, and any other invasive procedure that may cause mixing of maternal and fetal blood during pregnancy.

116. **Define premature rupture of membranes. How is it diagnosed?**

PROM is rupture of the amniotic sac before the onset of labor. Diagnosis of rupture of membranes (whether premature or not) is based on history, sterile speculum exam, and/or a positive Nitrazine test. The sterile speculum exam shows pooling of amniotic fluid and a ferning pattern when the fluid is placed on a microscopic slide. Nitrazine paper turns blue (indicating basicity) in the presence of amniotic fluid. Ultrasound should be done in cases of PROM to assess amniotic fluid volume as well as gestational age and any anomalies that may be present.

117. **What usually follows membrane rupture? What should you do if it does not occur?**

Spontaneous labor usually follows membrane rupture; for this reason, an amniotomy may be done in an attempt to induce labor if membranes do not rupture spontaneously. If labor does not occur within 18 hours of membrane rupture, the mother is term, and the cervix is favorable, labor should be induced.

Labor is induced because the main risk of PROM is infection, which may occur in the mother (chorioamnionitis) and/or the infant (neonatal sepsis, pneumonia, meningitis).

118. **Define preterm premature rupture of membranes (PPROM). How is it managed?**

PPROM is defined as premature rupture of membranes that occurs during the preterm period (i.e., <37 weeks of gestation). The risk of infection increases with the duration of ruptured membranes, especially if 18 hours have elapsed since membrane rupture. Order a culture and Gram stain of the amniotic fluid. If it is negative, management for a hemodynamically stable patient with reassuring fetal heart tones simply involves pelvic rest with frequent follow-up. Hemodynamic instability or nonreassuring fetal testing could deteriorate quickly with expectant management and should instead be managed with delivery. If the culture is positive for GBS, treat the mother with penicillin G or ampicillin, even if she is asymptomatic.

119. **How does chorioamnionitis present, and how is it treated?**

Patients with chorioamnionitis present with fever and a tender, irritable uterus, usually near and after delivery. Antepartum chorioamnionitis may occur in patients with PROM, especially if the time since membrane rupture exceeds 18 hours. Do a culture and Gram stain of the cervix and amniotic fluid, then treat with antibiotics such as ampicillin plus gentamicin while awaiting culture results.

120. **Define postpartum hemorrhage. What are the most common causes?**

Postpartum hemorrhage is defined as a blood loss greater than 500 mL during vaginal delivery or greater than 1 L during cesarean section. The most common cause is **uterine atony** (75%–80% of cases). Other causes include lacerations, retained placental tissue, coagulation disorders, low placental implantation, and uterine inversion. Retained placental tissue results from placenta accreta (penetration of the placenta through the endometrium into the myometrium), increta (deeper penetration of the placenta into the myometrium), or percreta (penetration of the placenta through the myometrium to the uterine serosa); in all three conditions, the placenta grows deeper into the uterine wall than it should. The major risk factors for this condition include previous uterine surgery, multiparity, or prior cesarean section, and the typical treatment is a total abdominal hysterectomy.

121. **What causes uterine atony? How is it managed?**
Uterine atony is caused by overdistention of the uterus (due to multiple gestation, polyhydramnios, or macrosomia), prolonged labor, oxytocin usage, grand multiparity (a history of five or more deliveries), chorioamnionitis, and precipitous labor (too fast or <3 hours). Manage uterine atony with a dilute oxytocin infusion to tighten the uterus, and use bimanual compression to massage the uterus while the oxytocin infusion is running. If this approach fails, use ergonovine (contraindicated with maternal hypertension), prostaglandin f_2-alpha (contraindicated with maternal history of asthma), or misoprostol. If these strategies also fail, the patient may need a hysterectomy. Ligation of the uterine vessels may be attempted to preserve fertility if the patient desires.

122. **What is the treatment for retained products of conception?**
With retained products of conception, the most common cause of a *delayed* postpartum hemorrhage, remove the placenta manually to stop the bleeding. Next, perform dilation and curettage in the operating room under anesthesia. If placenta accreta, increta, or percreta is present, total abdominal hysterectomy is usually necessary to stop the bleeding.

123. **What causes uterine inversion? How is it treated?**
When the uterus inverts, it usually can be seen outside the vagina and will not be palpable in the suprapubic region. Uterine inversion is usually iatrogenic, a result of *pulling too hard on the umbilical cord*. If it occurs, immediately manually replace the uterus; if you wait too long, the uterus may become edematous or swollen and become ischemic. Anesthesia may be required for pain management. Once the uterus is back in place, give IV fluids and oxytocin to anchor the uterus in place.

124. **Define postpartum fever. What are the common causes?**
Postpartum fever is a temperature greater than 100.4°F (38°C) for at least 2 consecutive days following delivery. It is classically due to endometritis. However, do not forget typical postoperative causes of fever, such as a urinary tract infection or atelectasis/pneumonia. Pulmonary problems are especially common after a cesarean section.

125. **What should you do if postpartum fever does not improve with antibiotics?**
If a postpartum fever does not resolve with broad-spectrum antibiotics such as clindamycin plus gentamicin, there are two main etiologies to consider: progression to pelvic abscess or pelvic thrombophlebitis. Computed tomography (CT) scan will identify a pelvic abscess, which needs to be drained. Pelvic thrombophlebitis presents with persistent spiking fevers, lack of response to antibiotics, and no abscess on CT. Give heparin or low-molecular-weight heparin to manage this diagnosis of exclusion.

126. **What should you consider if a postpartum patient goes into shock without evident bleeding?**
- Amniotic fluid embolism (minutes to hours postpartum)
- Uterine inversion
- Concealed hemorrhage (e.g., uterine rupture with bleeding into the peritoneal cavity)

127. **What typical physiologic changes of pregnancy may present with "abnormal" laboratory results if you don't recognize them?**
- Erythrocyte sedimentation rate (ESR) becomes markedly elevated. For this reason, measuring ESR during pregnancy is essentially worthless.
- Total thyroxine (T4) and thyroid-binding globulin (TBG) increase (stimulated by hCG), but free T4 remains normal.
- Red blood cell (RBC) mass increases, but plasma volume increases even more. The net result of these changes is a dilutional anemia, presenting as a decrease in hemoglobin and hematocrit. *Remember, hemoglobin and hematocrit are **ratios** whose denominators (plasma volume) become much larger during pregnancy.*
- Blood urea nitrogen (BUN) and creatinine decrease because of an increase in glomerular filtration rate. Therefore BUN and creatinine levels at the high end of normal suggest renal disease in pregnancy.
- Alkaline phosphatase increases markedly.
- Mild (1+) proteinuria and glycosuria are normal in pregnancy.
- Electrolytes and liver function tests remain normal.

128. **What cardiovascular and pulmonary changes occur in a normal pregnancy?**
Normal cardiovascular changes of pregnancy: blood pressure decreases slightly, heart rate increases by 10 to 20 beats/minute, stroke volume increases, and cardiac output increases (by up to 50%).
Normal pulmonary changes of pregnancy: minute ventilation increases because of increased tidal volume, but respiratory rate remains the same or increases only slightly. Functional residual capacity decreases as the uterus expands and the diaphragm displaces superiorly. Carbon dioxide decreases as the increased minute ventilation blows it off. Collectively, these changes cause the physiologic respiratory alkalosis of pregnancy.

129. What is the average weight gain during pregnancy? What commonly causes weight gain to be more or less?

The average weight gain in pregnancy is roughly 28 lb (12.5 kg), but goal weight gain should be less for overweight and obese women. A larger weight gain may mean maternal diabetes. A smaller weight gain may mean hyperemesis gravidarum, nutritional deficiencies, psychiatric disturbances, or major systemic diseases.

130. Define hyperemesis gravidarum. How do you recognize and treat it?

Hyperemesis gravidarum is intractable nausea and vomiting leading to dehydration and possible electrolyte disturbances. It presents in the first trimester, usually in younger patients with their first pregnancy while experiencing underlying social stressors or psychiatric problems. Treat hyperemesis gravidarum with supportive care along with small, frequent meals and antiemetic medications such as pyridoxine-doxylamine, diphenhydramine, meclizine, dimenhydrinate, prochlorperazine, metoclopramide, or ondansetron. Hyperemesis gravidarum can be a sign of trophoblastic disease, so be sure to rule it out with ultrasound. Dehydrated patients need IV fluids, and electrolyte abnormalities must be corrected. Remember that hyperemesis gravidarum plus severely elevated hCG or a uterus greater than gestational age is suggestive of a hydatidiform molar pregnancy.

131. Define cholestasis of pregnancy. How is it managed?

Cholestasis of pregnancy presents with itching (often severe) and/or abnormal liver function tests, usually in the second and third trimesters. In rare cases, jaundice may coexist. It is dangerous because of the associated risk of fetal demise. Heightened fetal surveillance and induction of labor at 37 weeks are typically recommended. The only known definitive treatment is delivery, but ursodeoxycholic acid or cholestyramine may help with symptoms.

132. What is acute fatty liver of pregnancy? How is it managed?

Acute fatty liver of pregnancy is a more serious disorder than cholestasis. It presents in the third trimester or after delivery and usually progresses to hepatic coma. Treat with IV fluids, glucose, and fresh frozen plasma to correct coagulopathies. Vitamin K does not work because the liver is in temporary failure. If the patient survives with supportive care, liver dysfunction usually resolves on its own with time.

133. True or False: Appendicitis during pregnancy may present with acute pain somewhere other than the lower right quadrant

True. Pregnant women can develop appendicitis, which may present with right upper quadrant pain due to displacement of the appendix by the pregnant uterus. Just as in nonpregnant patients, a laparotomy or laparoscopy is appropriate when the diagnosis is unsure and the patient has peritoneal signs. Note that purely elective surgical cases must be avoided during pregnancy.

134. How do you manage fetal malpresentation?

External cephalic version can be used to rotate the fetus from the breech to the cephalic position. Absolute contraindications to external cephalic version are placenta previa and history of classical (vertical) cesarian incision. Occiput posterior (OP) presentations can cause protraction of the second stage of labor. Most fetuses eventually rotate to occiput anterior (OA) presentations on their own or can be delivered OP, but providers may also attempt internal manual rotation. If this fails, the decision must be made whether to attempt vaginal delivery or do a cesarean section. Frank and complete breech presentations must be delivered by cesarean section, as should shoulder presentation or incomplete/footling breech. For face and brow presentations, watchful waiting is best, because most cases convert to vertex presentations. Cesarean section must be performed if they do not.

135. What is the "poor man's way" to distinguish between monozygotic and dizygotic twins?

If the sex or blood type is different, the twins are dizygotic (i.e., fraternal). If the placentas are monochorionic, the twins are monozygotic (i.e., identical). These three simple points differentiate monozygotic from dizygotic twins in 80% of cases. In the remaining 20%, human leukocyte antigen typing studies are required to determine the type of twins.

136. What are the maternal and fetal complications of multiple gestations?

Maternal complications: anemia, hypertension, premature labor, postpartum uterine atony, postpartum hemorrhage, and preeclampsia

Fetal complications: polyhydramnios, malpresentation, placenta previa, abruptio placentae, velamentous cord insertion/vasa previa, premature rupture of the membranes, prematurity, umbilical cord prolapse, IUGR, congenital anomalies, and increased perinatal morbidity and mortality

137. How are multiple gestations delivered?

With vertex-vertex presentations of twins (both infants are head first), you can try vaginal delivery for both infants, but with any other twin presentation combination or more than two infants, perform cesarean section.

CHAPTER 26

ONCOLOGY

1. What are the key differential points for the commonly tested blood dyscrasias?

Type	Age	What to Look for in Case Description/ Trigger Words
ALL	Children (peak age: 3–5 yr)	Pancytopenia (bleeding, fever, anemia), history of radiation therapy, Down syndrome
AML	>30 yr	Pancytopenia (bleeding, fever, anemia), Auer rods (Fig. 26.1), DIC
CML (Fig. 26.2)	30–50 yr	White blood cell count >50,000, Philadelphia chromosome (t[9;22]), blast crisis, splenomegaly
CLL	>50 yr	Male gender, lymphadenopathy, lymphocytosis, infections, smudge cells, splenomegaly
Hairy cell leukemia	Adults	Blood smear (hairlike projections), splenomegaly, tartrate-resistant acid phosphatase (TRAP) staining
Mycosis fungoides/ Sézary syndrome	>50 yr	Plaquelike, itchy skin rash that does not improve with treatment, blood smear (cerebriform nuclei known as "butt cells"), Pautrier abscesses in epidermis
Burkitt lymphoma (Fig. 26.3)	Children	Associated with Epstein-Barr virus (in Africa), (t[8;14]), "starry sky" on histology
CNS B-cell lymphoma	Adults	Seen in patients with HIV infection, AIDS
T-cell leukemia	Adults	Caused by HTLV-1 virus
Hodgkin disease	15–34 yr	Reed-Sternberg cell, painless cervical lymphadenopathy, night sweats, lymph nodes become painful with alcohol consumption
Non-Hodgkin lymphoma	Any age	Small follicular type has best prognosis, diffuse large type has worst prognosis; primary tumor may be located in gastrointestinal tract
Myelodysplasia/ myelofibrosis	>50 yr	Anemia, teardrop cells, "dry tap" on bone marrow biopsy, high MCV and RDW; associated with CML
Multiple myeloma	>40 yr	Bence-Jones protein (IgG = 50%, IgA = 25%), osteolytic lesions, high serum calcium, anemia, renal impairment
Waldenström macroglobulinemia	>40 yr	Hyperviscosity syndrome, IgM spike, cold agglutinins (Raynaud phenomenon with cold sensitivity)
Polycythemia vera	>40 yr	High hematocrit/hemoglobin, aquagenic pruritus; use phlebotomy
Primary thrombocythemia	>50 yr	Platelet count usually >1,000,000; may have bleeding or thrombosis

ALL, Acute lymphoblastic leukemia; *AML*, acute myelogenous leukemia; *CLL*, chronic lymphocytic leukemia; *CML*, chronic myelogenous leukemia; *CNS*, central nervous system; *DIC*, disseminated intravascular coagulation; *HTLV-1*, human T-cell leukemia virus type 1; *MCV*, mean corpuscular volume; *RDW*, red cell distribution width.

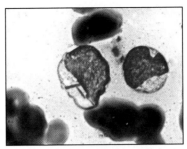

Fig. 26.1 Auer rods vary from prominent, as in this cell, to thin and delicate. (From McPherson RA. *Henry's Clinical Diagnosis and Management by Laboratory Methods.* 22nd ed. Philadelphia: Saunders; 2011 [fig. 33.25].)

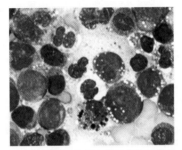

Fig. 26.2 Chronic myelogenous leukemia showing myeloid blast phase. (From Hoffman R. *Hematology: Basic Principles and Practice.* 5th ed. Edinburgh: Churchill Livingstone; 2008 [fig. 69.5].)

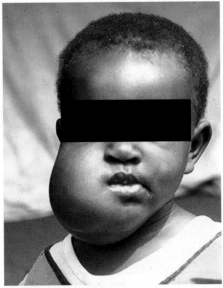

Fig. 26.3 A young boy from South America with typical endemic Burkitt lymphoma presenting in the mandible. (From Jaffe ES. *Hematopathology.* 1st ed. Philadelphia: Saunders; 2010 [fig. 24.1]. Courtesy Prof. Georges Delsol, Toulouse, France.)

2. Which cancers have the overall highest incidence and mortality rate in men and women in the United States?
Overall highest incidence:

Male	Female
1. Prostate	1. Breast
2. Lung	2. Lung
3. Colon	3. Colon

Overall highest mortality rate:

Male	Female
1. Lung	1. Lung
2. Prostate	2. Breast
3. Colon	3. Colon

3. What are the most common types of cancer in children and young adults (age <30 years)?
Leukemia and lymphoma.

4. What is the major risk factor for cancer? What is the major modifiable risk factor for cancer?
Age is the biggest risk factor (the incidence of cancer in the United States roughly doubles every 5 years after age 25), and smoking is the biggest modifiable risk factor.

5. What is the most common cancer in most organs?
Metastatic cancer (Fig. 26.4). On the Step 2 exam, do not assume that the question is looking for the most common primary cancer unless the word "primary" is specified.

6. Metastatic cancer to the spine can cause spinal cord compression. How do you recognize and treat this medical emergency?
Spinal cord compression causes local spinal pain and neurologic symptoms (reflex changes, weakness, sensory loss, paralysis, incontinence, urinary retention). In rare cases it may be the first indication of a malignancy. The first step is to start high-dose corticosteroids and order a magnetic resonance imaging (MRI) scan. Surgery, external beam radiation therapy, and stereotactic body radiotherapy are the treatment options for a tumor compressing the spinal cord. Prompt intervention is essential, and outcome is closely linked to pretreatment function.

7. Name the mode of inheritance and types of cancer found in the following conditions

Disease/Syndrome	Inheritance	Type of Cancer (In Order of Most Likely)/Other Information
Retinoblastoma	Autosomal dominant	Retinoblastoma, osteosarcoma (later in life)
MEN, type I	Autosomal dominant	Parathyroid, pituitary, pancreas (islet cell tumors)

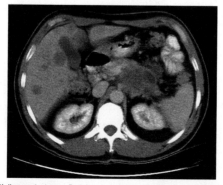

Fig. 26.4 Pancreatic carcinoma with liver metastases. Portal venous phase computed tomography shows poorly enhancing liver deposits from a primary mass in the pancreatic body. (From Adam A, et al. *Grainger & Allison's Diagnostic Radiology*. 5th ed. Edinburgh: Churchill Livingstone; 2008 [fig. 37.33].)

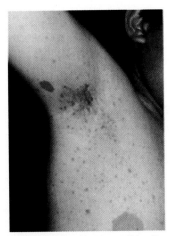

Fig. 26.5 Café au lait patches as well as multiple axillary freckles in a 14-year-old boy. (From Hoyt C. *Pediatric Ophthalmology and Strabismus.* 4th ed. Philadelphia: Saunders; 2012 [fig. 65.4].)

Disease/Syndrome	Inheritance	Type of Cancer (In Order of Most Likely)/Other Information
MEN, type IIa	Autosomal dominant	Thyroid (medullary cancer), parathyroid, pheochromocytoma
MEN, type IIb	Autosomal dominant	Thyroid (medullary cancer), pheochromocytoma, mucosal neuromas, marfanoid habitus
Familial polyposis coli	Autosomal dominant	Hundreds of colon polyps that always become cancerous
Gardner syndrome	Autosomal dominant	Familial polyposis plus osteomas and soft tissue tumors
Turcot syndrome	Autosomal dominant	Familial polyposis plus CNS tumors
Peutz-Jeghers syndrome	Autosomal dominant	Look for perioral freckles and multiple noncancerous GI polyps; increased incidence of GI (colorectal, stomach, small bowel, and pancreas) and extraintestinal malignancies (breast, ovary, cervix, Sertoli cell testicular tumors)
Neurofibromatosis, type 1 (Fig. 26.5)	Autosomal dominant	Multiple neurofibromas, café au lait spots; increased number of pheochromocytomas, bone cysts
Neurofibromatosis, type 2	Autosomal dominant	Bilateral acoustic neuromas (also known as vestibular schwannomas)
Tuberous sclerosis	Autosomal dominant	Adenoma sebaceum, ash-leaf spots, shagreen patches, seizures, intellectual disability, glial nodules in brain; increased renal angiomyolipomas and cardiac rhabdomyomas
Von Hippel-Lindau disease	Autosomal dominant	Hemangioblastomas in cerebellum, renal cell cancer; cysts in liver and/or kidney
Xeroderma pigmentosa	Autosomal recessive	Skin cancer
Albinism	Autosomal recessive	Skin cancer
Down syndrome	Trisomy 21	Leukemia

CNS, Central nervous system; *GI,* gastrointestinal; *MEN,* multiple endocrine neoplasia.

8. **What other conditions are associated with an increased risk of malignancy?**
Other diseases with an increased incidence of cancer include dermatomyositis, polymyositis, immunodeficiency syndromes, and Fanconi anemia. Breast, ovarian, and colon cancer are well known to have familial tendencies (as well as some other types of cancer), but rarely can a mendelian inheritance pattern be demonstrated. For example, *BRCA-1* and *BRCA-2* gene mutations account for about 5% of breast cancers.

9. **Cover the right-hand column and specify the major environmental risk factors for the following cancers**

Cancer Type	Environmental Risk Factors*
Lung	Smoking, asbestos (also nickel, radon, coal, arsenic, chromium, uranium)
Mesothelioma	Asbestos and smoking
Leukemia	Chemotherapy/radiotherapy, other immunosuppressive drugs, benzene
Bladder	Smoking, aniline dyes (rubber and dye industry), schistosomiasis (in immigrants)
Skin	Ultraviolet light exposure (e.g., sun), coal tar, arsenic
Liver	Alcohol, vinyl chloride (liver angiosarcomas), aflatoxins (Africa)
Oral cavity	Smoking, alcohol, HPV infection (often genotype 16)
Pharynx/larynx	Smoking, alcohol, HPV infection
Esophagus	Smoking, alcohol
Pancreas	Smoking, chronic pancreatitis
Renal cell	Smoking
Stomach	Alcohol, nitrosamines/nitrites (from smoked meats and fish)
Clear cell cancer[†]	In utero exposure to diethylstilbestrol (DES)
Colon/rectum	High-fat and low-fiber diet, smoking, alcohol, obesity
Breast	Chest radiation, hormone replacement therapy, alcohol
Cervix	HPV infection, smoking
Thyroid	Childhood neck or chest irradiation, low dietary iodine
Endometrium	Unopposed estrogen stimulation (e.g., PCOS), obesity, tamoxifen, high-fat diet
All cancer overall	Smoking (number two is probably alcohol)

HPV, Human papillomavirus; *PCOS*, polycystic ovary syndrome.
*The factor with the greatest impact is listed first.
[†]Of cervix and vagina.

10. **What clinical vignette should make you suspect lung cancer?**
The classic clue is a change in the chronic cough of a smoker. The greater the pack-years of tobacco use, the more suspicious you should be. Patients may also present with hemoptysis, pneumonia, or weight loss. The chest radiograph may show a mass or pleural effusion. Perform thoracentesis to examine for malignant cells. A less common presentation is recurrent or unresolving pneumonia in the same lung lobe, which would be suspicious for a postobstructive bronchogenic carcinoma.

11. **How do you diagnose and treat lung cancer?**
As with all cancers, you need a tissue biopsy (e.g., via bronchoscopy, computed tomography (CT)–guided biopsy, open lung biopsy) to confirm malignancy and to define the histologic type. Non–small cell lung cancer may be treated with surgery if the cancer remains within the lung parenchyma (i.e., without involvement of the opposite lung, pleura, chest wall, spine, or mediastinal structures) (Fig. 26.6). Small cell lung cancer is inoperable and is treated with chemotherapy. Extensive non–small cell lung cancer is treated with chemotherapy with or without radiation. Usually a platinum-containing chemotherapy regimen (e.g., cisplatin) is used, and bevacizumab can be added for non–small cell lung cancer.

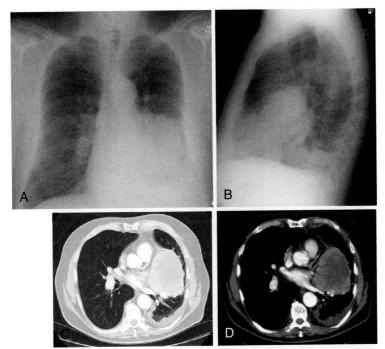

Fig. 26.6 Imaging non–small cell lung cancer (NSCLC). (A) Posteroanterior and (B) lateral chest radiogram of patients with NSCLC, which is locally advanced. (C) Computed tomography imaging using lung and (D) mediastinal windows. (From Abeloff M, et al. *Abeloff's Clinical Oncology.* 4th ed. Philadelphia: Churchill Livingstone; 2008 [fig. 76.12].)

12. **What consequences can result from an apical (Pancoast) lung cancer?**
    Horner syndrome: from invasion of the cervical sympathetic chain. Look for unilateral ptosis, miosis, and anhidrosis (no sweating).
    Superior vena cava syndrome: due to compression of superior vena cava with impaired venous drainage. Look for edema and plethora (redness) of the neck and face (Fig. 26.7) and central nervous system (CNS) symptoms (headache, visual symptoms, and altered mental status).
    Unilateral diaphragm paralysis: from phrenic nerve involvement (apical tumor not required), which will result in an elevated hemidiaphragm on chest x-ray
    Hoarseness: from recurrent laryngeal nerve involvement (apical tumor not required).

13. **What is a paraneoplastic syndrome? What are the commonly tested paraneoplastic syndromes of lung cancer?**
    A paraneoplastic syndrome is a condition caused by a malignancy but not due directly to destruction or invasion by the tumor. Classic examples in lung cancer include:

    Cushing syndrome: from production of adrenocorticotropic hormone (histologic type: small cell carcinoma).
    Syndrome of inappropriate antidiuretic hormone secretion (SIADH): from production of antidiuretic hormone (histologic type: small cell carcinoma).
    Hypercalcemia: from production of parathyroid-like hormone (histologic type: squamous cell carcinoma).
    Lambert-Eaton syndrome: myasthenia gravis–like disease from lung cancer that spares the ocular muscles. The muscles become stronger with repetitive stimulation, which is the opposite of myasthenia gravis (histologic type: small cell carcinoma).

14. **Over the course of their lifetime, how many women in the United States will develop breast cancer?**
    Roughly 1 in 8 women

15. **What are the risk factors for breast cancer?**
    - Personal history of breast cancer (major risk factor)
    - Female sex

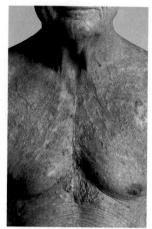

Fig. 26.7 A patient with superior vena cava syndrome and the characteristic venous dilation and facial edema. (From Abeloff M, et al. *Abeloff's Clinical Oncology*. 4th ed. Philadelphia: Churchill Livingstone; 2008 [fig. 54.3].)

- Family history in first-degree relatives
- Age >40 (rare before age 30, incidence steadily increases with age)
- Early menarche or late menopause (longer estrogen exposure)
- Late first pregnancy or nulliparity (more menstrual cycles = higher risk)
- Atypical hyperplasia of the breast
- Radiation exposure before age 30
- Inherited gene mutations (e.g., *BRCA1* and *BRCA2*)
- Dense breast tissue
- High-fat diet
- Diethylstilbestrol (DES) exposure
- Recent oral contraceptive use
- Combined postmenopausal hormone replacement therapy
- Excessive alcohol consumption
- Obesity

16. **What classic signs and symptoms suggest that a breast mass is cancer?**
    - Fixation of the breast mass to the chest wall or overlying skin
    - Satellite nodules or ulcers on the skin
    - Lymphedema (peau d'orange)
    - Matted or fixed axillary lymph nodes
    - Inflammatory skin changes ("peau d'orange" or red, hot thickened skin with enlargement of the breast due to inflammatory carcinoma)
    - Prolonged unilateral scaling erosion of the nipple with or without discharge (may be Paget disease of the nipple)
    - Microcalcifications on mammography
    - **Any new breast mass in a postmenopausal woman**

17. **What is the conservative approach to ensure that you do not miss a breast cancer?**
    When in doubt, biopsy every palpable breast mass in women over 35 that is not clearly a cyst (ultrasound is needed make the determination), especially if the patient has any of the risk factors mentioned in the previous question. If the Step 2 question does not want you to biopsy the mass, it will give clues that the mass is not a cancer (e.g., bilateral lumpy breasts that become symptomatic with every menses and have no dominant mass, patient age <30).

18. **What should you do with a breast mass in a woman under age 30?**
    In women under 30, breast cancer is rare. With a discrete breast mass in this age group, you should think of fibroadenoma. Consider ultrasound of the breast and observe the patient over a few menstrual cycles before considering biopsy unless the ultrasound is suspicious (e.g., solid mass or complex cyst). Fibroadenomas are usually roundish, rubbery, and mobile.

19. **What is the most common histologic type of breast cancer?**
    Invasive (infiltrating) ductal carcinoma (Fig. 26.8) accounts for about 70% of breast cancer.

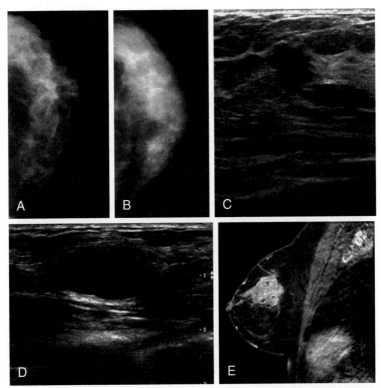

Fig. 26.8 Mammographic, ultrasonographic, and magnetic resonance imaging (MRI) findings in breast disease. (A) Stellate mass in the breast. A density with spiculated borders in combination with distortion of surrounding breast architecture suggests a malignancy. (B) Clustered microcalcifications. Fine, pleomorphic, and linear calcifications that cluster together suggest the diagnosis of ductal carcinoma in situ. (C) Ultrasound image of breast cancer. The mass is solid, contains internal echoes, and displays an irregular border. Most malignant lesions are taller than they are wide. (D) Ultrasound image of a simple cyst. The cyst is round with smooth borders, there is a paucity of internal sound echoes, and there is increased through-transmission of sound with enhanced posterior echoes. (E) Breast MRI showing gadolinium enhancement of a breast cancer. Rapid and intense gadolinium enhancement reflects increased tumor vascularity. (From Townsend C, et al. *Sabiston Textbook of Surgery*. 18th ed. Philadelphia: Saunders; 2008 [fig. 34.6].)

20. **What is the role of mammography in deciding whether to biopsy a breast mass?**
    When a palpable breast mass is detected, the decision to biopsy is made on clinical grounds. A mammogram that looks benign should not deter you from doing a biopsy if you are clinically suspicious. On the other hand, a lesion that is detected on mammography and looks suspicious should be biopsied, even if it is not palpable. Needle localization biopsy can be used.

21. **True or False: A mammogram should not be done in women under age 30**
    True in most cases. The breast tissue in women under age 30 is too dense for mammogram to be of value. First-line imaging in women under age 30 is breast ultrasound.

22. **What are the adjuvant therapies for breast cancer? How does each type of therapy work?**
    Tamoxifen is a selective estrogen-receptor modulator (SERM) that improves outcomes in premenopausal women with estrogen receptor–positive breast cancer. Tamoxifen has also been shown to decrease the risk of breast cancer in women at high risk of developing the disease.
    Aromatase inhibitors block the peripheral conversion of androgens to estrogens. Examples include anastrozole, exemestane, and letrozole.
    Ovarian suppression (with a gonadotropin-releasing hormone [GnRH] agonist such as goserelin) or ablation inhibits endogenous estrogen production from the ovaries.

23. **How are the adjuvant therapies used in nonmetastatic, hormone receptor–positive breast cancer?**
    The endocrine options for treatment depend on whether a woman is in menopause. A premenopausal woman at high risk of recurrence is usually treated with ovarian suppression and exemestane. A premenopausal woman not

at high risk of recurrence is usually treated with tamoxifen, which avoids the toxicities of ovarian suppression and endocrine therapy.

A postmenopausal woman is usually treated with an aromatase inhibitor (no ovarian suppression is needed because estrogen is not being produced by the ovaries).

24. **How is human epidermal growth factor receptor 2 (Her-2/neu) breast cancer treated?**
HER-2/neu breast cancer is treated with chemotherapy (usually doxorubicin and cyclophosphamide) with trastuzumab as adjuvant therapy. Trastuzumab targets the HER-2 protein.

25. **What is the recommended treatment for women at high risk of developing breast cancer who have not yet developed breast cancer?**
For women at high risk of developing breast cancer, endocrine therapy is generally preferred over observation. Postmenopausal women can be treated with a SERM (tamoxifen or raloxifene) or an aromatase inhibitor (anastrozole or exemestane). Premenopausal women at high risk are usually treated with tamoxifen.

26. **True or False: Mastectomy and breast-conserving surgery with radiation are considered equal in efficacy**
True. In either case, an axillary node dissection (or a sentinel node biopsy) is done to determine spread to the nodes. If nodes are positive, chemotherapy is warranted.

27. **What are the three main risk factors for prostate cancer?**
Age: prostate cancer is rare in men younger than 40 years old. The incidence increases with age, and about 60% of men older than 80 years have at least microscopic prostate cancer.
Race: black greater than white greater than Asian.
Family history: men who have a family history of prostate cancer are more likely to develop the disease at a younger age and to die from it than men who do not have a family history of prostate cancer.

28. **How do you recognize prostate cancer on the Step 2 exam?**
Look for patients over the age of 50 years. Patients often present late because early prostate cancer is asymptomatic. Look for symptoms typical of benign prostatic hyperplasia (hesitancy, dysuria, frequency) with hematuria and/or elevated prostate-specific antigen (PSA). Look for prostate irregularities (nodules) on rectal exam. Patients may also present with back pain from vertebral metastases, which are osteoblastic.

29. **How is prostate cancer treated?**
Local prostate cancer is treated with surgery (prostatectomy) or local radiation. For metastatic disease, treatment is androgen deprivation therapy (ADT) with surgical or medical orchiectomy to suppress serum testosterone levels. Options include orchiectomy or medical treatment with a GnRH agonist (leuprolide, goserelin, buserelin, triptorelin) combined with an antiandrogen such as an androgen-receptor antagonist (flutamide) or a GnRH antagonist (degarelix). Radiation therapy is used for local disease or pain from bony metastases. Chemotherapy can be combined with ADT for patients with extensive metastatic disease.

30. **List the primary risk factors for colon cancer**
Age: incidence begins to increase after age 40; peak incidence between 60 and 75 years
Family history: especially with familial polyposis or Gardner, Turcot, Peutz-Jeghers, or Lynch syndromes
Inflammatory bowel disease: ulcerative colitis more than Crohn disease, but both are associated with increased risk
Low-fiber, high-fat diet

31. **How do patients with colon cancer tend to present?**
Patients may present with asymptomatic blood in the stool (visible streaks of blood in stool or positive fecal occult blood test). Anemia is classic with right-sided colon cancer. Change in stool caliber ("pencil stool") or frequency (alternating constipation and frequency) is a classic presentation of left-sided colon cancer. Colon cancer is also a common cause of large bowel obstruction in adults. As with any cancer, look for unintentional weight loss.

32. **What is the rule about occult blood in the stool of a patient over age 40?**
Occult blood in the stool of a person older than 40 years should be considered colon cancer until proven otherwise. To rule out colon cancer, do a colonoscopy.

33. **How is colon cancer treated?**
Treatment is primarily surgical, with resection of involved bowel. Adjuvant chemotherapy is usually recommended if there is lymph node involvement. Distant metastases frequently go to the liver first (as with all gastrointestinal [GI] tumors). Surgical resection of a solitary liver metastasis is often attempted. With metastases elsewhere, chemotherapy is the only option, and prognosis is poor.

34. What is the classic tumor marker for colon cancer? How is it used clinically?

Carcinoembryonic antigen (CEA) may be elevated with colon cancer, and if a patient is found to have colon cancer, the CEA level is usually measured before surgery. If it is elevated preoperatively (not always), the CEA level should return to normal after surgical removal of the tumor. Periodic monitoring of CEA after surgery may help to detect recurrence before it is clinically apparent. CEA is not used as a screening tool for colon cancer; it is used only to follow known cancer because it is neither sensitive nor specific (can be elevated with other visceral tumors).

35. Describe the classic presentation of pancreatic cancer. How is it treated? What is the cell of origin?

The classic patient is a 40- to 80-year-old smoker who has lost weight and has painless jaundice. Other signs and symptoms include depression, epigastric pain, migratory thrombophlebitis (**Trousseau syndrome**, which may also be seen with other visceral cancers), and a palpable, nontender gallbladder (**Courvoisier sign**). Pancreatic cancer is more common in men than in women, in diabetics than in nondiabetics, and in blacks than in whites. Surgery (Whipple procedure) is rarely curative, and the prognosis is generally dismal. Chemotherapy is minimally successful at prolonging survival. The cell of origin in pancreatic cancer is ductal epithelium (Fig. 26.9).

36. What is the most common islet cell tumor of the pancreas? How is it diagnosed?

Insulinomas (beta cell tumor) are the most common islet cell tumors. Look for two-thirds of the **Whipple triad:** hypoglycemia (glucose <50 mg/dL) and central nervous symptoms due to hypoglycemia (confusion, stupor, loss of consciousness). As a good doctor, you provide the third part of the Whipple triad: administration of glucose or glucagon to relieve symptoms. Ninety percent of insulinomas are benign and can be cured with resection, if possible. In your workup, take a history and check the C-peptide level first to make sure that the patient is not a diabetic who is taking too much insulin or a patient with factitious disorder. C-peptide levels are high with insulinoma and low with the other disorders.

37. Define Zollinger-Ellison syndrome. What clues point to the diagnosis?

Zollinger-Ellison syndrome is a gastrinoma that causes acid hypersecretion (gastrin stimulates acid secretion) and peptic ulcer disease. Peptic ulcers are often multiple and resistant to therapy and may be found in unusual locations (distal duodenum or jejunum). More than one-half of these pancreatic islet cell tumors are malignant. Diagnosis is made with an elevated fasting serum gastrin level or a secretin stimulation test.

38. Name the other two islet cell tumors. What should islet cell tumors make you think about?

1. **Glucagonomas** (alpha cell tumor) cause hyperglycemia with high glucagon levels and necrolytic migratory erythema.
2. **VIPomas** (tumors that secrete vasoactive intestinal peptide [VIP]) cause watery diarrhea, hypokalemia, and achlorhydria.
   Watch for multiple endocrine neoplasia (MEN) syndromes in patients with islet cell tumors.

39. How does ovarian cancer classically present? How are ovarian masses evaluated?

Ovarian cancer classically presents late with weight loss, pelvic mass, ascites, and/or bowel obstruction. Any ovarian enlargement in a postmenopausal female is cancer until proven otherwise. In women of reproductive age, most ovarian enlargements are benign. Ultrasound is the first-line test to evaluate an ovarian lesion.

40. How is ovarian cancer treated? What is the cell of origin? What is the most common type of ovarian cancer?

Ovarian cancer is usually treated with debulking surgery and chemotherapy. The prognosis is usually poor due to a late presentation. Most ovarian cancers arise from ovarian epithelium. Serous cystadenocarcinoma is the most common type; histopathologic studies classically reveal psammoma bodies. Mucinous cystadenocarcinoma is also common. When clinicians use the term "ovarian cancer" without a qualifier, they are talking about epithelial malignancies (i.e., cystadenocarcinomas).

41. List the three commonly tested germ cell tumors. What clues suggest their presence?

1. **Teratoma/dermoid cyst** (most common and most tested type). Look for a description of the tumor to include skin, hair, and/or teeth or bone; it may show up with calcifications on radiograph.
2. **Sertoli-Leydig cell tumor**, which causes virilization (hirsutism, receding hairline, deepening voice, clitoromegaly).
3. **Granulosa-theca cell tumors**, which cause feminization and precocious puberty.
   Female patients with germ cell tumors of the ovary are classically under the age of 30.

42. What is Meigs syndrome?

An ovarian fibroma that causes ascites and right hydrothorax.

43. What is a Krukenberg tumor?

A stomach cancer (or other GI malignancy) with metastases to the ovaries.

44. What commonly used medication has been shown to reduce the risk of ovarian cancer?

Oral contraceptive pills, which also reduce the incidence of endometrial cancer.

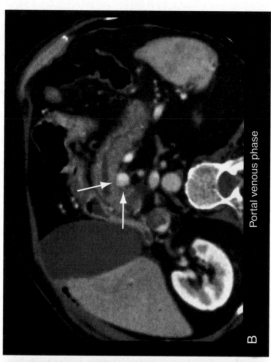

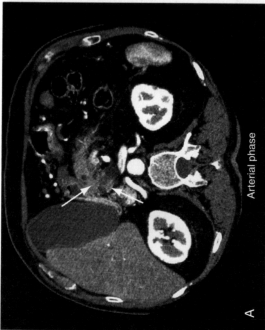

Fig. 26.9 Pancreatic computed tomography in a patient with pancreatic cancer. (A) Arterial phase showing a nonenhancing lesion in the head of the pancreas *(arrows)*. (B) Venous phase showing a noninvolved fat plane around the portal vein *(arrows)*. (From Feldman M, Friedman LS, Brandt LJ. *Sleisenger and Fordtran's Gastrointestinal and Liver Disease*. 10th ed. Philadelphia: Elsevier; 2016.)

Portal venous phase

B

Arterial phase

A

45. What is the best available screening method to reduce the incidence and mortality of cervical cancer?

Papanicolaou (Pap) smears. Perform a Pap smear on all female patients if they are due, even if they present for a totally unrelated complaint. Screening should start at age 21 regardless of sexual activity. The frequency of screening depends on whether human papillomavirus (HPV) testing is also being used as well as the patient's age and results of previous Pap smears. See Chapter 32 for additional details.

46. What should you do if a Pap smear is abnormal?

The follow-up for an abnormal Pap smear depends on the cervical cytologic results. Lower-grade lesions may be evaluated with HPV testing and colposcopy/endocervical curettage, if needed. Higher-grade lesions require colposcopy with biopsy and/or loop electrosurgical excision procedure (LEEP). Invasive cancer requires surgery (at least a hysterectomy) and includes radiation plus cisplatin-based chemotherapy.

47. List the main risk factors for cervical cancer

- HPV infection
- Early onset of sexual activity
- Multiple sexual partners
- A high-risk sexual partner (e.g., partner with multiple sexual partners or known HPV infection)
- Smoking
- History of sexually transmitted infection
- Immunosuppression
- Low socioeconomic status

48. Where does cervical cancer begin? How does it present? How is it treated?

Invasive cervical cancer begins in the transformation zone and usually presents with vaginal bleeding or discharge (postcoital bleeding, intermenstrual spotting, or abnormal menstrual bleeding). Treat with surgery and/or radiation.

49. What do you need to know about diethylstilbestrol (DES) and cancer?

Maternal exposure to DES during pregnancy increases a daughter's risk of developing clear cell cancer of the cervix and/or vagina.

50. What is the rule of thumb for postmenopausal vaginal bleeding?

Postmenopausal vaginal bleeding is cancer until proven otherwise. Endometrial cancer is the most common type to present in this fashion; it is also the fourth most common cancer overall in women. Do an endometrial biopsy (generally preferred) or a transvaginal ultrasound for any woman with postmenopausal bleeding (as well as a Pap smear).

51. List the main risk factors for endometrial cancer

- Obesity
- Nulliparity
- Late menopause
- Diabetes, hypertension, and gallbladder disease (probably related to obesity)
- Chronic, unopposed estrogen stimulation (e.g., polycystic ovary syndrome, estrogen-secreting neoplasm [granulosa-theca cell tumor], and estrogen replacement therapy without progesterone)

52. What is the most common type of endometrial cancer? How is it treated?

Most uterine cancers are adenocarcinomas and spread by direct extension. Treat with surgery and radiation.

53. Describe the common presentations of brain tumors

CNS tumors are the second most common tumors in children (second to leukemia); be suspicious in this age group. In adults, two-thirds of primary tumors are supratentorial (i.e., above the tentorium cerebelli, a portion of dura that separates the cerebellum from the cerebral hemispheres), whereas in children, two-thirds are infratentorial (i.e., lower brainstem or cerebellum [posterior fossa]). In either group, look for new-onset seizures, neurologic deficits, or signs of intracranial hypertension (headache, blurred vision, papilledema, nausea, projectile vomiting). In children, also look for hydrocephalus (manifested as an inappropriately increasing head circumference), new clumsiness, ataxia, loss of developmental milestones, or a change in school performance or personality.

54. What are the most common histologic types of primary CNS tumors in children and adults? How are primary brain tumors treated?

The most common primary type in **adults** is **glioma** (Fig. 26.10). Most gliomas are astrocytomas, which are intraparenchymal and have little or no calcification. The second most common type in adults is **meningioma**, which is often calcified and is external to the brain substance. In **children** the most common types are **cerebellar astrocytoma** (benign pilocytic astrocytoma) and **medulloblastoma**, followed by ependymoma. Treat with surgical removal (if possible), followed by radiation and/or chemotherapy, depending on the tumor.

55. Which cancers tend to metastasize to the brain?

Lung cancer, breast cancer, and melanoma are the most common; together they account for 75% of brain metastases.

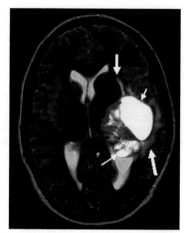

Fig. 26.10 A malignant glioma is seen on this T2-weighted magnetic resonance image demonstrating edema *(large arrows)* and necrosis (uniform high signal regions, *small arrows*). (From Goldman L, Ausiello D. *Cecil Medicine*. 23rd ed. Philadelphia: Saunders; 2008 [fig. 419.5].)

56. **What tumor is most likely in a young, obese woman with headaches, papilledema, vomiting, and a negative CT/MRI?**
A pseudotumor, as in **pseudotumor cerebri**. Pseudotumors are not actual tumors but reflect idiopathic increased intracranial pressure. Signs and symptoms include headache, papilledema, vision loss, elevated opening pressure on lumbar puncture with normal cerebrospinal fluid (CSF) findings, and no other evident cause of intracranial hypertension. Weight loss may help; acetazolamide or topiramate may also help. Serial lumbar punctures or a CSF shunt may be needed to prevent vision loss.

57. **What tumor should you suspect in an adult with signs of eighth cranial nerve damage and increased intracranial pressure?**
An acoustic neuroma (especially in the setting of neurofibromatosis). Coinvolvement of the facial nerve is common (Fig. 26.11).

58. **What tumor should you suspect in children with intracranial calcifications on skull radiographs?**
Craniopharyngioma (benign tumors that arise from remnants of the Rathke pouch and grow slowly from birth).

59. **What should you know about testicular cancer?**
It is the most common solid malignancy in adult men younger than 30 years old. The main risk factor is **cryptorchidism**. Transillumination and ultrasound help to distinguish a hydrocele (which is filled with fluid and transilluminates) from cancer (solid and does not transilluminate). The most common histologic type is seminoma, which is radiosensitive and highly curable. Use ultrasound to make the diagnosis.

60. **What tumor resembles "a bunch of grapes" coming out of the vagina?**
Sarcoma botryoides, a type of embryonal rhabdomyosarcoma usually seen in children.

61. **What is the classic physical finding of a pituitary tumor? What is the most common type?**
The classic physical finding is **bitemporal hemianopsia**. Order an MRI of the brain in any patient with this finding. Patients also may have signs and symptoms of increased intracranial pressure. The most common type is a prolactinoma, which is associated with high prolactin levels, galactorrhea, and menstrual or sexual dysfunction. Other types of pituitary tumors may cause hyperthyroidism, Cushing disease, or acromegaly, or they may be nonfunctional (i.e., they do not secrete hormones).

62. **What two points do you need to know about nasopharyngeal cancer?**
It usually is seen in Asians (particularly those who are from Asia), and it is associated with **Epstein-Barr virus**.

63. **Describe the classic presentation of esophageal cancer. What is the most common cell type?**
The presentation depends on the histologic type. The classic patient with squamous cell carcinoma is a chronic smoker and alcohol drinker between the ages of 40 and 60 years (blacks more than whites) who presents with weight loss, anemia, and the complaint that "food is sticking in my throat," which progresses to dysphagia for liquids. The other cell type is adenocarcinoma, which is typically due to malignant degeneration of Barrett

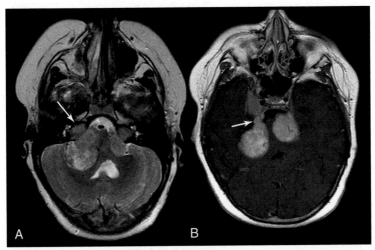

Fig. 26.11 Neurofibromatosis type 2 (NF-2). (A) Bilateral cerebellopontine angle masses extending into the internal auditory meatus and causing expansion *(arrow)* in a child with NF-2 and bilateral acoustic neuromas. (B) Trigeminal schwannomas extending into the cavernous sinus on the right. The arrow indicates the cisternal segment of the right trigeminal nerve. (From Adam A, et al. *Grainger & Allison's Diagnostic Radiology.* 5th ed. Edinburgh: Churchill Livingstone; 2008 [fig. 70.24].)

esophagus (columnar metaplasia of esophageal squamous epithelium due to acid reflux); thus patients typically have a long history of acid reflux and heartburn. Prognosis is usually quite poor in either type due to late presentation. Squamous cell carcinomas used to predominate, but squamous cell carcinoma and adenocarcinoma now occur with almost equal frequency.

64. **What physical and laboratory findings suggest thyroid cancer? What is the most common type of thyroid cancer? What historical point is of concern with thyroid cancer?**
Patients often have a single, stony-hard nodule or mass in the thyroid gland that may be rapidly enlarging. The nodule is "cold" on a nuclear scan (i.e., it fails to take up radioactive tracer). The most common type is papillary thyroid cancer. Other worrisome findings are hoarseness, which indicates recurrent laryngeal nerve invasion, and increased calcitonin level, which indicates the rare medullary thyroid cancer. Patients with medullary thyroid cancer may have a MEN syndrome. Historically, irradiation to the head or neck is of concern due to its association with thyroid cancer.

65. **How should you evaluate a thyroid mass for possible malignancy?**
To evaluate a nodule in the thyroid, order thyroid function tests and a thyroid ultrasound. Thyroid-stimulating hormone (TSH) is the best screening test; "toxic" or functional nodules are unlikely to be cancer. If the TSH is normal/elevated or the ultrasound has suspicious findings, obtain a fine-needle aspiration of the mass. If the TSH is decreased, then order a nuclear scan. A "cold" nodule or area of decreased uptake is more suspicious than a nodule with normal or increased uptake ("hot" nodule). Fine-needle aspiration and biopsy should be performed for almost all thyroid nodules.

66. **What clinical vignette is suspicious for bladder cancer?**
Persistent, painless hematuria, especially in patients older than 40 years who smoke or work in the rubber or dye industry (exposure to aniline dye). CT scan to evaluate the upper urinary tract and cystoscopy should be performed to evaluate for potential bladder cancer (as well as other causes of hematuria, including renal cell carcinoma).

67. **What increases the risk for hepatocellular cancer? What is the classic tumor marker for liver cancer?**
The same factors that increase the risk for cirrhosis. The "big three" are alcohol, chronic hepatitis (hepatitis C is now a more likely culprit than hepatitis B), and hemochromatosis. **Alpha-fetoprotein** is often elevated and can be measured postoperatively to detect recurrences. It can also be used for screening, along with ultrasound, in high-risk populations (e.g., those with cirrhosis).

68. **How do patients with liver cancer present? How is liver cancer treated?**
Patients often have a history of alcoholism, hepatitis, and/or hemochromatosis or other causes of cirrhosis. They present with weight loss, right upper quadrant pain, and an enlarged liver. Surgery (e.g., resection, transplantation) is the only hope for cure. The prognosis is poor.

69. **What other tumors of the liver may appear on the USMLE? What clues suggest their presence?**
Hemangioma: most common primary tumor of the liver; benign and generally left alone. Surgery is done only if symptomatic (pain, bleeding).
Hepatic adenoma: benign tumor in women of reproductive age who take **birth control pills.** Stop the birth control pills, and the tumor may regress. If not, surgery is usually preferred to prevent hemorrhage and rare malignant transformation.
Cholangiocarcinoma: malignant. Fifty percent of patients have inflammatory bowel disease (especially ulcerative colitis). Liver flukes (*Clonorchis* sp.) increase the risk in some immigrant populations (China, Japan, Taiwan, Vietnam, Korea, far eastern Russia).
Angiosarcoma: malignant. Look for industrial exposure to vinyl chloride.
Hepatoblastoma: malignant; the most common primary liver malignancy in children.

70. **What is the significance of adrenal tumors?**
Most are benign, but they may be functional and cause primary hyperaldosteronism (Conn syndrome) or hypercortisolism (Cushing syndrome). Another possibility is pheochromocytoma, which is associated with intermittent, severe hypertension, mental status changes, headaches, and diaphoresis.

71. **What are the risk factors for stomach cancer? What are the symptoms?**
Risk factors include Asian race, increasing age, smoking history, ingestion of smoked meat, and *Helicobacter pylori* infection. Signs and symptoms include anemia, weight loss, early satiety, abdominal pain, and a nonhealing gastric ulcer. All gastric ulcers must be biopsied to exclude malignancy. Consider follow-up endoscopy to document resolution of an ulcer, though this is somewhat controversial. Be especially suspicious if the question describes a nonhealing ulcer in a patient with weight loss.

72. **What is a Virchow node?**
A Virchow node is a left supraclavicular node enlargement due to the spread of visceral cancer (classically stomach cancer).

73. **What do you need to know about osteosarcomas for the Step 2 exam?**
Osteosarcomas are most commonly seen around the knee in 10- to 30-year-old patients. The classic x-ray finding is a "sunburst" periosteal reaction (Fig. 26.12) in the distal femur or proximal tibia associated with a mass. In older adults, the risk is increased in bones with long-standing Paget disease or osteomyelitis.

74. **What are the symptoms of carcinoid tumors? Where are they most commonly found?**
Carcinoid tumors secrete serotonin-like products that can cause symptoms, but the liver breaks down serotonin and other vasoactive secretions to make the tumor initially asymptomatic. Once a carcinoid tumor metastasizes to the liver and vasoactive products reach the systemic circulation, symptoms begin (carcinoid syndrome): episodic cutaneous flushing, abdominal cramps, diarrhea, and right-sided heart valve damage. The most common location is in the small bowel, but carcinoid tumors are also the most common appendiceal tumor (sometimes found at the time of appendectomy in patients with appendicitis).

75. **What lab test detects carcinoid tumors?**
Urinary levels of 5-hydroxyindoleacetic acid (5-HIAA; a serotonin breakdown product) are increased.

76. **What is the classic clinical manifestation of Kaposi sarcoma?**
A rash that does not respond to multiple treatments in an HIV-positive patient. Kaposi sarcoma is a vascular skin tumor that commonly begins as a papule or plaque on the upper body or in the oral cavity (Fig. 26.13). It is highly associated with human herpesvirus 8 (HHV-8) infection.

77. **What is the main risk factor for skin cancer?**
Ultraviolet light exposure

78. **Explain the ABCDEs of melanoma. What should you do if they are present?**
The ABCDEs of melanoma (Fig. 26.14) are characteristics of a mole that should make you suspicious of malignant transformation: **a**symmetry, **b**orders (irregular), **c**olor (change in color or multiple colors), **d**iameter (lesions ≥6 mm are more likely to be malignant), and **e**volving changes (lesions that change over time). Do an excisional biopsy of a lesion with any of these characteristics because melanomas commonly metastasize if not caught early. The risk of metastasis correlates most closely with depth of invasion into the skin.

79. **What do you need to know about basal cell and squamous cell skin cancers?**
Both of these cancers usually appear on sun-exposed areas (classically the head and neck area). The classic description of a basal cell cancer is a pearly, umbilicated nodule with telangiectasias; it is extremely common and almost never metastasizes (see Chapter 6). Squamous cell cancer sometimes metastasizes and often has a red, scaly, inflamed appearance or presents as an area of skin ulceration (see Fig. 6.19 in Chapter 6). Excisional biopsy is appropriate for all suspicious lesions.

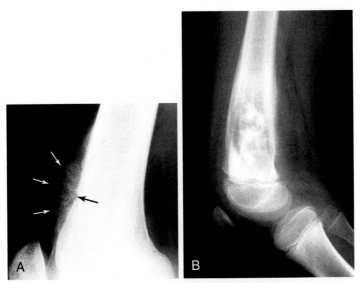

Fig. 26.12 Osteogenic sarcoma of the knee. A lateral view of the knee (A) in a 19-year-old man shows a sunburst-type periosteal reaction *(arrows)*. Knowing that the distal femur is the most common site of osteogenic sarcoma, that periosteal reaction is a feature, and that this patient is a teenager should make osteogenic sarcoma very high on your differential diagnostic list. A destructive central lesion (B) is seen here in the distal femur of an 8-year-old girl. (From Mettler F. *Essentials of Radiology.* 2nd ed. Philadelphia: Saunders; 2004 [fig. 8.113].)

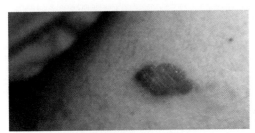

Fig. 26.13 Kaposi sarcoma. (From Hoffman R. *Hematology: Basic Principles and Practice.* 5th ed. Edinburgh: Churchill Livingstone; 2008 [fig. 121.35].)

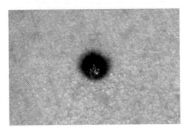

Fig. 26.14 Primary nodular malignant melanoma found on back of patient. (From Yanoff M, Sassani JW. *Ocular Pathology.* 6th ed. St. Louis: Mosby; 2008 [fig. 17.8].)

80. How can you differentiate a Wilms tumor from a neuroblastoma?

Both present as flank masses in children (peak age: ~2 years). Neuroblastomas most commonly arise from the adrenal gland and often contain calcifications, whereas Wilms tumors arise from the kidney and rarely calcify; thus imaging (CT scan) can usually distinguish the two. In addition, neuroblastomas can cross the midline, but Wilms tumors are always unilateral. In rare cases, neuroblastomas regress spontaneously (for unknown reasons).

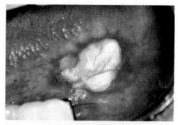

Fig. 26.15 A thick, sharply marginated focal leukoplakia of the ventral/lateral tongue with a uniform erythematous periphery. (From Flint PW. *Cummings Otolaryngology: Head & Neck Surgery.* 5th ed. St. Louis: Mosby; 2010 [fig. 91.5].)

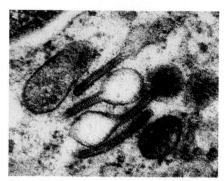

Fig. 26.16 Birbeck granules. These characteristic racquet-shaped cytoplasmic inclusions are a marker for Langerhans cells of the skin. (From du Vivier A. *Atlas of Clinical Dermatology.* 3rd ed. New York: Churchill Livingstone; 2002:27. With permission.)

81. **What factors increase the risk for oral cancers? Describe the typical appearance**
    Smoking or chewing tobacco, alcohol consumption, and HPV infection are the main risk factors for oral cancer, and their effects are synergistic. Also look for poor oral hygiene. Lesions often begin as leukoplakia (white patch) (Fig. 26.15) or malakoplakia (red patch). Oral hairy leukoplakia can resemble leukoplakia somewhat but is an unrelated condition affecting HIV-positive patients that is associated with the Epstein-Barr virus (which is the main risk factor for nasopharyngeal cancer).

82. **What are the two major cytologic clues for histiocytosis?**
    CD1-positive cells and Birbeck granules (cytoplasmic inclusion bodies that look like tennis rackets) (Fig. 26.16)

83. **What is a unicameral bone cyst? Who gets it? Describe the classic presentation**
    It is an expansile, lytic, well-demarcated benign lesion in the proximal portion of the humerus in children and adolescents (Fig. 26.17). Although benign, it may weaken bone enough to cause a pathologic fracture of the humerus (the classic presentation).

84. **Describe the classic presentation of a retinoblastoma**
    Retinoblastoma classically presents in a child younger than age 3 years with leukocoria (the pupillary red reflex changes to white) and/or unilateral exophthalmos. It may be bilateral in the inherited form.

85. **True or False: All patients with metastatic cancer should be encouraged to receive chemotherapy**
    False. The risks and side effects of chemotherapy can be significant, and sometimes minimal prolongation of life is achieved. The risks and benefits must be weighed. Patients with cancer (like all other patients) have the right to refuse any treatment. However, watch for and treat depression, even in terminal patients.

86. **Cover the right-hand column and name the cancer(s) associated with the following tumor markers**

Marker	Cancer(s)
Alpha-fetoprotein (AFP)	Liver (hepatocellular carcinoma), gonad (yolk-sac tumors)
Carcinoembryonic antigen (CEA)	Colorectal, lung, breast, ovary, pancreas, thyroid, liver, stomach, bladder, prostate

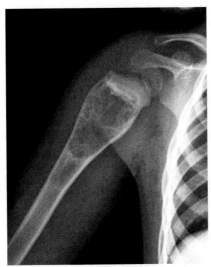

Fig. 26.17 Plain film of unicameral bone cyst manifesting as a large expansile, completely cystic intermedullary lesion that has well-defined focally sclerotic borders. (From Gilbert-Barness E. *Potter's Pathology of the Fetus, Infant and Child*. 2nd ed. St. Louis: Mosby; 2007 [fig. 34.1.2].)

Marker	*Cancer(s)*
Prostate-specific antigen (PSA)	Prostate
Human chorionic gonadotropin (hCG)	Hydatidiform moles, choriocarcinoma, testicular
CA-125	Ovary
S-100	Melanoma
CA 19-9	Pancreas, colorectal
CA 27-29	Breast
CA15-3	Breast
Hormone receptors (estrogen and progesterone)	Breast
HER-2	Breast
Beta$_2$-microglobulin	Multiple myeloma, chronic lymphocytic leukemia (CLL), and some lymphoma
Bladder tumor antigen (BTA)	Bladder
Calcitonin	Medullary thyroid carcinoma

87. What are the clinical manifestations of Beckwith-Wiedemann syndrome?
    The clinical manifestations include hemihyperplasia, macrosomia, macroglossia, and abdominal wall defects (such as omphalocele, umbilical hernia, or diastasis recti). Patients are also at high risk of Wilms tumors.

88. What malignancies are associated with tumor lysis syndrome (TLS)? What sort of electrolyte abnormalities would you expect?
    TLS typically develops in patients with rapidly progressive hematologic malignancies (e.g., aggressive non-Hodgkin lymphomas and acute lymphoblastic leukemia, especially Burkitt lymphoma) after initiation of cytotoxic chemotherapy. Due to massive lysis of tumor cells, high amounts of intracellular electrolytes are released into the circulation, causing hyperphosphatemia, hyperkalemia, hyperuricemia, and hypocalcemia.

89. **What clinical and laboratory abnormalities are associated with multiple myeloma?**

    A useful mnemonic to remember the abnormalities associated with multiple myeloma is **CRAB**: hypercalcemia, renal insufficiency, anemia, and bone lesions (osteolytic, often chest or back pain). Another often overlooked clue is a protein gap (Total protein - Albumin > 4) due to excessive production of a monoclonal protein.

90. **Name some common agents for the treatment of cancer-related anorexia/cachexia syndrome (CACS)**

    First-line agents for treatment of CACS include progesterone analogs (e.g., megestrol acetate, medroxyprogesterone acetate) and corticosteroids. Studies have not shown any benefit with the use of synthetic cannabinoids.

91. **How do you differentiate between a leukemoid reaction and chronic myelogenous leukemia (CML)?**

    Leukemoid reaction is associated with a high leukocyte alkaline phosphatase (LAP) score and predominance of mature neutrophils, whereas CML is associated with a low LAP score, predominance of immature neutrophil precursors, and absolute basophilia.

92. **How do giant cell tumors of the bone commonly present?**

    Giant cell tumors present in young adults with pain, swelling, and limited range of joint movement. It most commonly affects the epiphyseal region of long bones, especially the distal femur and proximal tibia. An x-ray will typically show osteolytic lesions characterized by a "soap bubble" appearance.

CHAPTER 27

OPHTHALMOLOGY

1. **What is the hallmark of conjunctivitis?**
   Hyperemia of the conjunctival vessels (Fig. 27.1)

2. **Distinguish between allergic, viral, and bacterial conjunctivitis.**

Etiology	Signs and Symptoms	Treatment
Allergic	Itching, bilateral, seasonal, long duration	Vasoconstrictors or topical antihistamines/mast cell stabilizers
Viral*	Preauricular adenopathy, highly contagious (look for affected contacts); clear, watery discharge	Supportive, hand washing to prevent spread
Bacterial**	Purulent discharge; classic in neonates	Topical antibiotics ± systemic antibiotics

*The number-one viral cause is adenovirus.
**The number-one bacterial cause in adults is *Staphylococcus aureus*.

3. **What are three common causes of neonatal conjunctivitis?**
   Chemical, *Neisseria gonorrhoeae*, and *Chlamydia trachomatis*

4. **What causes chemical conjunctivitis? How do you recognize it?**
   Silver nitrate (or erythromycin) drops, which are given to all newborns to prevent gonorrhea conjunctivitis, can cause chemical conjunctivitis. The drops may cause a chemical conjunctivitis (with no purulent discharge) that appears within 12 hours of instilling the drops and resolves within 48 hours. Chemical conjunctivitis is always the best guess if the conjunctivitis develops in the first 24 hours of life.

5. **How can you distinguish gonorrheal from chlamydial conjunctivitis?**
   In cases of suspected **gonorrheal conjunctivitis**, look for symptoms of gonorrhea in the mother. The infant has an extremely purulent discharge starting between 2 and 5 days after birth. Infants who were given prophylactic drops should not develop gonorrheal conjunctivitis. Treatment involves systemic ceftriaxone or cefotaxime.

   In cases of **chlamydial (inclusion) conjunctivitis**, the mother often reports no symptoms. The infant has mild-to-severe conjunctivitis beginning between 5 and 14 days after birth. Oral erythromycin is recommended for chlamydial conjunctivitis or pneumonia; topical therapy for chlamydial conjunctivitis is not effective.

6. **If you forget everything else about neonatal conjunctivitis, what point should you remember to help you distinguish among the three discussed causes?**
   The varying time frames during which they present.

7. **True or False: Conjunctivitis frequently causes loss of vision.**
   False. Other than transient blurriness (due to tear film debris) that resolves with blinking, conjunctivitis should not affect vision. If vision is affected, think of other, more serious conditions.

8. **Define glaucoma. What are the risk factors for developing it? What are the two general types?**
   Glaucoma is best thought of as ocular hypertension (or elevated intraocular pressure, measured with a tonometer). Effects of glaucoma include visual field defects and blindness. The risk factors are age over 40, black race, and positive family history. The two main types are open-angle and closed-angle glaucoma.

9. **Describe physical findings of open-angle glaucoma. How common is it? How is it treated?**
   Open-angle glaucoma causes 90% of the cases of glaucoma; it is painless and does not have acute attacks. The only signs are elevated intraocular pressure (usually 20–30 mm Hg), a gradually progressive visual field loss, and optic nerve changes (increased cup-to-disc ratio "cupping" on funduscopic exam). Treatment may involve several different classes of medications, including beta-blockers, prostaglandins, alpha-adrenergic agonists, carbonic anhydrase inhibitors, and cholinergic agonists, as well as laser therapy and surgery.

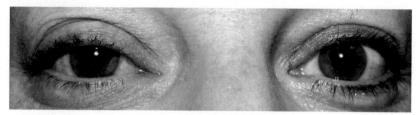

Fig. 27.1 Acute conjunctivitis of the right eye with watery discharge. (From Alfonso SA, Fawley J. Conjunctivitis. *Prim Care.* 2015;42[3]: 325-345. Courtesy Emory Eye Center, Emory University School of Medicine, Atlanta, GA.)

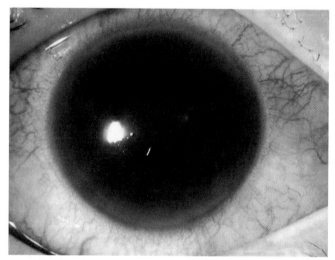

Fig. 27.2 Slit lamp photograph of an eye in acute primary angle closure. The cornea displays edema. The iris is middilated and there is conjunctival injection. (From Perera S, et al. Angle closure glaucoma. In: Levin LA, et al., eds. *Ocular Disease: Mechanisms and Management.* Philadelphia: Saunders; 2010:193-199 [fig. 25.3].)

10. How does closed-angle glaucoma present? What should you do if you recognize it?
    Closed-angle glaucoma presents with sudden ocular pain, seeing halos around lights, red eye, high intraocular pressure (>30 mm Hg), nausea and vomiting, sudden decreased vision, and a fixed, middilated pupil (Fig. 27.2). Patients aged 55 to 70 years are most commonly affected. Dark environments, such as movie theaters, that trigger pupillary dilation are commonly the trigger in USMLE Step 2 question stems. It is an ophthalmologic emergency. Treat the patient immediately with **pilocarpine**, timolol, brimonidine, and/or acetazolamide to abort the attack. If these therapies fail, you can consider intravenous (IV) mannitol or oral glycerin. Definitive surgery (peripheral iridectomy) is used to prevent further attacks. In rare cases, anticholinergic medications can trigger an attack of closed-angle glaucoma in a susceptible, previously untreated patient. Medications do not cause acute attacks in patients with open-angle glaucoma or in patients with surgically treated closed-angle glaucoma.

11. How do steroids affect the eye?
    Steroids, whether topical or systemic, can cause glaucoma and cataracts. Topical ocular steroids can worsen ocular herpes and fungal infections. For Step 2, do not give topical ocular steroids—especially if the patient has a dendritic corneal ulcer that stains green by fluorescein. Such an ulcer represents herpes.

12. Define ultraviolet keratitis. How is it treated?
    Excessive exposure to ultraviolet light can cause keratitis (corneal inflammation) with pain, foreign body sensation, red eye, tearing, and temporarily decreased vision. Patients have a history of welding, using a tanning bed or sunlamp, or snow-skiing ("snow-blindness"). Treat with an eye patch (for 24 hours) and topical antibiotic. You can reduce pain with an anticholinergic eye drop that causes paralysis of the ciliary muscle (cycloplegia).

13. What pediatric rheumatologic condition is commonly associated with uveitis?
    Juvenile idiopathic arthritis (especially the pauciarticular form). Patients with juvenile idiopathic arthritis need periodic ophthalmologic examination to check for uveitis.

14. **What is the most common cause of painless, slowly progressive loss of vision?**
Cataracts, especially in the elderly. Treatment is surgical removal of the affected lens(es) and replacement with an artificial lens.

15. **What should cataracts in a neonate suggest?**
Cataracts in a neonate may indicate a TORCH (**t**oxoplasmosis, **o**ther, **r**ubella, **c**ytomegalovirus, and **h**erpes simplex virus) infection or an inherited metabolic disorder (the classic example is galactosemia).

16. **What changes in the retina and fundus are seen in diabetes and hypertension?**
Diabetes is associated with dot-blot hemorrhages, microaneurysms, and neovascularization of the retina.
Hypertension is associated with arteriolar narrowing, copper/silver wiring, and cotton-wool spots. Papilledema may be seen with severe hypertension and should alert you to the presence of a hypertensive emergency.

17. **What is the most common cause of blindness in patients under and over the age of 55? In black patients?**
Diabetes is the number-one cause of blindness in younger adults in the United States, and senile macular degeneration (look for macular drusen) is the most common cause of blindness in adults over age 55. Glaucoma is the number-one cause of blindness in blacks of any age and the third overall cause of blindness in the United States.

18. **Define proliferative diabetic retinopathy. How is it treated? How is nonproliferative diabetic retinopathy treated?**
Proliferative diabetic retinopathy occurs after many years of established diabetes and is defined by the development of neovascularization (new, abnormal growth of vessels in the retina). Treatment involves application of a laser beam to the periphery of the entire retina (**panretinal photocoagulation**). Surgical or medical vitrectomy is used in some cases. Medical therapy for proliferative diabetic retinopathy is investigational but is used in some circumstances. The most promising are the vascular endothelial growth factor (VEGF) inhibitors (bevacizumab, ranibizumab, pegaptanib).
  Focal laser treatment and anti-VEGF is common for nonproliferative (background) retinopathy when macular edema is present; the laser is applied only to the affected area. In severe cases, panretinal photocoagulation may be used. Otherwise, nonproliferative retinopathy is treated supportively—primarily with tight control of blood glucose and follow-up eye exams to watch for development of macular edema or neovascularization.

19. **Distinguish between preorbital (preseptal) and orbital cellulitis.**
Both conditions may present with swollen lids; fever; a history of facial laceration, trauma, insect bite, or sinusitis; and chemosis (edema of the conjunctiva). Orbital cellulitis can mimic preorbital cellulitis early in its course. However, if ophthalmoplegia, proptosis, severe eye pain, double vision, decreased eye movements, or decreased visual acuity is present, the patient has orbital cellulitis (Fig. 27.3). Orbital cellulitis is an ophthalmologic emergency because it may extend into the skull, causing meningitis, venous thromboses, and/or blindness. Computed tomography scan of the orbits and sinuses is the imaging modality of choice for evaluation of suspected orbital cellulitis.

20. **What are the common bacterial causes of preorbital and orbital cellulitis? How are they treated?**
The most common bugs in both are *Streptococcus pneumoniae, Haemophilus influenzae* type b, and *Staphylococcus aureus* or streptococcal species (in patients with a history of trauma). Treat orbital cellulitis with blood cultures and administration of broad-spectrum IV antibiotics until culture results are known. In preorbital cellulitis, blood cultures are not routinely collected, as they are rarely positive, and cultures from the site are difficult to obtain. Empiric oral antibiotics for preorbital cellulitis consist of monotherapy with trimethoprim-sulfamethoxazole or combination therapy with clindamycin plus either amoxicillin or amoxicillin-clavulanic acid or cefpodoxime or cefdinir. A typical regimen for orbital cellulitis is vancomycin plus either ceftriaxone or cefotaxime or ampicillin-sulbactam, or piperacillin-tazobactam. Although preorbital cellulitis may be treated on an outpatient basis with close follow-up, orbital cellulitis requires hospital admission and IV antibiotics.

21. **What is the key to managing chemical burns to the eye? Which is worse—acid or alkaline burns?**
With chemical burns to the eye (acid or alkaline), the key to management is copious irrigation with the closest source of water. The longer you wait, the worse the prognosis. Do not wait to get additional history. Alkali burns have a worse prognosis because they go through liquefactive necrosis and tend to penetrate more deeply into the eye.

22. **Distinguish between a hordeolum (stye) and a chalazion. How are they treated?**
A hordeolum is a painful, red lump near the lid margin. A chalazion is a painless lump away from the lid margin (Fig. 27.4). Treat both with warm compresses. For chalazions, use intralesional steroid injection or incision and drainage if warm compresses do not work.

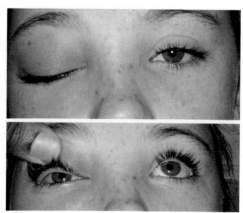

Fig. 27.3 A 12-year-old boy with orbital cellulitis. Note the poor elevation of the affected eye. (From Hoyt C. *Pediatric Ophthalmology and Strabismus.* 4th ed. Philadelphia: Saunders; 2012 [fig.13.10].)

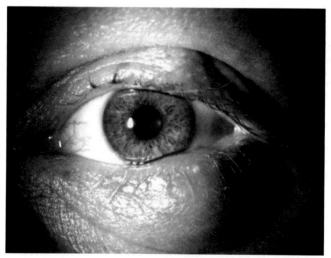

Fig. 27.4 Upper eyelid chalazion. Note the focal swelling in the upper eyelid without significant erythema. (From Foulks G. Meibomian gland disease: treatment. In: Holland EJ, et al., eds. *Ocular Surface Disease: Cornea, Conjunctiva and Tear Film.* Philadelphia: Elsevier; 2013:67-76.)

23. How do you recognize and treat herpes simplex keratitis?

Herpes simplex keratitis usually begins with conjunctivitis and vesicular lid eruption, then progresses to the classic dendritic keratitis (seen with fluorescein stain) (Fig. 27.5). Treat with topical antivirals (e.g., idoxuridine, trifluridine). Corticosteroids are generally contraindicated with dendritic keratitis because they may make the condition worse.

24. What findings suggest an ophthalmic herpes zoster infection?

Ophthalmic herpes zoster infection should be suspected in patients with involvement of the tip of the nose (Hutchinson sign) and/or medial eyelid, a typical zoster dermatomal skin rash, and eye complaints. Treat with oral acyclovir. Complications include loss of vision, uveitis, keratitis, and glaucoma.

25. How do you recognize a central retinal artery occlusion? What causes it?

Central retinal artery occlusion presents with sudden (within a few minutes), painless, unilateral loss of vision. The classic funduscopic appearance includes a pale, opaque fundus with a cherry red spot in the fovea (center) of the macula. The most common cause is emboli (from carotid plaque or heart), but watch for temporal arteritis as a cause on Step 2. No satisfactory treatment is available. However, treatment options include ocular massage, timolol, hyperventilation, and surgical therapies.

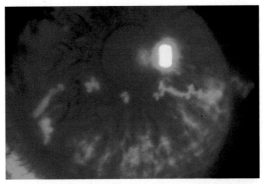

Fig. 27.5 Varicella dendritic keratitis. Numerous dendrites are seen in this slit lamp photograph with fluorescein staining of the dendritic lesions from active viral growth in the corneal epithelium. (From Krachmer JH. *Cornea*. 3rd ed. St. Louis: Mosby; 2010 [fig. 80.2].)

26. Describe the symptoms of temporal arteritis (giant cell arteritis). What should you do if you suspect it?

Temporal arteritis is a vasculitis seen in individuals over 50 years of age. Symptoms include jaw claudication, unilateral headache, loss of vision (due to central retinal artery occlusion), tortuous temporal artery (as seen or palpated on exam), markedly elevated erythrocyte sedimentation rate, and coexisting **polymyalgia rheumatica** (in 50%; causes proximal muscle pain and stiffness). If temporal arteritis is suspected in the setting of vision complaints, administer high-dose corticosteroids immediately before confirming the diagnosis with a temporal artery biopsy. Withholding treatment until a formal diagnosis can be made may cause the patient to lose vision in the other eye.

27. How do you recognize central retinal vein occlusion? Describe the cause and treatment.

Central retinal vein occlusion also presents with sudden (within a few hours), painless, unilateral loss of vision. The classic funduscopic appearance includes distended, tortuous retinal veins, retinal hemorrhages, cotton wool exudates, and a congested, edematous fundus. No satisfactory treatment is available. The most common causes are hypertension, diabetes, glaucoma, and increased blood viscosity (e.g., leukemia). Complications are related to neovascularization, which commonly develops and leads to vision loss and glaucoma.

28. Describe the classic history of a patient with retinal detachment.

The classic history of a patient with retinal detachment includes a sudden (instant), painless, unilateral loss of vision with "floaters" (little black spots that are seen no matter where the patient looks), and flashes of light. It is sometimes described as "a curtain or veil coming down in front of my eye." This history should prompt immediate referral to an ophthalmologist. On exam, you may see a gray, elevated retina. Risk factors include trauma, diabetes, and cataract surgery. Surgery may save the patient's vision by reattaching the retina.

29. True or False: Cataracts and macular degeneration are common causes of bilateral, painless loss of vision in the elderly.

True. Although one side may be worse than the other, bilateral complaints are not uncommon. The red reflex typically becomes black with a significant cataract. Those with macular degeneration typically have focal yellow-white deposits called **drusen** in and around the macula on funduscopic exam. Treat cataracts with surgery; most cases (90%) of macular degeneration are the "dry" or nonexudative subtype, which is treated supportively (e.g., magnification aids). "Wet" or exudative macular degeneration is treated with IV VEGF inhibitors, thermal laser photocoagulation in selected patients, and photodynamic therapy.

30. How do optic neuritis and papillitis present? What are the common causes?

Optic neuritis and papillitis typically present with a fairly quick (over hours to days), painful, unilateral or bilateral loss of vision. The pain is exacerbated with eye movements. Patients with optic neuritis will fail a red desaturation test and see red objects as pink or lighter red. The optic disc margins may appear blurred on funduscopic exam with papillitis, just as in papilledema.

Multiple sclerosis (which can also cause internuclear ophthalmoplegia) is a very common cause of optic neuritis, especially in 20- to 40-year-old women. Lyme disease, malignancy, and syphilis are other causes.

31. What causes bitemporal hemianopsia until proven otherwise?

A pituitary tumor (or other neoplasm) pressing on the optic chiasm

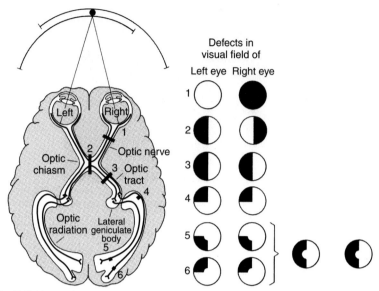

Fig. 27.6 Visual field defects produced by lesions at various levels of the visual pathway. *1,* Right optic nerve; *2,* optic chiasm; *3,* optic tract; *4,* Meyer loop; *5,* cuneus; *6,* lingual gyrus; bracket, occipital lobe (with macular sparing). (From Berne R. *Physiology.* 5th ed. Philadelphia: Mosby; 2003 [fig. 8.10].)

32. Use the visual field defect to localize the sight of the brain lesion (Fig. 27.6).

Visual Field Defect	Location of Lesion
Right anopsia (monocular blindness)	Right optic nerve
Bitemporal hemianopsia	Optic chiasm
Left homonymous hemianopsia	Right optic tract
Left upper quadrant anopsia	Right optic radiations in the right temporal lobe
Left lower quadrant anopsia	Right optic radiations in the right parietal lobe
Left homonymous hemianopsia with macular sparing	Right occipital lobe (from posterior cerebral artery occlusion)

33. What two diseases commonly cause isolated palsies of cranial nerves III, IV, and VI? How do you recognize them?

Isolated palsies of cranial nerves III, IV, and VI are usually due to vascular complications from diabetes mellitus and hypertension. Symptoms generally resolve on their own within 2 months. In patients over the age of 40 with a history of diabetes or hypertension and no other neurologic deficits or pain, observation is generally all that is required because hypertension and/or diabetes is the most likely cause. If resolution does not occur within 8 weeks, if the patient is under the age of 40, if neither hypertension nor diabetes is present, if the pupil is dilated and unreactive, or if the patient starts to develop pain or other neurologic deficits, order magnetic resonance imaging (MRI) of the head to rule out tumor or aneurysm (i.e., benign cause less likely).

34. What are the physical exam findings of a third cranial nerve palsy? What should you remember when trying to determine the cause?

With an oculomotor (cranial nerve III) lesion, the eye is down and out, and the patient can move the eye only laterally. If a third cranial nerve palsy is due to benign vascular causes (i.e., hypertension or diabetes), the pupil is normal, and close observation is all that is needed, as the condition typically resolves on its own in several weeks. A "blown" (dilated, nonreactive) pupil is a medical emergency. The most likely cause is an aneurysm or tumor. Order MRI and/or a cerebral angiogram.

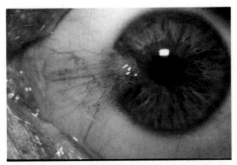

Fig. 27.7 Pterygium. (From Hirst LW. Prospective study of primary pterygium surgery using pterygium extended removal followed by extended conjunctival transplantation. *Ophthalmology.* 2008;115[10]:1663-1672.)

35. **What are the physical findings in palsies of cranial nerves IV and VI? How do lesions of cranial nerves V and VII affect the eye?**
    With a trochlear (cranial nerve IV) lesion, the affected eye cannot look down when the gaze is medial because of superior oblique muscle paralysis. With an abducens (cranial nerve VI) lesion, the patient cannot look laterally with the affected eye because of lateral rectus muscle paralysis. Cranial nerves V (afferent, sensory limb) and VII (efferent, motor limb) are involved in the corneal blink reflex. Lesions can produce corneal drying, which can be treated with saline eye drops.

36. **What is strabismus? Beyond what age is it abnormal in children?**
    Strabismus is the medical term for a "lazy eye." The affected eye deviates, most commonly inward. Strabismus is normal only if intermittent and during the first 3 months of life. When strabismus is constant or persistent beyond 3 months, it requires ophthalmologic referral to prevent blindness (known as amblyopia) in the affected eye.

37. **Why does blindness develop in patients with strabismus?**
    The visual system is still developing until the age of 7 or 8 years. For this reason, visual screening of both eyes is important in children. If one eye does not see well or is turned outward, the brain cannot fuse the two different images that it sees. Thus it suppresses the "bad" eye, which does not develop the proper neural connections. This eye will never see well and cannot be corrected with glasses because the problem is neural rather than refractive. This condition is called amblyopia and is treatable with special glasses, eye patching of the unaffected eye, or surgery if it is caught in time; the goal of treatment is to allow normal neural connections (and thus vision) to develop.

38. **What is presbyopia? When does it occur?**
    Presbyopia is the loss of the lenses' ability to accommodate; it is why aging adults need reading glasses for near vision. Presbyopia occurs between the ages of 40 and 50 years and is a normal part of aging.

39. **What is pterygium? How is it treated?**
    Pterygium is a fleshy benign growth that begins at the nasal edge of the conjunctiva and can extend over the cornea (Fig. 27.7). It usually is caused by irritation such as ultraviolet light or dust. It typically is not treated until it causes visual disturbance and is treated by surgical removal.

40. **What is trachoma? Which organism causes it?**
    Trachoma is the most common cause of infectious blindness worldwide. Patients have conjunctivitis-like symptoms with conjunctival follicles that look like white lumps on the inner upper eyelid (Fig. 27.8). Trachoma is caused by *Chlamydia trachomatis* serotypes A, B, and C and is spread by direct contact and fomites. In chronic cases, infection can lead to blindness through eyelid scarring and eyelash inversion with resultant ulceration of the cornea (trichiasis). Treat with oral (azithromycin) or topical (tetracycline) antibiotics. For those with trichiasis, eyelid surgery is required.

41. **What should you include in your differential for a patient with signs and symptoms concerning for orbital cellulitis with prominent, early cranial nerve VI palsy?**
    Cavernous sinus thrombosis. Facial, sinus, and dental infection may spread contiguously to the cavernous sinus through the valveless facial and ophthalmic veins. Cranial nerve VI is affected first due to its course medially through the cavernous sinus. Cranial nerves III, IV, V1, and V2 also course through the cavernous sinus and become affected as the condition progresses. This results in an inability to move the eye in any direction, numbness or paresthesia (around the eyes, nose, forehead), and loss of corneal blink reflex (afferent limb). The diagnostic imaging study of choice is MRI with MR venography. *Staphylococcus aureus* is the most common causative organism. Treatment is IV vancomycin plus a third- or fourth-generation cephalosporin. Anaerobic coverage with IV metronidazole should be added if dental or sinus infection is suspected.

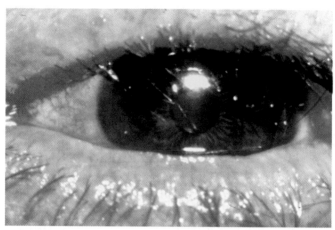

Fig. 27.8 Conjunctival scarring of trachoma. (From Bear NAV, Bastawrous A. *Manson's Tropical Diseases*. Elsevier; 2014:952-944.)

CHAPTER 28

ORTHOPEDIC SURGERY

1. **What orthopedic fractures are associated with the highest mortality rate?**
   Pelvic fractures, because patients can bleed to death. If the patient is unstable, consider heroic measures such as military antishock trousers (MAST trousers) and an external fixator.

2. **Why should areas distal to the fracture site be assessed by physical exam?**
   Areas distal to the fracture site should be assessed for neurologic and vascular compromise, either of which may be an emergency.

3. **Distinguish between an open and a closed fracture.**
   With an open (compound) fracture, the skin is broken over the fracture site. Suspect an open fracture with any overlying wound; the fractured bone does not have to be obviously exposed. In closed fractures, the skin is intact over the fracture site.

4. **Explain the difference in management of open and closed fractures.**
   With closed fractures, closed reduction (setting the bone without surgery) and casting can generally be done. With open fractures, prophylactic antibiotics are chosen based on the size of the wound, contamination, type of fracture, and vascular injury. Cefazolin is appropriate for lower-risk fractures; vancomycin if the patient is at risk for methicillin-resistant *Staphylococcus aureus* (MRSA); ceftriaxone plus gentamicin for higher-risk fractures with the addition of metronidazole if there has been soil contamination. Do surgical debridement, give a tetanus vaccine booster, lavage fresh wounds (if <8 hours old), and perform **open reduction and internal fixation** (ORIF). The main risk in open fractures is infection, which is usually not a problem with closed fractures because the skin is intact.

5. **What are the indications for open reduction other than an open fracture?**
   - Intraarticular fractures or articular surface malalignment
   - Nonunion or failed closed reduction
   - Neurovascular compromise
   - Multiple trauma (to allow mobilization at the earliest possible point)
   - Need for perfect reduction to optimize extremity function (e.g., professional athletes)

6. **What type of radiographs should you order if you suspect a fracture?**
   For any suspected fracture, order two views (usually anteroposterior and lateral) of the site, and consider radiographs of the joints above and below the fracture site.

7. **How should you treat a patient with severe pain after trauma and negative x-rays?**
   Rule out compartment syndrome. Treat the patient conservatively. Assume there is a fracture and have the patient rest the injured area. Splinting may be appropriate for distal extremity injuries. Obtain follow-up radiographs 7 to 14 days after the injury if symptoms persist; many occult fractures will become visible at this time. The exception to waiting is a suspected hip fracture in an elderly person—proceed to computed tomography (CT) or magnetic resonance imaging (MRI) of the hip to allow earlier diagnosis and treatment (Fig. 28.1), which decrease operative morbidity and length of hospital stay compared with delayed diagnosis and treatment. In the pediatric population, x-rays may not always reveal fractures (because the growth plate is cartilaginous rather than bone, so it is not radiopaque), so if a child has pain over a growth plate, consider this a fracture (Salter-Harris type I) and immobilize.

8. **Define compartment syndrome. What is the cause?**
   Compartment syndrome is a problem of muscle compartments, which are limited by the fascia in which they are contained. It is seen in the extremities (most commonly in the calf) when edema or hemorrhage causes swelling inside a muscle compartment. Rising pressure inside the fascial compartment can lead to decreased perfusion that can result in permanent muscle and nerve damage.
   The three common clinical scenarios in which compartment syndrome is seen are fractures (classically midshaft tibial fractures or supracondylar fractures of the humerus in children), burns (especially electrical and circumferential burns), and vascular compromise (or after vascular surgery procedures due to reperfusion injury).

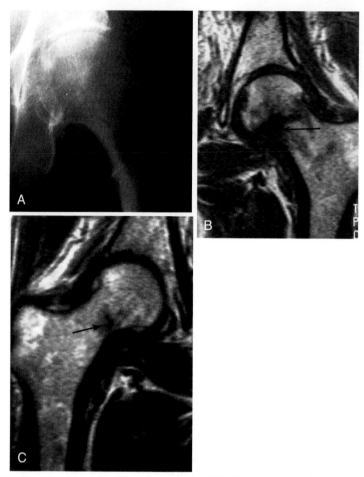

Fig. 28.1 Imaging of occult hip fracture. Anteroposterior radiograph of the left hip (A) demonstrates no evidence of fracture. Coronal T1-weighted magnetic resonance image (MRI) (B) clearly shows a well-demarcated line of decreased signal in the subcapital region of the left femoral neck consistent with a nondisplaced fracture *(arrow)*. MRI of the right hip (C) shows a subtle medial femoral neck fracture *(arrow)* not demonstrated on the conventional radiograph. (From Adam A, et al. *Grainger & Allison's Diagnostic Radiology.* 5th ed. Edinburgh: Churchill Livingstone; 2008 [fig. 46.73].)

9. What are the signs and symptoms of compartment syndrome? How is it treated?
   The seven Ps are as follows:
   • **P**ain (especially pain on passive movement that is out of proportion to the injury)
   • **P**aresthesias, hypoesthesia, and numbness (decreased sensation and two-point discrimination)
   • Cyanosis or **p**allor
   • **P**alpable swelling and firm-feeling muscle compartment
   • **P**aralysis (late, ominous sign)
   • Absent peripheral **p**ulses (late, ominous sign)
   • Elevated compartment **p**ressure (>30–40 mm Hg)
      On the USMLE, the diagnosis of compartment syndrome often has to be made clinically without a pressure reading. Although pulses may be slightly decreased, they are usually palpable (or detectable with Doppler ultrasound) with compartment syndrome. Lack of palpable pulses is an ominous, late sign. Compartment syndrome is an emergency, and quick action can save an otherwise doomed limb. Treatment is immediate fasciotomy; incising the fascial compartment relieves the pressure.

10. Cover the right-hand columns and specify the nerve root origin and the motor and sensory functions of the following peripheral nerves. In what common clinical scenarios are they often damaged?

Nerve	Nerve Roots	Motor Function	Sensory Function	Clinical Scenario
Radial	C5-T1	Wrist, thumb, and finger extension (watch for wrist drop)	Back of forearm, back of hand (first 3 digits)	Supracondylar humeral fracture with anterolateral displacement
Ulnar	C8-T1	Finger abduction (watch for "claw hand")	Front and back of last 2 digits	Elbow dislocation or fracture; supracondylar humeral fracture with posterior displacement
Median	C5-T1	Pronation of forearm, wrist flexion, thumb opposition	Palmar surface of hand (first 3.5 digits)	Carpal tunnel syndrome, humeral fracture, supracondylar humeral fracture with anteriomedial displacement (also consider brachial artery injury)
Axillary	C5-C6	Abduction and lateral rotation of arm	Lateral shoulder	Upper anterior humeral dislocation or fracture
Musculocutaneous	C5-C7	Flexion of the upper arm at the shoulder and elbow, supination of the forearm	Anterolateral forearm	Uncommon injury; penetrating trauma to the axilla
Peroneal	L4-S2	Dorsiflexion and eversion of foot (watch for foot drop)	Dorsal foot and lateral leg	Knee dislocation, fibula fracture

11. **What is the difference between fatigue stress fracture and insufficiency stress fracture? How are stress fractures diagnosed and treated?**
A stress fracture (Fig. 28.2) is an incomplete or small fracture that develops because of repeated or prolonged forces against the bone. Stress fractures are much more common in the lower extremities than the upper extremities because of weight-bearing forces. In fatigue stress fractures, abnormal stresses are applied to normal bones (e.g., overuse injury, as in military recruits or marathon runners). In insufficiency stress fractures, normal/physiologic stresses are applied to an abnormal bone (e.g., osteoporotic bone). Diagnosis is made using x-rays, though it may take weeks to months to see on x-ray; MRI or nuclear medicine scan may be utilized if x-rays are negative but strong clinical suspicion remains. The treatment is rest to allow healing and to prevent progression to a complete fracture. In the setting of insufficiency fractures, treatment of osteoporosis (e.g., alendronate, calcium, vitamin D) is also needed to help prevent future fractures. Fatigue stress fractures are treated with activity restriction.

12. **What fracture is usually diagnosed in trauma patients with pain in the anatomic snuff-box? Why is it concerning?**
Scaphoid bone fracture (Fig. 28.3), classically after a fall onto an outstretched hand ("FOOSH"). The scaphoid is the most commonly fractured carpal bone. X-rays may not show a fracture initially, so if the patient has a fall onto an outstretched hand and has pain in the anatomic snuff-box, treat these injuries as a fracture. Repeat x-rays can be performed 1 to 2 weeks later. Complications include nonunion of the fracture, chronic arthritis, and avascular necrosis due to its unidirectional blood supply.

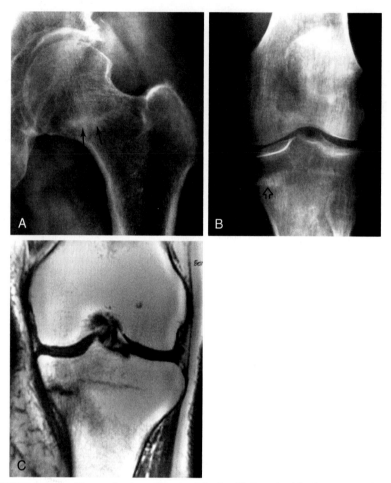

Fig. 28.2 (A) Stress fracture involving cancellous bone of the subcapital region of the femoral neck has the appearance of a band of sclerosis *(arrows)*. (B) A more subtle stress fracture at the medial tibial plateau *(open arrow)*. (C) Magnetic resonance imaging was ordered to confirm the fracture, clearly showing the low signal fracture line. (From Katz DS, Math KR, Groskin SA, eds. *Radiology Secrets.* Philadelphia: Hanley & Belfus; 1998:438. With permission.)

13. What are the most common locations of intervertebral disc herniations? What symptoms do they cause?

   Lumbar disc herniation is a common, often correctable cause of low back pain. The most common location is the L5-S1 disc, which affects the S1 nerve root. Symptoms include low back pain, buttock pain, and leg pain (worse with sitting and improved by standing). On exam, look for decreased ankle jerk, weakness of plantar flexors in the foot, pain from the midgluteal area to the posterior calf, and a positive straight leg-raise test. The second most common location for herniation is the L4-L5 disc, which affects the L5 nerve root. Look for decreased biceps femoris reflex, weakness of foot extensors, and pain in the hip or groin.

   After the lumbar area, the second most common location is the cervical spine. The classic symptom of cervical disc disease is neck pain. Herniation is most common at the C6-C7 disc, which affects the C7 nerve root. Look for decreased triceps reflex and weakness of the triceps and wrist flexion.

14. How is intervertebral disc herniation diagnosed and treated?

   Diagnosis is made with an MRI scan (preferred) or by a CT scan (use myelography if the patient has contraindications to MRI). Conservative treatment, including bed rest and analgesics, is usually tried first, as roughly 75% of cases will resolve with conservative management. Epidural steroid injection may help. Surgery (discectomy) may be required if conservative treatment fails or significant neurologic deficit is present (to prevent permanent nerve damage).

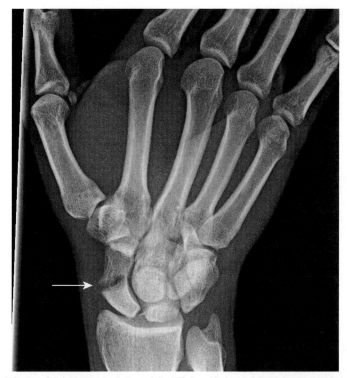

Fig. 28.3 Scaphoid fracture. Scaphoid view x-ray (anteroposterior [AP] view with ulnar deviation) is important to obtain in addition to standard wrist views (AP, lateral, and oblique) when scaphoid fracture is suspected. This scaphoid fracture was not seen on the x-rays on the day of the injury. The patient continued to have wrist pain and then presented 10 weeks later, when x-rays were obtained demonstrating the scaphoid fracture. (From Bope E, Kellerman R. *Conn's Current Therapy.* Elsevier; 2017:829-873.)

15. Define Charcot joint. What causes it? How is it managed?
    Charcot joints (neuropathic joints) are seen in patients with diabetes mellitus or other conditions causing peripheral neuropathy (e.g., tertiary syphilis). Due to decreased sensation, joints are subject to repetitive microtrauma, causing gradual arthritis or arthropathy and joint deformity. Patients should get radiographs for any (even minor) trauma because they may not feel even a severe fracture.

16. What is the most common bacterial cause of osteomyelitis? In what clinical scenarios should you think of other causes?
    Osteomyelitis is caused most commonly by *Staphylococcus aureus.* Think of gram-negative bacteria in immunocompromised patients or intravenous drug abusers. *Salmonella* species is the most likely cause in patients with sickle cell disease. Think *Pseudomonas aeruginosa* if there is a puncture wound through a tennis shoe. Diabetic patients who develop a "diabetic foot" with subsequent osteomyelitis usually have a polymicrobial infection. The gold standard for selecting antibiotic therapy is aspiration or biopsy of the affected joint or bone, respectively. Order a Gram stain, culture, and cell count of the fluid or tissue if osteomyelitis is suspected. Check a serum white blood cell (WBC) and erythrocyte sedimentation rate (ESR) or C-reactive protein.

17. Which bacteria are the most common cause of septic arthritis? In what scenario should you think of another cause?
    Septic arthritis is most commonly due to *Staphylococcus aureus,* but in sexually active adults (especially when young and/or promiscuous), suspect *Neisseria gonorrhoeae.* In immunocompromised, elderly, or neonatal patients, also consider gram-negative organisms. Aspirate the joint and order a Gram stain, culture, and cell count with differential if infection is suspected.

18. What is complex regional pain syndrome? How do patients present?
    Complex regional pain syndrome is a poorly understood disorder that generally occurs in an extremity and is characterized by pain, swelling, and signs of autonomic dysfunction (vasomotor instability with alternating warmth and coolness and/or sweating and dryness of the area). Type 1 does not involve a nerve injury, whereas type 2 develops after a known nerve injury. In most (but not all) cases, complex regional pain syndrome occurs after

trauma or surgery. The associated trauma is classically mild, and symptoms may begin days or several weeks after the injury. Patients classically have severe, intermittent pain, often described as burning, with associated temperature changes and sweating during episodes. A minor stimulus (e.g., light touch) may trigger severe pain symptoms. The diagnosis can be confirmed with radiographs or nuclear medicine scan. A presumptive diagnosis is often made in the appropriate setting if a sympathetic nerve block (i.e., injection of local anesthetic into the involved nerve) relieves symptoms. This procedure can be repeated as part of therapy if it is initially successful.

19. True or False: There is a high incidence of vascular injury with posterior knee dislocations.
True. Posterior displacement of the tibia is associated with popliteal artery injury. Order an angiogram if pulses are asymmetric (i.e., weaker or absent on the affected side) to check for injury.

20. What is the most common type of bone tumor?
Metastatic (especially from breast, lung, or prostate cancer).

21. What is a pathologic fracture? What is the most common cause of a pathologic fracture?
A pathologic fracture is one that occurs in bone previously weakened by another disease. Osteoporosis (especially in elderly, thin women) is the most common cause, but you should always think about the possibility of malignancy.

22. To what site is pain from hip inflammation or dislocation/fracture classically referred?
The knee (especially in children)

23. Specify age at presentation, epidemiology, signs and symptoms, and treatment for the three classically tested pediatric hip disorders

Name	Age	Epidemiology	Symptoms/Signs	Treatment
DDH	At birth	Female, firstborns, breech delivery	Barlow and Ortolani signs	Observation, abduction splint, or open or closed reduction
LCPD	4–8 yr	Short male with delayed bone age	Knee, thigh, groin pain, limp	Orthoses
SCFE	9–13 yr	Overweight male adolescent	Knee, thigh, groin pain, limp	Surgical pinning

DDH, Developmental dysplasia of the hip; *LCPD,* Legg-Calvé-Perthes disease; *SCFE,* slipped capital femoral epiphysis.
Note: All of these conditions may present in an adult as arthritis of the hip.

24. If you forget everything else about differentiating the three pediatric hip disorders, what historical point will help you the most on the USMLE?
Age at onset of symptoms.

25. Define Osgood-Schlatter disease. How is it recognized and treated?
Osgood-Schlatter disease is osteochondritis (aseptic ischemic necrosis) of the tibial tubercle. It is often bilateral and usually presents in boys between 10 and 15 years of age. It is mainly caused by overuse of the quadriceps muscles, leading to excess strain of the patellar ligament on the tibial tuberosity, resulting in traction apophysitis at the bony attachment. Signs and symptoms include pain, swelling, and tenderness in the knee (remember, the pediatric hip problems mentioned earlier have referred pain in the knee but no knee swelling or tenderness upon palpation of the knee). Treat with rest, activity restriction, and nonsteroidal antiinflammatory drugs. Most cases resolve on their own.

26. How do you check for scoliosis? Who is usually affected? What is the treatment?
Check for scoliosis by having patients touch their toes while you look at the spine. If scoliosis is present, you will see an abnormal lateral curvature of the spine. An imaginary straight line should run from C7 through the gluteal cleft. Scoliosis usually affects prepubertal girls and is idiopathic. Treat with a brace for anything other than very minor (<15 degrees) curvature. If the deformity is severe (e.g., respiratory compromise, rapid progression), surgery should be considered.

27. What are genu varum and genu valgum? At what ages do they present? When are they considered normal or abnormal?
Genu varum, or bowleg, is when the ankles come together but the knees do not. Genu valgum, or knock-knee, is when the knees come together but the ankles do not. Bowleg is normal in infants and toddlers, and it generally resolves by age 4 years. Knock-knee is generally normal within the 2- to 8-year age range. They are more likely to be pathologic if they are asymmetric. Both can be a sign of rickets, Blount disease, physeal deformity, or other bone conditions.

28. What is clubfoot? How is it treated?

    Clubfoot, or talipes equinovarus, is the most common congenital deformity of the lower extremity. It is an inward rotation of the forefoot with upward retraction of the heel that infants have at birth. Clubfoot is most commonly treated with serial casting beginning at diagnosis, but surgery is also an option if casting is unsuccessful.

29. What are the common findings with ligament injuries of the knee? How do you distinguish injuries of the anterior cruciate, posterior cruciate, medial collateral, and lateral collateral ligaments on physical exam?

    Ligament injuries in the knee commonly cause pain, joint effusions, instability of the joint, and history of the joint popping, buckling, or locking up.

    - **Anterior cruciate ligament** (**ACL**) tears are the most common. Watch for the *anterior* drawer test. With the patient supine, the knee is placed in 90 degrees of flexion and the tibia is pulled forward (like opening a drawer). If the tibia pulls forward more than normal (e.g., more than the unaffected side), the test is positive, and the patient has an ACL tear. Alternatively, use the Lachman test.
    - **Posterior cruciate ligament** (**PCL**) tears can be diagnosed with the *posterior* drawer test. Push the tibia back with the knee in 90 degrees of flexion. If the tibia pushes back more than the unaffected side, the test is positive and a PCL tear is present.
    - **Medial collateral ligament** (**MCL**) tears are suggested during the *abduction* or *valgus* stress test. With the patient supine and the knee in 30 degrees of flexion, place a hand on the lateral knee and push the lower leg laterally at the ankle. If the knee joint abducts to an abnormal degree, the test is positive and a medial compartment injury is present.
    - **Lateral collateral ligament** (**LCL**) tears are suggested during the *adduction* or *varus* stress test. This is the opposite of valgus stress. With the patient supine and the knee in 30 degrees of flexion, place a hand on the medial knee and push the lower leg medially at the ankle. If the knee joint adducts to an abnormal degree, the test is positive, and a lateral compartment injury is present.

    MRI (Fig. 28.4) and/or arthroscopy can be used to confirm suspected tears and look for other injuries.

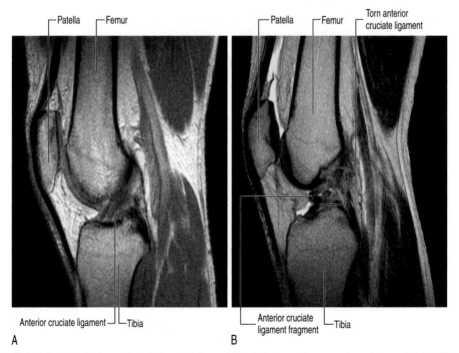

Fig. 28.4 (A) Knee joint showing an intact anterior cruciate ligament. T2-weighted magnetic resonance image in the sagittal plane. (B) Knee joint showing a torn anterior cruciate ligament. T2-weighted magnetic resonance image in the sagittal plane. (From Drake R, Vogl AW. *Gray's Anatomy for Students.* Elsevier; 2020:525-670.)

30. What is avascular necrosis (AVN) and what are the risk factors? What is the best test to make the diagnosis?

AVN describes interruption of blood supply with subsequent bone ischemia and necrosis of cancellous bone and marrow. Patients present with pain in the affected area. There are many potential risk factors, including:

- Trauma (usually in the setting of a fracture)
- Corticosteroid excess (endogenous or iatrogenic)
- Sickle cell disease or other hemoglobinopathy
- Alcohol abuse
- Lupus and other connective tissue disorders
- Decompression sickness
- Slipped capital femoral epiphysis
- Pancreatitis

The best test to make the diagnosis is MRI (Fig. 28.5), which becomes positive before regular x-rays.

31. What is plantar fasciitis and what are some common causes? How does it most commonly present?

Plantar fasciitis is the most common cause of pain at the bottom of the heel. The plantar fascia attaches the calcaneus to the front of the foot and supports the arch. Common causes include obesity, high arches, repetitive impact activity, and tight calf muscles. Plantar fasciitis most commonly presents as pain on the bottom of the foot near the heel. Pain is typically worse in the morning or after periods of rest.

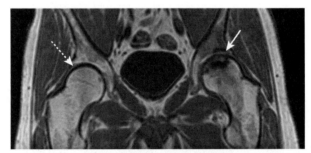

Fig. 28.5 Avascular necrosis of the hip. A T1-weighted coronal view of both hips demonstrates normal high signal from the fatty marrow in the right femur *(dotted white arrow)* but decreased signal in the left femoral head extending to the subchondral bone of the left hip joint *(solid white arrow)*. The joint space is preserved. Magnetic resonance imaging is the most sensitive method of detecting avascular necrosis of the hip. (From Herring W. *Learning Radiology: Recognizing the Basics.* Saunders; 2020:229-249.)

CHAPTER 29

PEDIATRICS

1. What is the first task you must complete when assessing a newborn immediately after delivery?
Stimulate respirations. Suction the **m**outh then **n**ose (i.e., in alphabetical order) if secretions appear to be impairing respiration.

2. When should positive pressure ventilation (PPV) be initiated?
Begin PPV if the neonate's heart rate drops below 100 beats/minute or if the neonate is experiencing respiratory difficulty (e.g., gasping, irregular breathing pattern).

3. How many blood vessels does a normal umbilical cord have? What disorder should be suspected if one of the vessels is absent?
The umbilical cord is checked at birth for the presence of **three** blood vessels: two arteries and one vein. If only one artery is present, investigate with ultrasound for congenital renal malformations (e.g., renal agenesis).

4. When should you initiate cardiopulmonary resuscitation (CPR) on a newborn? What is the appropriate compression-to-ventilation ratio?
CPR should be initiated if the newborn's heart rate drops below 60 beats/minute. Perform CPR at a ratio of 3:1 chest compressions to ventilations.

5. How can transient tachypnea of the newborn (TTN) be distinguished from respiratory distress syndrome (RDS)?
Look at the gestational age when delivery occurred and look at the infant's chest x-ray. When TTN occurs, it is often in term or near-term infants delivered by cesarean section. When RDS occurs, it will be in a premature infant due to insufficient surfactant production. The chest x-ray of TTN will show *hyper*expanded lungs, possibly with pulmonary edema (caused by fluid retention); the chest x-ray of RDS will show *hypo*expanded lungs that may be described as having a "ground-glass" appearance (due to atelectasis and decreased alveolar recruitment).

6. How does the management of TTN differ from managing RDS?
TTN management is more conservative, typically resolving after simple oxygen administration and occasionally requiring PPV. RDS, on the other hand, may require intubation with positive end-expiratory pressure (PEEP). Giving antenatal steroids to the mother may help reduce the severity of RDS if premature delivery is anticipated.

7. What are the potential sequelae of extended oxygen delivery by PEEP in a premature neonate?
Retinopathy of prematurity (caused by neovascularization and treated by laser ablation), intraventricular hemorrhage, and bronchopulmonary dysplasia are the three main sequelae to watch for that may be caused by excessive PEEP.

8. What is an Apgar score? At which time points should an Apgar score be measured? Explain the scoring criteria for each Apgar category.
The Apgar score is a general measure of newborn well-being, with five categories worth 2 points each for a total of 10 possible points. A score of 8 or above is considered acceptable. An Apgar score should be assessed at minutes 1 and 5 postpartum. Additional Apgar scores should be recorded every 5 minutes only if a score of 8 or higher has not been achieved. Use **APGAR** as a mnemonic to remember the five categories: **a**ppearance (skin color), **p**ulse (heart rate), **g**rimace (reflex irritability), **a**ctivity (muscle tone), and **r**espiratory effort (breathing).

	Number of Points Given		
Category	0	1	2
Appearance (color)	Completely cyanotic	Acrocyanosis: body pink, extremities blue	Completely pink
Pulse (heart rate)	Absent	<100 beats/min	>100 beats/min
Grimace (reflex irritability)[a]	None	Excessive stimulation required	Grimace and strong cry, cough, and sneeze

	Number of Points Given		
Category	**0**	**1**	**2**
Activity (muscle tone)	Flaccid limbs	Limbs are flexed but do *not resist* active extension	Active motion or able to partially resist active extension
Respiratory effort	Apneic	Irregular respirations or a slow, weak cry	Good, strong cry

[a]Reflex irritability usually is measured by the infant's response to stimulation of the sole of the foot or a catheter put into the nose.

9. True or False: The Apgar score may be used to predict long-term outcomes.
False. The Apgar score tells you what is happening *right now* but does not predict long-term outcomes.

10. Which two shots should all newborns receive?
All newborns should receive intramuscular vitamin K and the hepatitis B vaccine within 24 hours following delivery. If the mother is positive for the hepatitis B surface antigen (HBsAg), also give HBV immunoglobulin to the newborn. If the mother's HBV status is unknown, draw a serum HBsAg level to decide if the newborn needs immunoglobulin or if just giving the vaccine will be sufficient.

11. Why is a vitamin K injection given to the neonate immediately following delivery?
The neonate's gut flora is not yet mature enough to produce its own vitamin K. Giving an intramuscular injection of vitamin K is prophylactic against hemorrhagic disease of the newborn.

12. What are the commonly performed screening tests for metabolic and congenital disorders?
States vary widely in their policies regarding newborn screening, but there are a few nearly universal screens to know. All states screen for hypothyroidism and phenylketonuria at birth; these screens must be done within the first month of life. Most states also screen for galactosemia, cystic fibrosis, and hemoglobinopathies such as sickle cell disease. Less common screening tests that may still appear on the USMLE include homocystinuria, maple syrup urine disease, congenital adrenal hyperplasia, cystic fibrosis, biotinidase deficiency, tyrosinemia, and toxoplasmosis. Remember that screening tests are highly sensitive, so if any of these screens come back positive, your next step should be to order a confirmatory test with high specificity to rule out a false-positive result.

13. Compare and contrast gastroschisis vs. omphalocele. How do they present clinically? Which is enclosed in a membrane? What is the appropriate management for each condition?
Gastroschisis and omphalocele are two types of bowel extrusion that may be present at birth. Gastroschisis is typically extruding to the right of the umbilicus and is *not* covered in membrane. Omphalocele typically extrudes directly through the umbilicus (i.e., midline) and *is* covered by a membrane. Both are managed the same way: wrapped in a saline-soaked sterile dressing and covered (also called siloed) to prevent infection or desiccation as the intestines slowly return where they belong. A nasogastric tube may be considered to decompress the bowel.

14. How is imperforate anus diagnosed?
Imperforate anus is diagnosed with an upside-down x-ray, to allow colonic gas to rise and show exactly how far the imperforate lesion is from the anus.

15. Once imperforate anus has been diagnosed, which studies do you order next? Explain why?
Imperforate anus is associated with the VACTERL anomalies. **VACTERL** is an acronym for **v**ertebral anomalies, imperforate **a**nus, **c**ardiac malformations, **t**racheal-**e**sophageal malformation, **r**enal dysfunction, and **l**imb malformation (especially the thumbs). Order a spinal x-ray, fetal echocardiogram, and renal ultrasound, and attempt to pass a nasogastric tube to work up each potential VACTERL complication before diving straight into management for imperforate anus.

16. How does the management of imperforate anus differ if the lesion is distal (e.g., closer to the anus) vs proximal (e.g., further from the anus)?
After additional VACTERL complications have been ruled out, distal lesions can be corrected as soon as they are identified: either by dilation or minor surgery. Proximal lesions require further neonatal development before they can be corrected, so your management *right now* should be to place a colostomy and defer surgical correction for the future (but before the infant begins to toilet train).

17. A neonatal abdominal x-ray shows a double-bubble sign. What is on your differential? What clinical or imaging clues can be used to distinguish between these possibilities?
A neonatal abdominal x-ray with a double-bubble sign is not as narrow of a differential diagnosis as you may think. The most testable diagnoses include malrotation, intestinal atresia, duodenal atresia, and annular pancreas.

These can be distinguished by looking at what is going on with the air-fluid levels: A double-bubble sign with normal air-fluid levels suggests malrotation, a double-bubble sign with multiple air-fluid levels suggests intestinal atresia, and a double-bubble sign with no distal air-fluid levels indicates either duodenal atresia or annular pancreas. In clinical practice it is difficult to tell duodenal atresia and annular pancreas with from imaging alone, but on the USMLE, look for mentions of **D**own syndrome to indicate **d**uodenal atresia as the most likely etiology rather than annular pancreas.

18. How does Hirschsprung disease present? What is its pathophysiology?
   Hirschsprung disease presents as constipation in a newborn with explosive diarrhea on digital rectal exam (squirt sign). Less severe conditions may not present until the child is 2 to 3 years old. Hirschsprung disease is caused by a lack of neural crest cell migration, resulting in no Meissner plexus or Auerbach plexus in the rectum. Because of this, the sphincter cannot relax, resulting in fecal retention. Hirschsprung disease is associated with trisomy 21 (Down syndrome).

19. How is Hirschsprung disease worked up, diagnosed, and managed?
   If suspected, Hirschsprung disease is worked up with anorectal manometry (which would show increased rectal tone). Diagnosis is made by suction biopsy, taking care to include the **submucosa** (i.e., where the absent neurons *should* be found). Hirschsprung disease is managed with surgical resection of the affected colon.

20. What clinical presentation and physical exam findings would make you suspect pyloric stenosis in an infant? How is it managed once diagnosed?
   Pyloric stenosis is characterized by nonbilious projectile vomiting with possibly visible peristaltic waves or a palpable olive-shaped mass in the infant's abdominal right upper quadrant. Surgically correct with pyloromyotomy; be sure to give intravenous fluids and electrolytes to reduce the risk of postoperative apnea.

21. What three characteristic acid-base and electrolyte abnormalities are typically present in infants with pyloric stenosis? Explain why these occur.
   Expect to see hypochloremic hypokalemic metabolic alkalosis in these infants. Pyloric stenosis causes projectile vomiting of gastric acid, meaning your patient is actively losing H$^+$, Cl$^-$, and fluid. The body acts to prevent fluid-related dehydration by releasing aldosterone, which exchanges K$^+$ for Na$^+$ to facilitate water retention. The ultimate result of this physiologic cascade is hypochloremic hypokalemic metabolic alkalosis.

22. What is the leading diagnosis for a prematurely born infant now presenting with bloody stool? What is your next step?
   A premature infant with bloody stool will almost always have necrotizing enterocolitis (NEC). If you see pneumatosis intestinalis (air in the bowel wall), you have confirmed NEC. This patient needs to become NPO (*nil per os*, "nothing by mouth") immediately, with feeding provided by total parenteral nutrition and intravenous fluids. Decompress the bowel with a nasogastric tube and start broad-spectrum antibiotics to prevent shock. Surgery is only necessary if clinical deterioration or perforation occurs; perforation will present as air under the diaphragm on imaging studies.

23. How is infant colic defined and treated?
   Infant colic is described as crying/fussing for no apparent reason lasting 3 or more hours per day for at least 3 days per week in a healthy infant younger than 3 months. Parents should be educated regarding feeding and soothing techniques and reassured that the condition is self-limited.

24. How is neonatal hypoglycemia diagnosed and managed?
   Serum glucose levels below 40 mg/dL are considered diagnostic for neonatal hypoglycemia. There are four management options for neonatal hypoglycemia, depending on the level of severity. Asymptomatic hypoglycemia is managed with simple oral feeding. Symptomatic hypoglycemia (e.g., lethargic, tremulous, excessively irritable infants) should be managed with a bolus of dextrose (typically D10W): 2 L per kg body weight. If that bolus does not resolve the hypoglycemia, refractory hypoglycemia should be treated with a dextrose infusion. In the most severe cases, where serum glucose is either unmeasurable or the infant appears obtunded, administer intramuscular glucagon.

25. How can conjunctivitis caused by *Neisseria gonorrhoeae* be distinguished from conjunctivitis caused by *Chlamydia trachomatis*? How is each conjunctival infection treated?
   Conjunctivitis caused by *Neisseria gonorrhoeae* will occur during the first week of life (day 2–7), while conjunctivitis caused by *Chlamydia trachomatis* will occur during the second week of life (day 5–14). Either conjunctival infection may present bilaterally, but if the infection is unilateral only, it is *C. trachomatis*. Treat gonorrheal conjunctivitis with topical erythromycin drops; treat chlamydial conjunctivitis with oral erythromycin.

26. Which infants should receive iron supplementation? At what age?
   Iron supplements are recommended for exclusively breastfed infants beginning at 4 months of age. Infants receive enough iron during the third trimester of pregnancy to last for the first 4 months of life, but because breast milk contains so little iron, supplements are needed after 4 months. Formula-fed infants receive adequate iron for the first 12 months of life with standard infant formula.

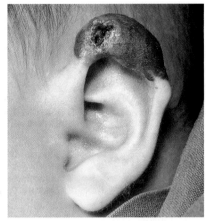

Fig. 29.1 Infantile hemangioma. Lesions grow rapidly during the first few months of life once they appear (20% at birth), but they are asymptomatic unless they bleed, become infected, or obstruct a vital structure. Complete resolution is typical before the age of 7, and no treatment is usually required. (From du Vivier A. *Atlas of Clinical Dermatology*. 3rd ed. New York: Churchill Livingstone, 2002, p. 117, with permission)

27. True or False: Breastfed infants are more likely to require vitamin D supplements than formula-fed infants.
    True. The American Academy of Pediatrics recommends that exclusively and partially breastfed infants receive **oral** vitamin **D** supplementation (neonates **d**rink vitamin **D** but receive an inje[k]tion of vitamin **K**) shortly after birth and continue until they are weaned and begin consuming formula or whole milk. Formula-fed infants do not require vitamin D supplements in the United States because all formulas are already supplemented with vitamin D.

28. Distinguish between caput succedaneum and cephalohematoma. How are these conditions treated?
    Both conditions are noted in newborns after vaginal delivery. **Caput succedaneum** defines diffuse swelling or edema of the scalp that crosses the midline, is benign, and requires no further investigation or treatment. A **cephalohematoma** is a subperiosteal hemorrhage that does not cross suture lines and is usually benign and self-resolving but in rare cases may indicate an underlying skull fracture. Order a radiograph or computed tomography (CT) scan of the head to rule out a fracture.

29. How are cavernous hemangiomas treated?
    Cavernous hemangiomas are benign vascular tumors that are often first noticed a few days after birth. They tend to increase in size after birth (sometimes becoming quite large) and gradually resolve within the first 2 years of life (Fig. 29.1). The best treatment is to do nothing but observe and follow.

30. When does the anterior fontanelle usually close? What disorder should you suspect if it fails to close?
    The anterior fontanelle is usually closed by **18 months** of age. Delayed closure or an unusually large anterior fontanelle may indicate hypothyroidism, hydrocephalus, rickets, or intrauterine growth restriction (IUGR).

31. When should the Moro and palmar grasp reflexes disappear?
    These primitive reflexes should disappear by 6 months of age.

32. Name the commonly tested gross motor, fine motor, social, and verbal/cognitive childhood milestones for each age of development listed.

Age	Gross Motor	Fine Motor	Social	Verbal/ Cognitive
3 mo	Roll	Grab	Smile	Laugh
6 mo	Sit up	Scraping/raking grasp Switch hands; move objects from one hand to the other	Stranger anxiety	Schmooze/coo incoherently

Age	Gross Motor	Fine Motor	Social	Verbal/ Cognitive
9 mo	Pull self up to standing position	Pincer grasp Able to play pat-a-cake	Parent/ separation anxiety	Can say single words ("papa") Personal: recognizes own name Object permanence
12 mo	Stand tall under own power "Walk by 1" may not follow the "T" mnemonic, but it's a nice memory hook	Track/point at objects	Nothing special	Nothing special
18 mo	Climb stairs	Uses cups and cutlery	Complains: starts throwing tantrums	Calls objects by name ("book," "dog") Potty training begins
2 yr	Uses 2 legs to run	Nothing special	2 people: will leave and return to parent but may not engage with peers yet ("two people" = child and parent)	200-word vocabulary 2-word sentences Follows 2-step commands
3 yr	Tricycle: able to ride it	Can draw a circle Rides tricycle	Three people: start playing with peers ("three people" = child, parent, child's friend)	Toilet trained: successful potty training complete Thousand (1000) word vocabualry Constantly asks W-H-Y (three letters)
4 yr	Four-limb dexterity: able to hop and balance on one leg	Draw square and cross (four sides in a square, four lines make a cross)	Figments: may have imaginary friends	Full sentences and storytelling Names at least two colors
5 yr	Uses five fingers to play with a jump rope	Uses five fingers to dress and groom self (e.g., tie shoes, button a shirt)	Nothing special	Uses five fingers to start counting (to 10)

Miscellaneous Milestone Pearls

The "appropriate" number of stacked blocks is 3x their age starting at age 1 year (i.e., a toddler should be able to stack 3 blocks by age 1, 6 by age 2, etc.).

For **premature infants** in their first 2 years of life, adjust their expected milestones by the number of weeks early they were delivered. For example, an infant born at a gestational age of 28 weeks (i.e., 12 weeks early) should be expected to reach their 6-month milestones around age 9 months (i.e., 12 weeks later), 12-month milestones around age 15 months, and so on until 2-year milestones around age 2 years, 3 months.

33. True or False: The overall trend or pattern of development is more important than the particular age at which any individual milestone is reached.
   True. The exact age is not as important as the overall pattern when monitoring for dysfunctional development. When in doubt, use a formal developmental test, such as the M-CHAT (**M**odified **Ch**ecklist for **A**utism in **T**oddlers).

34. What screening and preventive care measures should be done at every pediatric visit?
   Height, weight, blood pressure, and developmental/behavioral assessment should be performed during every pediatric clinic visit. Also be prepared to provide anticipatory guidance (e.g., counseling/discussion about age-appropriate concerns) to the child's parents during each visit.

35. **Define failure to thrive. What causes it?**
There is no consensus definition for failure to thrive, but commonly used definitions include a head circumference, height, or weight less than the 5th percentile for age; a weight less than 80% of ideal weight for age; or a weight that drops two or more major lines on the growth curve. Failure to thrive is most commonly due to psychosocial or functional problems. Watch for signs of neglect and child abuse. Organic causes usually have specific clues to trigger your suspicion.

36. **What conditions are suggested by obesity in children?**
Obesity is usually due to overeating and too little activity (>95% of cases). Less than 5% of cases are due to organic causes (e.g., Cushing syndrome, Prader-Willi syndrome).

37. **True or False: Screening and preventive care do not have to be addressed during a pediatric clinic visit if the chief complaint is unrelated to well-child development.**
False. Screening and preventive care are an important part of every patient encounter—adult or child. Your exam questions may try to fool you on this point. For example, consider a mother who complains that her 4-year-old child sleeps 11 hours every night. The answer to the question, "What should you do next?" may not be about sleep patterns at all, but rather should be to perform any routine screening procedure that you would expect a 4-year-old child to receive (e.g., an objective hearing exam).

38. **What are the frequently tested items under the umbrella of primary prevention using "anticipatory guidance"?**
Tell parents the following:
- Keep the water heater under 120°F.
- Have functional smoke detectors in the home.
- Have the phone number for poison control handy.
- Advise smoking cessation if anyone in the home uses tobacco or vape products.
- Use proper car restraints (e.g., child safety seat until 2 years, booster seat until height is 4'9").
- Put the infant to sleep on the side or back ("Back to Sleep") to help prevent sudden infant death syndrome (SIDS).
- Advise against sharing a bed with the infant due to risk of SIDS or accidental smothering.
- Do not use infant walkers (they cause injuries).
- Watch out for small objects (they may be aspirated).
- Do not give honey before 1 year of age (risk of unintended *botulinum* poisoning).
- Do not give cow's milk before 1 year of age.
- Introduce solid foods gradually, starting at 4 to 6 months of age.
- Supervise children in bathtubs and swimming pools.
- Minimize screen time (televisions, computers, portable devices).
- Get plenty of physical activity (at least 60 minutes daily).

39. **How often should height, weight, and head circumference be measured? What do they signify? Which measurements will be the first and last to become abnormal if the child is not developing appropriately?**
Height and weight should be measured routinely during every clinic visit, well into adulthood. Head circumference should be measured at every visit until the patient is 2 years old. All three parameters are markers of general well-being; abnormal values may suggest disease. The first measurement to become abnormal is weight (a child can lose weight but cannot shrink); the last measurement to become abnormal is head circumference because you are essentially waiting for the child's body to outgrow the head.

40. **What if a child has low height, weight, or head circumference compared to peers?**
The trend or pattern over time along a plotted growth curve will tell you more than any single measurement. You may be asked to interpret these growth curves on the USMLE. If a child has always tended low or high compared to their peers, the pattern is generally benign. A patient who crosses two or more growth curves is more worrisome. Parents commonly bring in a child who they believe is experiencing delayed physical growth or delayed puberty. You need to know when to reassure and when to do further testing and questioning.

41. **What conditions should you consider in a child with an abnormal head circumference?**
Increased head circumference may indicate hydrocephalus or tumor, whereas decreased head circumference may indicate microcephaly (e.g., TORCH infections: congenital **t**oxoplasmosis, **o**ther [e.g., syphilis, HIV], **r**ubella, **c**ytomegalovirus, **h**erpes simplex infection or Zika virus; aneuploidy). Again, the pattern of head circumference over time (plotted on a growth curve) is most helpful in defining pathology.

42. **True or False: Children have the same range of normal vital signs as adults.**
False. Children have *lower* baseline blood pressure and *higher* baseline heart and respiratory rates than do adults. In addition, children often have different acceptable ranges of lab values. For example, a healthy child's hemoglobin/hematocrit value is normally higher at birth and lower throughout childhood compared with that of an adult. In addition, the renal, pulmonary, hepatic, and central nervous systems are not fully mature or functional at birth.

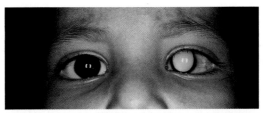

Fig. 29.2 Leukocoria (white pupillary reflex) is the most common presenting feature of retinoblastoma and may be first noticed in family photographs. (From Kanski JJ. *Clinical Diagnosis in Ophthalmology.* 1st ed. St. Louis: Mosby; 2006 [fig. 9.94.] Courtesy U. Raina.)

43. **When are hearing and vision screened?**
Hearing and vision should be measured objectively at least once by 4 years of age. After that initial screen, measure every few years until adulthood or more often if the history so dictates.

44. **In what clinical situations should you worry about hearing loss in pediatric patients?**
    - Bacterial meningitis, especially by *Hemophilus influenzae,* which may cause sensorineural hearing loss of the vestibulocochlear nerve (cranial nerve 8)
    - Congenital TORCH infections
    - Measles or mumps
    - Chronic middle ear effusions or chronic or recurrent otitis media
    - Use of ototoxic drugs (e.g., aminoglycosides, furosemide)

45. **What is the red reflex? What does an abnormal red reflex suggest?**
When a penlight is shined at the pupil, you usually see red because of the underlying fundus. Check for the red reflex at birth and routinely thereafter to detect congenital cataracts, strabismus, or ocular tumors. If a cataract, strabismus, or ocular tumor is present, the red reflex disappears. For cataracts and tumors, you may see white instead of red—this finding is known as leukocoria and is classically due to retinoblastoma (Fig. 29.2).

46. **True or False: Before a certain age intermittent strabismus is normal.**
True. It is normal for infants to have occasional ocular misalignment (strabismus) until 4 months of age. After 4 months (or with constant eye deviation), strabismus should be evaluated and managed by an ophthalmologist to prevent possible blindness in the affected eye.

47. **How is strabismus managed if it persists beyond age 3 months?**
Patch the **good eye** to force the abnormal eye to develop. Severe strabismus may require surgical intervention.

48. **How and when should pediatric patients be screened for iron-deficiency anemia?**
According to AAP guidelines, a risk assessment for iron-deficiency anemia should begin at 4 months of age, with hemoglobin and hematocrit measured at 1 year of age. Risk factors to assess for include prematurity, low birth weight, excessive ingestion of cow's milk before 1 year of age, low dietary iron intake, and low socioeconomic status.

49. **True or False: Screening children for renal disease with a urinalysis is not recommended.**
True. However, you should screen for congenital/anatomic abnormalities (e.g., vesicoureteral reflux) after a febrile urinary tract infection in children between the ages of 2 months and 2 years by getting an ultrasound plus either voiding cystourethrogram (VCUG) or radionuclide cystogram (RNC). Screening after 2 years of age is more controversial and likely will not be asked on the USMLE.

50. **How and when do you screen for lead exposure?**
Screening for lead toxicity is controversial. Routine screening is no longer recommended. However, all Medicaid-eligible children must be screened. Consider screening high-risk children (those who live in old buildings, have a sibling or playmate with lead toxicity, eat paint chips, live near a battery-recycling plant, or have a parent who works at a battery recycling plant). Screen for lead exposure by ordering a serum lead level. If the initial lead level is abnormally high, closer follow-up and intervention are needed. The best first step is to stop the exposure.

51. **When should children be screened for tuberculosis?**
Universal screening for tuberculosis is not recommended. There is no need to screen children who have no risk factors. Risk assessment should occur regularly until 2 years of age, then annually. Test those at high risk (family member with tuberculosis or a positive tuberculosis test, a child born in a high-risk country, a child who has traveled to a high-risk country, or a child who has consumed unpasteurized milk or cheese).

52. True or False: A diagnosis of encopresis or enuresis cannot be made before a certain age.
True. Encopresis is considered normal until age 4 years and enuresis is normal until age 5 years. This diagnostic point is obviously important when the parent complains because both are normal findings in a 3-year-old child. If the problem persists, rule out physical problems (e.g., Hirschsprung disease, urinary tract infection) and treat with behavioral modification (e.g., "gold star for being good" charts, alarms, biofeedback) as the first-line treatment. Desmopressin and imipramine may be used for refractory cases of enuresis.

53. What are some complications of constipation in young children?
Common complications include encopresis, enuresis, anal fissures, and hemorrhoids. Constipation can be associated with toilet training, entry to daycare/school, transition to solid diet, and introduction or excessive consumption of cow's milk.

54. What should you always consider when a question mentions that a child with flulike symptoms was given aspirin?
Reye syndrome. Reye syndrome causes encephalopathy and/or liver failure after aspirin is given for influenza or varicella infection. Use acetaminophen in children to avoid this rare (but often tested) condition.

55. What high-yield information do you need to know about immunizations for the USMLE Step 2 exam?
High-yield information includes the recommendations for special patient populations (e.g., give pneumococcal vaccine to patients with sickle cell disease or splenectomy) and notable vaccine contraindications (no live vaccines such as measles-mumps-rubella or varicella for immunocompromised patients or pregnant patients).

56. Which vaccine is contraindicated in pediatric patients with a history of intussusception?
The **rotavirus** vaccine is contraindicated for pediatrics with a history of intussusception.

57. True or False: Pediatric immunizations for preterm infants should be given based on chronologic age.
True. The only exception is for the hepatitis B vaccine. If the birth weight is less than 2 kg, the infant should be immunized by hospital discharge or 1 month of age (whichever event is earlier).

58. True or False: Most children need fluoride supplementation.
False. Because most water is fluoridated, supplementation is not needed. However, if a child lives in an area where the water is inadequately fluoridated (rare) or the child is fed exclusively from premixed, ready-to-eat formulas (which use nonfluoridated water), fluoride supplements should be given.

59. When should you recommend that a child see a dentist for the first time?
The AAP and American Academy of Pediatric Dentistry (AAPD) both recommend that a child see a dentist within 6 months of first tooth eruption or at 12 months of age, whichever comes first.

60. What clinical findings would you expect in milk protein allergy? How do you manage it?
Milk protein allergy is the most common food allergy in young children and typically presents in the first few months of life with failure to thrive, regurgitation, atopic dermatitis, and occasionally bloody stools. Management involves avoidance of any dairy or soy in the maternal diet for breastfed infants and use of hydrolyzed formula in formula-fed infants. The condition typically self-resolves eventually.

61. True or False: Button battery ingestion in an asymptomatic, clinically stable child requires immediate endoscopic removal.
False. In a clinically stable patient, the first step involves obtaining a chest x-ray to determine the location of the ingested button battery. If the battery is located in the esophagus, endoscopic removal is warranted. If the battery is located beyond the esophagus, it is safe to observe for excretion of the object via stool and follow-up x-ray.

62. What are clinical signs of a breath-holding spell in a child?
In a breath-holding spell, the child has an episode of apnea followed by collapse, limpness, and loss of consciousness with a quick return to baseline. Triggers are often minimal and include anger/frustration (cyanotic type) or minor fall/head injury (pallid type). Breath-holding spells are self-limited and do not affect neurologic development.

63. What are the clinical findings associated with growing pains? How is the condition managed?
Growing pains occurs in children ages 3 to 12 years and typically causes bilateral lower extremity pain, primarily at night. Parents should be reassured that the condition self-resolves. Symptoms can be managed with leg massages, heat, stretching exercises, and nonopioid analgesics (e.g., acetaminophen, ibuprofen).

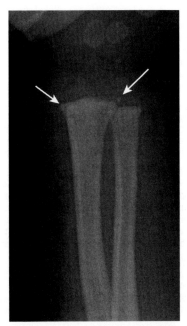

Fig. 29.3 Metaphyseal corner fractures *(solid white arrows)* and small avulsion-type fractures of the distal radius are findings characteristic of child abuse. (From Herring W. *Learning Radiology: Recognizing the Basics.* Saunders; 2020:324-338.)

64. **What findings should make you suspect child abuse?**
    - Failure to thrive
    - Multiple fractures, bruises, or injuries in different stages of healing
    - Concentric cigarette-shaped burns
    - Signs of intentional burns (e.g., scald injuries from intentional immersion that are symmetric with sharp lines of demarcation)
    - Metaphyseal "bucket handle" or "corner" fractures (Fig. 29.3)
    - Shaken baby syndrome (retinal hemorrhages or subdural hematomas with no external signs of trauma)
    - Behavioral, emotional, or interactional problems
    - Sexually transmitted diseases
    - Dissociative identity disorder (previously known as multiple personality disorder; classically due to sexual abuse)
    - Whenever a parent's story does not fit the child's injury

65. **True or False: You must have proof before you can report child abuse.**
    False. In fact, reporting any suspicion of child abuse is mandatory. You do not need proof and cannot be sued for reporting your suspicion.

66. **What are the Tanner stages? When do they occur?**
    The Tanner stages measure the stages of puberty. Stage 1 is preadolescent; stage 5 is adult. Advancing stages are assigned for testicular and penile growth in boys and breast growth in girls. Both male and female stages also use pubic hair development. The average age of puberty (when a patient first has changes from the preadolescent stage 1) is earlier for girls than boys (10.5 years in girls compared to 11.5 years in boys). The classic first events of puberty are testicular enlargement in boys and breast development in girls.

67. **True or False: A 1-month history of a painful nipple mass in a 13-year-old boy with Tanner stage 3 genitalia and who is otherwise healthy warrants further workup.**
    False. This situation is a common description of pubertal gynecomastia, which occurs in over 50% of male adolescents. It usually presents with a palpable mass or lump behind one or both nipples and can be painful. It can be safely observed, as the condition typically regresses substantially or self-resolves by 1 year.

68. Define delayed puberty. What is the most common cause?

In boys, delayed puberty is defined as no enlargement of the testicles by age 14 or a time lapse of more than 5 years from the start to the completion of growth of the genitals. In girls, delayed puberty is defined as no breast development (thelarche) by age 13, a time lapse of more than 5 years from the beginning of breast growth to the first menstrual period, or no menstruation by age 16. The most common cause is **constitutional delay**, a normal variant. Watch for parents with a similar history of being "late bloomers." The child's growth curve consistently lags behind that of peers, but the line representing the child's growth curve is parallel to the normal growth curve. Treatment is reassurance only.

69. What are other potential causes for delayed puberty?

Rarely, delayed puberty is due to primary testicular failure (Klinefelter syndrome, cryptorchidism, history of chemotherapy, gonadal dysgenesis) or ovarian failure (Turner syndrome, gonadal dysgenesis). Even more rarely, delayed puberty is due to a hypothalamic/pituitary defect, such as Kallmann syndrome or tumor.

70. What causes precocious puberty?

Precocious puberty is usually idiopathic but may be due to the **McCune-Albright syndrome** (triad includes precocious puberty, fibrous dysplasia of the bone, and the "coast of Maine" café au lait spots), ovarian tumors (e.g., granulosa, theca cell, or gonadoblastoma), testicular tumors (e.g., Leydig cell tumors), central nervous system disease or trauma, adrenal neoplasm, or congenital adrenal hyperplasia (CAH). CAH causes precocious puberty in boys only (due to elevated androgen levels) and is usually due to 21-hydroxylase deficiency. Obesity may also lead to precocious puberty in girls due to elevated adipose-related estrone levels.

71. True or False: If the underlying cause for precocious puberty is uncorrectable or idiopathic after diagnostic workup, patients should still receive treatment.

True. Most patients are given long-acting gonadotropin-releasing hormone (GnRH) agonists (e.g., leuprolide) to modulate the hypothalamic-pituitary-gonadal axis and ultimately suppress the progression of puberty. Among other benefits, this approach helps to prevent the short stature that may result from premature epiphyseal closure.

72. True or False: Sexually active teenaged girls need screening for chlamydial infection and gonorrhea.

True. There are high numbers of reported cases of chlamydia and gonorrhea in younger women. The Centers for Disease Control and Prevention (CDC) recommends annual screening for chlamydia for all sexually active females ages 25 and under. The CDC recommends screening high-risk sexually active females for gonorrhea.

CHAPTER 30

PHARMACOLOGY

1. On the USMLE, bizarre, unique, and fatal side effects are tested as well as common side effects of common drugs. Cover the right-hand column and name the side effects of the listed drugs.

Drug or Drug Class	Side Effect(s)
Acetaminophen	Liver toxicity (in high doses)
Acetazolamide	Normal anion gap metabolic acidosis
Aminoglycosides	Hearing loss, renal toxicity
Amiodarone	Thyroid dysfunction, pulmonary toxicity, liver toxicity (mnemonic: TFTs, PFTs, LFTs), bradyarrhythmias, corneal microdeposits, blue-gray skin discoloration
Angiotensin-converting enzyme inhibitors	Cough, angioedema
Angiotensin receptor blockers	Angioedema
Aspirin	Gastrointestinal bleeding, hypersensitivity, early respiratory alkalosis with late high anion gap metabolic acidosis
Bleomycin	Pulmonary fibrosis
Bupropion	Seizures
Busulfan	Pulmonary fibrosis
Chloramphenicol	Aplastic anemia, gray-baby syndrome
Chlorpropamide	Syndrome of inappropriate antidiuretic hormone (SIADH)
Cisplatin	Nephrotoxicity
Clindamycin	Pseudomembranous colitis (can be caused by any broad-spectrum antibiotic)
Clofibrate	Increased gastrointestinal neoplasms
Clozapine	Agranulocytosis
Cyclophosphamide	Hemorrhagic cystitis
Cyclosporine	Renal toxicity
Demeclocycline	Diabetes insipidus
Didanosine (ddI)	Pancreatitis, peripheral neuropathy
Digitalis	Gastrointestinal disorders, hyperkalemia, vision changes, arrhythmias
Doxorubicin	Cardiomyopathy
Ethambutol	Optic neuritis
Halogen anesthesia	Malignant hyperthermia
Halothane	Liver necrosis
Heparin	Thrombocytopenia, thrombosis
HMG-CoA reductase inhibitors (e.g., simvastatin)	Liver and muscle toxicity

Drug or Drug Class	Side Effect(s)
Hydralazine	Lupuslike syndrome
Hydroxychloroquine	Retinopathy
Isoniazid	Vitamin B_6 deficiency (leading to intractable seizures, neuropathy), lupuslike syndrome, liver toxicity
Isotretinoin	Terrible teratogen
Lithium	Diabetes insipidus, thyroid dysfunction
Local anesthetic	Seizures, cardiac arrhythmia
Methotrexate	Hepatotoxicity, pulmonary toxicity, and myelosuppression
Methyldopa	Hemolytic anemia (positive Coombs test)
Metronidazole	Disulfiram-like reaction with alcohol
Minoxidil	Hirsutism
Monoamine oxidase inhibitors (MAOIs)	Tyramine crisis (after eating cheese or wine)
Morphine	Sphincter of Oddi spasm
Niacin	Skin flushing, pruritus
Opiates	SIADH
Oxytocin	SIADH
Penicillins	Anaphylaxis; rash with Epstein-Barr virus
Phenytoin	Folate deficiency, teratogen, hirsutism
Procainamide	Lupuslike syndrome
Quinine	Cinchonism (tinnitus, vertigo), thrombocytopenia, QT prolongation
Quinolones	Teratogens (cartilage damage), QT prolongation, delirium
Rifampin	Orange-red body secretions
Selective serotonin reuptake inhibitors (e.g., fluoxetine)	Anxiety, agitation, insomnia, sexual dysfunction, serotonin syndrome
Succinylcholine	Malignant hyperthermia; do not use in the presence of hyperkalemia
Sulfa drugs	Rash, acute interstitial nephritis, kernicterus in neonates
Tetracyclines	Photosensitivity, teeth staining in children
Thioridazine	Retinal deposits, cardiac toxicity
Trazodone	Priapism
Valproic acid	Neural tube defects in offspring
Vancomycin	Red man's syndrome (related to infusion rate)
Vincristine	Peripheral neuropathy
Warfarin	Skin necrosis, teratogen, increased risk for clots early (that is why heparin bridging is needed)
Zidovudine (AZT)	Bone marrow suppression

2. What are the side effects of diuretics?

Thiazide diuretics cause calcium retention, hyperglycemia, hyperuricemia, hyperlipidemia, hyponatremia, hypokalemic metabolic alkalosis, and hypovolemia; because they are sulfa drugs, watch out for sulfa allergy. Think of the acronym **hyperGLUC** for high **g**lucose, **l**ipids, **u**ric acid, and **c**alcium.

Loop diuretics cause hypokalemic metabolic alkalosis, hypovolemia (more potent than thiazides), ototoxicity, and calcium excretion; with the exception of ethacrynic acid, they also are sulfa drugs.
Carbonic anhydrase inhibitors cause metabolic acidosis.
Potassium-sparing diuretics (e.g., spironolactone) may cause hyperkalemia.

3. What are the side effects of beta-blockers?
Like many antihypertensive agents, beta-blockers can cause sedation, depression, and sexual dysfunction. They also cause bradycardia and heart block in susceptible patients and should be avoided in patients with these conditions, as should central-acting calcium channel blockers (e.g., verapamil and diltiazem). Beta-blockers can also precipitate asthmatic attacks (via $beta_2$-receptor) and mask the symptoms of hypoglycemia and sepsis; thus they should be avoided or used with caution in asthmatics and those with chronic obstructive pulmonary disease (COPD). A $beta_1$ selective beta-blocker (atenolol, metoprolol) or a combined beta- and alpha-blocker (carvedilol) is preferred if a beta-blocker is needed to treat another condition such as heart disease. Use in diabetic patients requires an analysis of the risks and benefits; if other equivalent medications are available, use them instead.

4. What class of antihypertensive agents is best known for severe, first-dose orthostatic hypotension?
$Alpha_1$-antagonists (e.g., tamsulosin, which is now often used in benign prostatic hyperplasia and nephrolithiasis)

5. What antihypertensive is best known for causing depression?
Methyldopa. Beta-blockers may also cause depression.

6. Cover the right-hand column and give the antidote(s) for overdose or toxic exposure to the drugs in the left-hand column.

Poison or Medication	Antidote
Acetaminophen	N-acetylcysteine
Benzodiazepines	Flumazenil (can precipitate benzodiazepine withdrawal and seizure)
Beta-blockers	Glucagon, high-dose insulin, intralipid/fat emulsion therapy
Calcium channel blockers	Calcium, glucagon, high-dose insulin, intralipid/fat emulsion therapy
Carbon monoxide	Oxygen (hyperbaric in cases of severe poisoning)
Cholinesterase inhibitors	Atropine, pralidoxime
Copper or gold	Penicillamine
Cyanide	Hydroxocobalamin, nitrates, or sodium thiosulfate
Digoxin	Normalize potassium and other electrolytes; digoxin antibodies (Fab)
Heparin	Protamine sulfate
Iron	Deferoxamine
Isoniazid	Vitamin B_6
Lead	Edetate (EDTA); use succimer in children
Methanol or ethylene glycol	Fomepizole, ethanol
Methemoglobin	Methylene blue
Muscarinic blockers	Physostigmine
Opioids	Naloxone (just enough to maintain respiratory drive)
Quinidine or tricyclic antidepressants	Sodium bicarbonate (cardioprotective)
Salicylates	Activated charcoal, sodium bicarbonate, dialysis
Warfarin	Vitamin K, 4-factor prothrombin complex concentrate (PCC), fresh frozen plasma (FFP)

7. If the following medications are given at the same time, what may happen?

Medications	Possible Effect of Simultaneous Administration
MAOI plus meperidine	Serotonin syndrome
Aminoglycoside plus loop diuretic	Enhanced ototoxicity
Thiazide plus lithium	Lithium toxicity
MAOI plus SSRI	Serotonin syndrome (hyperthermia, rigidity, myoclonus, and autonomic instability)

MAOI, Monoamine oxidase inhibitor; *SSRI*, selective serotonin reuptake inhibitor.

8. What prophylactic medication should be given to contacts of a patient with *Neisseria* meningitis?
Rifampin, ciprofloxacin, or ceftriaxone

9. Name three medications that cause hepatic enzyme induction and two that cause hepatic enzyme inhibition.
Barbiturates, antiepileptics (AEDs), and rifampin are the classic enzyme inducers; cimetidine, erythromycin, and ketoconazole are classic enzyme inhibitors. The end result may be ineffectiveness or toxicity of other administered drugs (e.g., warfarin, oral contraceptives, and AEDs).

10. True or False: If a patient responds to placebo, a psychosomatic condition can be diagnosed.
False. Response to placebo means only that the patient responded to placebo. Normal people with real diseases often have an improvement in symptoms with a placebo medication or treatment.

11. Describe the mechanism of action for aspirin and other nonsteroidal antiinflammatory drugs (NSAIDs). How do they differ?
Aspirin and other NSAIDs inhibit cyclooxygenase centrally and peripherally, an action that gives them antiinflammatory, antipyretic, analgesic, and antiplatelet effects. The difference between aspirin and other NSAIDs is that aspirin binds to and inhibits cyclooxygenase irreversibly, whereas the cyclooxygenase inhibition of other NSAIDs is reversible. The net result of this difference is in platelets, which cannot make new cyclooxygenase. One dose of aspirin causes antiplatelet effects for the entire life of the platelet (~10 days), whereas the antiplatelet effects of other NSAIDs last only for several hours.

12. How is acetaminophen different from aspirin and other NSAIDs?
Acetaminophen is thought to inhibit cyclooxygenase primarily in the brain; it does not act well in the periphery of the body. Thus it has analgesic and antipyretic effects but no antiplatelet or significant antiinflammatory effects.

13. What are the side effects and toxic effects of aspirin?
Aspirin causes gastrointestinal (GI) upset and bleeding; it is the most important preventable risk factor for the development of gastric ulcers. Always consider GI bleeding and ulcers in any patient taking aspirin. In addition, aspirin can cause renal damage or aggravate gout. Toxic doses of aspirin can cause tinnitus, vertigo, respiratory alkalosis and metabolic acidosis (this is a classic Step 2 question), hyperthermia, coma, and death. Severe overdoses of aspirin can be removed by dialysis.

14. What are the side effects of nonaspirin NSAIDs?
NSAIDs also cause GI upset, bleeding, and ulcers. Consider GI bleeding and ulcer in all patients taking aspirin or other NSAIDs. NSAIDs may also cause renal damage (interstitial nephritis, acute tubular necrosis, and/or papillary necrosis), especially in patients who take them chronically and have preexisting renal disease.

15. What two developments in NSAID therapy may reduce GI and bleeding complications?
Cyclooxygenase 2 (COX-2) inhibitors and new combinations of NSAIDs with prostaglandin E_1. Normal NSAIDs inhibit COX-1 (in addition to COX-2), which is thought to be the main culprit in causing GI problems. Prostaglandin E_1 protects the stomach by supplying what NSAIDs take away. COX-2 inhibitors avoid the problem altogether but are not as protective against GI bleeding as initially thought.

16. What happens with an overdose of acetaminophen?
High doses of acetaminophen cause liver toxicity due to the toxic metabolite NAPQI, which causes depletion of glutathione by overloading glutathione stores. Treat with ***N*-acetylcysteine** to decrease liver injury by regenerating glutathione.

17. **What age group should not be given aspirin? What finding on physical exam is a contraindication to aspirin use?**

Children younger than 15 years of age (especially with a fever or viral infection) should not be given aspirin because of concern about causing Reye syndrome. Do not give aspirin to people with **nasal polyps** because hypersensitivity reactions involving an asthmatic attack are extremely common. People with asthma may have an asthma attack after taking aspirin even in the absence of nasal polyps. One exception is patients with Kawasaki disease, who are usually younger than age 5 years and are treated with high-dose aspirin and intravenous immunoglobulin (IVIG) to prevent coronary artery aneurysms.

18. **What is the relationship between aspirin and myocardial infarction (MI)?**

Low-dose aspirin has been proven to be of benefit in reducing the risk of MI in both patients who have had a previous MI and patients with stable or unstable angina who have not had an infarction. The 2012 American College of Chest Physicians (ACCP) clinical practice guidelines on antithrombotic and thrombolytic therapy recommends that all patients with chronic stable angina or other clinical or laboratory evidence of coronary artery disease receive aspirin indefinitely.

There is strong medical literature support for the net benefit of aspirin for the primary prevention of first MI in individuals at moderate to high risk. Aspirin is recommended in all diabetics with cardiovascular disease and for primary prevention in diabetics with one or more risk factors (e.g., age >40 years, cigarette smoking, hypertension, hyperlipidemia, obesity, albuminuria, or family history of cardiovascular disease). The risks of aspirin prophylaxis may outweigh the benefits in patients with a history of liver disease, kidney disease, peptic ulcer disease or GI bleeding, poorly controlled hypertension, or a bleeding disorder.

High-dose aspirin during an acute MI has been shown to decrease mortality by 23%. In addition, low-dose (81 mg) aspirin prophylaxis is recommended in pregnant patients with high risk of preeclampsia and should be started between 12 and 28 weeks of gestation.

19. **Discuss the relationship between aspirin and strokes.**

Low-dose aspirin is of proven benefit in reducing strokes in patients with transient ischemic attacks (TIAs) and/or known carotid artery stenosis. However, always weigh the risks and benefits, as mentioned in question 18, especially in patients with uncontrolled hypertension who can have an increased risk of a hemorrhagic stroke when taking aspirin.

20. **True or False: Patients should be given an aspirin as soon as possible in the emergency department for a suspected MI or unstable angina.**

True, but beware the patient who presents with chest pain and ends up having an aortic dissection (aspirin should be avoided in such patients).

21. **True or False: In the setting of an acute neurologic deficit, you should give aspirin before ordering brain imaging.**

False. When patients present with an acute neurologic deficit, you do not know whether they are having a stroke or TIA. TIA is a retrospective diagnosis made once the symptoms clear and imaging has ruled out tissue injury. First you should order a noncontrast computed tomography (CT) scan or magnetic resonance imaging (MRI) to rule out hemorrhagic stroke. If the CT scan or MRI is negative for blood, the patient should be given aspirin (160–325 mg) within 24 to 48 hours of TIA or stroke onset.

CHAPTER 31

PREVENTIVE MEDICINE

1. Cover all but the left-hand column, and give the appropriate screening recommendations for healthy, asymptomatic patients with average risk for the related cancers. Although other guidelines for cancer screening are in clinical use, the recommendations from the American Cancer Society (in table) are a good guideline to use for the USMLE. Controversial topics are typically not tested on the USMLE.

Cancer	Procedure	Age to Begin Screening	Age to Stop Screening	Frequency
Breast	Mammography **Note:** Clinical breast exam is no longer recommended.	45 yr **Note:** Interested patients may begin annual screening at age 40 yr.	Life expectancy <10 yr. No age specified.	Annually (age 45–54 yr) Every 2 yr (age ≥55 yr)
Cervical	Pap smear only (age 21–29 yr) **or** Pap and HPV cotest (age 30–65 yr) **Note:** HPV cotest only performed in age 21–29 yr if Pap is abnormal. **Note:** A woman with prior total hysterectomy should not be screened unless she has other risk factors.	21 yr regardless of sexual activity	65 yr **Note:** Women with cervical precancer should continue screening for at least 20 more yr, even if they pass age 65 yr.	Every 3 yr (if screened by Pap only) Every 5 yr (if Pap and HPV cotest is used)
Colorectal	Colonoscopy **or** Flexible sigmoidoscopy (FS) **or** CT colonography **or** Multitarget stool DNA test (mt-sDNA) **or** Guaiac-based fecal occult blood test (gFOBT) **or** Fecal immunochemical test (FIT)	45 yr (qualified recommendation) **or** 50 yr (strong recommendation)	75 yr **or** Life expectancy <10 yr	Every 10 yr (colonoscopy) **or** Every 5 yr (FS or CT colonography) **or** Every 3 yr (mt-sDNA) **or** Annually (gFOBT or FIT)
Endometrial	Endometrial biopsy			Routine screening is not recommended unless the patient is symptomatic (e.g., unexplained vaginal bleeding)
Lung	Low-dose CT scan	55 yr **and** 30-pack-year smoking history **and** Currently smokes or quit within the last 15 yr	80 yr	Annually

Cancer	Procedure	Age to Begin Screening	Age to Stop Screening	Frequency
Prostate	Prostate-specific antigen test (with or without DRE) **Note:** Have a risk/benefit discussion with patients before screening. Shared decision making. Consider DRE for PSA between 2.5 and 4 ng/mL.	50 yr **Note:** Start screening at age 45 yr for all black men or men with a first-degree relative diagnosed before age 65 yr. Start at age 40 years for men at even higher risk (those with more than one first-degree relative with prostate cancer at an early age).	75 yr **or** Life expectancy <10 yr	PSA ≥2.5 ng/mL screened annually PSA <2.5 ng/mL screened every 2 yr

CT, Computed tomography; *DRE*, digital rectal exam; *HPV*, human papillomavirus; *Pap*, Papanicolaou.

2. True or False: Tumor markers are generally not used for cancer screening.
True. Prostate-specific antigen is the exception to this rule. Alpha-fetoprotein (liver and testicular cancer), carcinoembryonic antigen (CEA), CA-125, and other serum markers are not used for screening the general population, though they may be used to monitor for cancer recurrence. While they may not be used for screening in clinical practice, look for abnormal lab values to show up in questions as a clue to diagnosis.

3. True or False: Urinalysis should not be used to screen the general population for bladder cancer.
True. Screening with urinalysis for urinary tract cancer (which causes hematuria) is not recommended. However, look for persistent, painless hematuria as a clue that urinary tract cancer may be present. On the USMLE, a mention of painless hematuria after extended use of the alkylating agent cyclophosphamide or exposure to the parasite *Schistosoma haematobium* should also make you suspect bladder cancer.

4. Cover the right-hand column and give the indications for each of the following vaccines.

Vaccine	Who Should Receive (and Other Information)
Hepatitis B	Recommended for adults at increased risk of hepatitis B virus infection (e.g., health care workers, diabetics, patients with HIV, end-stage renal disease, chronic liver disease, or MSM). Infants should be vaccinated in a three-step series, starting the day they are born.
Influenza (inactivated)	Everyone ≥6 mo, including pregnant women, adults age >50 yr, people with chronic medical conditions or immunocompromised status (and their caregivers), and health care workers should be vaccinated annually. **Note:** The live attenuated influenza vaccine is contraindicated during pregnancy and in patients with HIV, asplenia, complement deficiencies, or immunocompromised status. The inactivated vaccine has no contraindications.
Pneumococcus	13-valent pneumococcal conjugate vaccine (PCV13) and 23-valent pneumococcal polysaccharide vaccine (PPSV23) is recommended for all adults age ≥65 yr. A four-step series of PCV13 is recommended for infants, starting at age 2 mo. Minimum age to receive PPSV23 is 2 yr. PPSV23 is recommended for adults ages 19–64 yr with chronic heart disease, chronic lung disease, chronic liver disease, diabetes mellitus, alcoholism, or cigarette use. Both PCV13 and PPSV23 should be given to immunocompromised adults ages 19–64 yr. Immunocompromised status includes HIV, chronic renal failure, asplenia, leukemia, lymphoma, Hodgkin disease, generalized malignancy, multiple myeloma, and solid organ transplantation. **Note:** When both are indicated, give PCV13 first. PCV13 and PPSV23 should not be given during the same visit.
Rubella	All nonpregnant women of childbearing age and health care workers. Women of childbearing age who lack immunity or history of immunization. Do not give to pregnant women or immunocompromised patients, including those with HIV and CD4 <200 cells/mm^3. Women should avoid pregnancy for 4 wk after receiving the vaccine.

Vaccine	Who Should Receive (and Other Information)
Tetanus	A five-step series of DTaP is recommended for children starting at age 2 mo, with the fifth dose received between age 4 and 6 yr. At age 11 yr, one dose of Tdap followed by a Td booster every 10 yr is recommended. Tdap should be given to women with every pregnancy regardless of their prior immunization history (preferably in the late second or the third trimester).
	When deciding whether a wound requires tetanus prophylaxis, first ask the patient about immunization history, then consider the severity of the wound. Patients with unknown or incomplete immunization status (i.e., fewer than three doses in their lifetime) should **always** be given a tetanus booster (preferably Tdap) no matter how clean or minor the wound. Patients with complete immunization history (i.e., three or more doses in their lifetime) should only receive a tetanus booster with clean, minor wounds if their last dose was >10 yr ago, or with unclean or major wounds (including burns) if their last dose was >5 yr ago. Coadministration of tetanus immune globulin is only recommended for patients with unknown or incomplete vaccination **and** unclean or major wounds.

DTaP, Diphtheria tetanus acellular pertussis; *HIV*, human immunodeficiency virus; *MSM*, men who have sex with men; *Tdap*, tetanus diphtheria acellular pertussis.

5. Which immunizations are contraindicated during pregnancy?
The live attenuated influenza, varicella, live zoster, and measles, mumps, rubella (MMR) vaccines are all contraindicated during pregnancy. Note that these same vaccines are also contraindicated in immunocompromised individuals and HIV patients with CD4 counts below 200 cells/mm^3.

6. Define the following rates that are commonly seen on the USMLE. Note that each rate is compared to 1000 members of a related population, except for maternal mortality rate (100,000 live births).

Rate	Definition
Birth rate	Live births/1000 population
Fertility rate	Live births/1000 population of women age 15–45 yr
Death rate	Deaths/1000 population
Neonatal mortality rate	Neonatal deaths (first 28 days of life)/1000 live births
Perinatal mortality rate	Neonatal deaths + stillbirths/1000 total births
Infant mortality rate	Deaths (from birth–1 yr)/1000 live births
Maternal mortality rate	Maternal pregnancy-related deaths (deaths while pregnant or in the first 42 days after delivery)/100,000 live births

7. Define stillbirth. How does it differ from miscarriage?
A stillbirth (fetal death) is defined as a prenatal or natal (during delivery) death after 20 weeks of gestation. A miscarriage (spontaneous abortion) is prenatal death at or before gestational age 20 weeks.

8. Name the major cause of neonatal mortality. What is the neonatal mortality rate in the United States?
The major cause of neonatal mortality is prematurity. The neonatal mortality rate in the United States is roughly 6/1000 and is higher in blacks due to higher rates of premature births.

9. List the top three causes of infant mortality in the United States.
- Congenital abnormalities
- Prematurity/low birth weight
- Sudden infant death syndrome (SIDS)

10. List the top three causes of maternal mortality in the United States on the day of delivery, 1 to 6 days after delivery, and 7 to 42 days after delivery.

Day of delivery:
- Hemorrhage
- Amniotic fluid embolism

- Preexisting cardiovascular conditions*

1–6 days after delivery:
- Hemorrhage
- Hypertensive disorders of pregnancy (preeclampsia/eclampsia)
- Infection

7–42 days after delivery:
- Infection
- Preexisting cardiovascular conditions*
- Stroke

*Preexisting cardiovascular conditions include congenital heart disease, ischemic heart disease, cardiac valvular disease, hypertensive heart disease, and congestive heart failure.

Note: Maternal mortality rate increases with age and is higher among black women and American Indian/ Alaskan Native women.

11. What is the basic difference between Medicare and Medicaid?

Medicare is health insurance for people who are eligible for Social Security (primarily people who are age >65 years, those who are permanently or totally disabled, and those who have end-stage renal disease). Nursing home fees are paid by Medicare only for a short time after a hospital admission; then they are paid by the patient. If the patient has no money, the state usually pays.

Medicaid covers the indigent and poor who are deemed eligible according to the criteria of individual states.

---

*Preexisting cardiovascular conditions include congenital heart disease, ischemic heart disease, cardiac valvular disease, hypertensive heart disease, and congestive heart failure.

CHAPTER 32

PSYCHIATRY

1. **What are the differential diagnoses to consider in a patient presenting with psychosis?**
There are primary and secondary etiologies to consider when evaluating a patient exhibiting psychotic behavior. Primary causes include psychiatric illnesses such as acute psychotic disorder, schizophrenia, schizoaffective disorder, schizophreniform disorder, or a mood disorder with psychotic symptoms. Secondary causes include substance-induced psychosis (e.g., prescription or illicit drug use) or comorbid medical conditions (e.g., hepatic encephalopathy, uremic encephalopathy, electrolyte abnormalities, infection, or endocrine disturbances). Secondary causes should be ruled out before pursuing a primary cause.

2. **Why is the duration of symptoms important with psychosis?**
The time frame is important because given the exact same symptoms, a patient is given one of three different diagnoses based only on the duration:
   - Less than 1 month: acute psychotic disorder
   - 1–6 months: schizophreniform disorder
   - More than 6 months: schizophrenia

3. **What are the five main diagnostic criteria for schizophrenia?**
According to the fifth edition of the *Diagnostic and Statistical Manual of Mental Disorders* (DSM-V), the five main diagnostic symptoms of schizophrenia are:
   1. Delusions
   2. Hallucinations
   3. Disorganized speech
   4. Grossly disorganized or catatonic behavior
   5. Negative symptoms (i.e., flat affect, avolition)
   A minimum of two criteria must be present, one of which must be either a delusion, hallucination, or disorganized speech pattern. The impairment must last for a minimum of 6 months to establish this diagnosis.

4. **List the positive symptoms of schizophrenia.**
   - Delusions (e.g., severe paranoia, grandiosity)
   - Hallucinations (auditory is the most common; visual is second most common)
   - Disorganized speech patterns (e.g., tangentiality, circumstantiality, clanging)
   - Abnormal psychomotor behavior
   Positive symptoms are extreme distortions or severe exaggerations of normal behavior. Positive symptoms respond well to all currently used antipsychotics.

5. **List the negative symptoms of schizophrenia.**
   - Flat affect
   - Anhedonia (lack of pleasure)
   - Alogia (no speech)
   - Poor attention
   - Avolition (apathy)
   - Asociality
   Negative symptoms are symptoms for which patients have lost some form of normal behavior; they no longer exhibit behaviors that normal individuals typically have. Negative symptoms respond poorly to typical antipsychotics (e.g., haloperidol) but may respond to atypical antipsychotics such as risperidone, olanzapine, aripiprazole, paliperidone, quetiapine, or ziprasidone. Note that the atypical antipsychotic clozapine is not used as a first-line treatment for schizophrenia due to its side effect profile that includes the risk of agranulocytosis. Strict additional criteria must be met to consider using clozapine in treatment-resistant schizophrenia.

6. **What features of schizophrenia suggest a poor prognosis?**
   - Poor premorbid functioning (most important)
   - Family history of schizophrenia
   - Early onset
   - Negative symptoms
   - No precipitating factors
   - Poor support system
   - Single, divorced, or widowed status

7. What features of schizophrenia suggest a good prognosis?
   - Good premorbid functioning (most important)
   - Family history of mood disorders
   - Late onset
   - Positive symptoms
   - Obvious precipitating factors
   - Good support system
   - Married status

8. What is the difference in age of onset for schizophrenia in males and females?
   The typical age of onset is 15 to 25 years for males (look for someone going to college and deteriorating) and 25 to 35 years for females.

9. True or False: Roughly 1% of the population has schizophrenia in almost every country in the world.
   True

10. True or False: In the United States, most schizophrenic people are born in the summer months.
    False. Most schizophrenic patients in the United States are born in the winter (reason unknown).

11. Roughly what percentage of patients with schizophrenia commit suicide?
    In the United States, roughly 10% of patients with schizophrenia eventually commit suicide (a past attempt is the best predictor of eventual success).

12. True or False: Psychosocial treatment has been shown to improve outcomes in schizophrenia.
    True. Antipsychotic medications are the mainstay of therapy, but psychosocial treatment has been shown to improve outcomes. Medications are needed first, but the best treatment (as in most psychiatric illnesses) is medications plus therapy.

13. Differentiate among the classes of antipsychotics drugs.

	High-Potency Typical Agents	Low-Potency Typical Agents	Atypical Agents*
Prototype drug	Haloperidol	Chlorpromazine	Cariprazine, risperidone, olanzapine, aripiprazole, paliperidone, quetiapine, ziprasidone
EPS side effects	High incidence	Low incidence	Low incidence
ANS side effects†	Low incidence	High incidence	Medium incidence
Positive symptoms	Works well	Works well	Works well
Negative symptoms	Works poorly	Works poorly	Works fairly well

ANS, Autonomic nervous system; *EPS,* extrapyramidal system.
*Atypical antipsychotics are generally first-line treatment and maintenance therapy due to reduced extrapyramidal side effects and efficacy with negative symptoms. Choose them over older agents. A 2017 study showed cariprazine to be the most efficacious agent against negative symptoms. Remember that although it is an atypical antipsychotic, clozapine is not used first-line due to the low but possible risk of agranulocytosis.
†ANS side effects include anticholinergic effects (dry mouth, urinary retention, blurry vision, mydriasis), alpha₁-blockade (orthostatic hypotension), and antihistamine effects (sedation).

14. What are the four commonly tested extrapyramidal side effects of antipsychotics?
    Acute dystonia, akathisia, parkinsonism, and tardive dyskinesia

15. Define acute dystonia. How is it treated?
    Acute dystonia is an extrapyramidal movement disorder that occurs in the first few hours or days of treatment. Patients develop prolonged muscle spasms or stiffness such as torticollis (disfiguring neck muscle spasms; literally *twisted column*), trismus (lockjaw), tongue protrusions and twisting, opisthotonos (back muscle spasm causing extension of the head, neck, and spine), and/or oculogyric crisis (forced sustained deviation of the head and eyes). Acute dystonia is most common in young men. Treat with antihistamines such as diphenhydramine or anticholinergics such as benztropine.

16. Define akathisia. How is it treated?
    Akathisia occurs in the first few days to weeks of treatment. The patient has a subjective feeling of restlessness and may pace constantly, alternate sitting and standing, and be unable to sit still. Beta-blockers such as propranolol are first-line treatment, with benztropine used as second line.

17. Describe the relationship between antipsychotics and parkinsonism. How is secondary parkinsonism treated?

Parkinsonism usually occurs in patients taking antipsychotics within the first few days to months of treatment. It is thought that parkinsonism develops because of dopamine depletion, but that psychosis develops because of too much dopamine in the brain (a gross oversimplification). Thus antipsychotics create an iatrogenic decrease in effective dopamine in the brain by blocking dopamine receptors. The patient develops classic parkinsonian symptoms such as stiffness, cogwheel rigidity, a shuffling gait, masklike facies, and resting tremor. It is most common in older women. Treat with benztropine or consider the dopamine agonist amantadine if the patient cannot tolerate benztropine.

18. Define tardive dyskinesia. When does it occur?

Tardive dyskinesia appears after years of treatment with antipsychotics. Most commonly, the patient develops painless perioral movements (darting, protruding movements of the tongue, chewing, grimacing, and puckering). The patient may also have involuntary, choreoathetoid movements of the head, limbs, and trunk. There is no known treatment for tardive dyskinesia. If you are asked to make a choice when the patient develops tardive dyskinesia, discontinue the current antipsychotic and consider switching to a second-generation antipsychotic such as clozapine or quetiapine. Anticholinergic medications or decreasing the antipsychotic may initially worsen the tardive dyskinesia.

19. What is neuroleptic malignant syndrome? How do you recognize and treat it?

Neuroleptic malignant syndrome is a life-threatening condition that can occur at any time during antipsychotic treatment. Patients classically develop "lead pipe" rigidity, tachycardia, profuse diaphoresis, mutism, obtundation, agitation, high fever (up to 107°F), very **high levels of creatine phosphokinase** (more than four times the normal upper limit), and myoglobinuria. Treat first by discontinuing the antipsychotic; then give supportive care for fever and potential renal failure caused by myoglobinuria (primarily intravenous [IV] fluids). Lastly, consider dantrolene (just as in malignant hyperthermia, which is thought to be a similar condition).

20. Describe the relationship between antipsychotics and prolactin levels.

Dopamine blockade increases serum prolactin levels because dopamine is a prolactin-inhibiting factor in the tuberoinfundibular tract of the brain. The end result may be high serum prolactin levels, resulting in **galactorrhea** and impotence, menstrual dysfunction, and/or decreased libido.

21. What are the classic side effects of the low-potency typical antipsychotics thioridazine and chlorpromazine?
- Thioridazine: retinal pigment deposits
- Chlorpromazine: jaundice and photosensitivity

22. List the atypical antipsychotics associated with each of the side effects

Side Effect	Associated Atypical Antipsychotic(s)
Agranulocytosis	Clozapine
Increased prolactin	Risperidone
Weight gain	Olanzapine, quetiapine, clozapine
Extrapyramidal symptoms (EPS)	Paliperidone, aripiprazole
QT prolongation	Ziprasidone, paliperidone, risperidone
Sedation	Olanzapine, quetiapine, clozapine
Orthostatic hypotension	Olanzapine, quetiapine, clozapine
Dry mouth	Olanzapine, quetiapine
Constipation	Clozapine, aripiprazole
Nausea	Ziprasidone, aripiprazole
Weakness	Ziprasidone

23. How do you distinguish schizoaffective disorder from a mood disorder with psychotic symptoms?

Schizoaffective disorder and mood disorder with psychotic features each have a mix of schizophrenic features and mood disturbance (either major depressive or bipolar). The difference is that schizoaffective disorder has *consistent* schizophrenic features with *occasional* mood disturbances, while mood disorder with psychotic features has *consistent* mood disturbances with *occasional* schizophrenic features. Patients with schizoaffective disorder will never show signs of the mood disturbance outside of the context of their schizophrenic features; conversely, patients with a mood disorder with psychotic symptoms will never display purely schizophrenic symptoms without features of the underlying mood disturbance (either major depressive or bipolar).

24. Define bipolar I disorder. What are the classic symptoms?

Mania is the only criterion required for a diagnosis of bipolar disorder, but a history of depression is commonly present as well. Remember the mnemonic **DIG FAST** for classic symptoms of mania: **d**istractibility, **i**nsomnia and **i**mpulsivity, **g**randiosity and **g**oal-directed activity, **f**light of ideas, **a**gitation, **s**pending sprees and **s**exual promiscuity, and **t**alking with pressured speech. Look for initial onset between the ages of 16 and 30 years.

25. Psychosis and mania may present with similar features, including erratic behavior, speech disturbances, agitation, and grandiosity. How do you distinguish between the two?

The erratic behavior in mania is fundamentally goal oriented, but psychosis is not. Hallucinations typical of psychosis will not be present in mania.

26. How is bipolar I disorder treated?

Both lithium and valproic acid are mood stabilizers and first-line agents. Typical antipsychotics (haloperidol), atypical antipsychotics (risperidone, quetiapine, clozapine, ziprasidone, and aripiprazole), carbamazepine, and gabapentin are second-line agents. Antipsychotics or antidepressants may be needed if the patient becomes psychotic or depressed; use at the same time as the mood stabilizer.

27. What are the side effects of lithium, valproic acid, and carbamazepine?

- Lithium: thyroid dysfunction, diabetes insipidus, tremor (**u**nintentional **m**ovements; lith**ium**, get it?), and central nervous system (CNS) effects at toxic levels. Lithium exposure is also teratogenic and is associated with the Ebstein anomaly if used during pregnancy.
- Valproic acid: liver dysfunction, tremor, and gastrointestinal (GI) distress. It is contraindicated in pregnancy due to its association with neural tube defects.
- Carbamazepine: bone marrow suppression, diplopia, ataxia, agranulocytosis, aplastic anemia, syndrome of inappropriate antidiuretic hormone (SIADH), Stevens-Johnson syndrome.

28. Define bipolar II disorder.

Bipolar II disorder is hypomania (mild mania without psychosis that does not cause occupational dysfunction) plus major depression. Note that major depression is not required to diagnose bipolar I disorder but *is* required to diagnose bipolar II disorder.

29. List the major risk factors for suicide.

- Age greater than 45 years
- Prior psychiatric history
- Alcohol or substance abuse
- Depression
- History of rage or violence
- Recent loss or separation
- Prior suicide attempts
- Loss of health
- Male gender (men commit suicide three times more often than women, but women attempt it four times more often than men)
- Unemployed or retired status
- Single, widowed, or divorced status
- Access to weapons
- Organized plan

30. What is the strongest predictor of a future suicide attempt?

A past attempt

31. True or False: Some psychiatric patients can be hospitalized against their will.

True. Patients can be hospitalized against their will if they are a danger to themselves (suicidal or unable to take care of themselves) or others (homicidal).

32. True or False: Be careful in asking about suicide because you may plant the idea in the patient's head.

False. Always ask patients about suicidal thoughts; it does not make them more likely to commit suicide. If necessary, you should temporarily hospitalize acutely suicidal patients against their will.

33. True or False: When patients are just emerging from a deep depression, they are at an increased risk of suicide.

True. When the antidepressant begins to work, the patient gets a little more energy—possibly just enough to carry out a suicide plan.

34. True or False: The highest suicide rates are in people aged 15 to 24 years.

False. Suicide rates are rising most rapidly in 15- to 24-year-olds, but the highest absolute suicide rate is in people older than 65 years.

35. Define depression.

Depression, or major depressive disorder as it is technically called, is defined as a depressed mood or a loss of interest or pleasure in daily activities for 2 weeks or longer. There is impaired function in social, occupational, or educational roles. A depressed mood, decreased interest, or lack of pleasure, along with at least five of the following symptoms, are required to diagnose major depressive disorder. The symptoms can be remembered by the mnemonic **SIGECAPS**.

- **S**leep disturbance
- **I**nterest loss
- **G**uilt, worthless, or hopeless feelings
- **E**nergy loss
- **C**oncentration difficulty
- **A**ppetite disturbance
- **P**sychomotor agitation or retardation
- **S**uicidality

You can remember that five of the SIGECAPS criteria must be present by mentally replacing the letter S with the number 5 in 5IGECAPS.

36. True or False: Patients with depression often do not complain about it directly.

True. Patients often do not come out and say, "I'm depressed." You must watch for the clues by recognizing SIGECAPS or vague somatic complaints. The history may or may not reveal obvious precipitating factors, such as loss of loved one, divorce or separation, unemployment or retirement, or chronic or debilitating disease.

37. How do you treat depression?

As with most psychiatric illnesses, the ideal treatment plan includes both medications (antidepressants) and psychotherapy. The addition of psychotherapy is more effective than medications alone. Selective serotonin reuptake inhibitors (SSRIs) are usually the preferred first-line agents. Other options include serotonin-norepinephrine reuptake inhibitors (SNRIs) and the tricyclic antidepressants. Bupropion and mirtazapine have unique modes of action and are more commonly used in treatment-resistant depression than as first-line agents. Be careful when prescribing bupropion, as it is known to lower the seizure threshold.

38. Is depression more common in males or females?

Depression is more common in females.

39. What is an adjustment disorder with depressed mood?

A diagnosis that you must be able to distinguish from major depressive disorder. In adjustment disorder, a patient goes through a normal life experience (e.g., relationship breakup, failing grade, job loss) but does not handle it well. There is marked distress that is exceeds what would be expected from exposure to the stressor or that causes significant impairment in social or occupational functioning. Although patients may have a depressed mood, they do not meet the criteria for full-blown major depressive disorder, and symptoms do not last longer than 6 months. An example is a woman who divorces her husband, seems to cry a lot for the next few weeks, and leaves work early on most days. Another example is a high-school boy who doesn't make the basketball team and mopes around the house, crying, and not wanting to go to school or out with his friends for a few weeks.

40. Define persistent depressive disorder (dysthymia) and cyclothymia. What features distinguish one from the other?

Both disorders involve a moderate mood disturbance that persists for at least 2 years. Persistent depressive disorder (dysthymia) is a depressed mood on most days for more than 2 years without episodes of major depression, mania/hypomania, or psychosis, while cyclothymia involves at least 2 years of hypomania alternating with depressed mood with no full-blown episodes of mania or major depression.

41. True or False: Antidepressants can trigger mania or hypomania.

True—especially in bipolar patients. Remember to ask about any history of manic episodes when considering treatment for depression.

42. How do SSRIs work? Why are they preferred over tricyclics?

SSRIs (e.g., fluoxetine, citalopram, paroxetine, sertraline, fluvoxamine, escitalopram) prevent reuptake of serotonin only. They have less serious side effects (insomnia, anorexia, jitteriness, headache, sexual dysfunction) and are not dangerous with overdose compared to tricyclics.

43. What are the signs and symptoms of serotonin syndrome? Which medications may interact with SSRIs to precipitate serotonin syndrome? How is serotonin syndrome treated?

Serotonin syndrome may present with a combination of GI upset, hyperreflexia, clonus, flushing of the skin, hyperthermia, or diaphoresis. Be careful when prescribing SSRIs to patients taking other antidepressants, including SNRIs, monoamine oxidase (MAO) inhibitors, and tricyclics. Less obvious medications that may also interact with SSRIs to cause serotonin syndrome include linezolid, ondansetron, tramadol, triptans, dextromethorphan, meperidine, and nonprescription drugs such as MDMA (ecstasy) or St. John wort. Serotonin syndrome is treated with cyproheptadine, a 5-HT receptor antagonist.

44. How do SNRIs work?

SNRIs (e.g., venlafaxine, duloxetine, desvenlafaxine) prevent reuptake of serotonin and norepinephrine. The side effects of SNRIs are similar to those of SSRIs but also include noradrenergic symptoms such as sweating, dizziness, increased blood pressure, and sedation.

45. How do tricyclic antidepressants work? What are their side effects?

Tricyclic antidepressants (e.g., nortriptyline, amitriptyline) prevent reuptake of norepinephrine and serotonin, similar to SNRIs. They also block alpha-adrenergic receptors (which may cause orthostatic hypotension, dizziness, or falls), muscarinic receptors (watch for anticholinergic effects, such as dry mouth, blurred vision, constipation, and urinary retention), and histamine receptors (causing sedation), and lower the seizure threshold. Tricyclic antidepressants are dangerous in overdose primarily because of **cardiac arrhythmias,** which may respond to bicarbonate. Remember the three Cs of tricyclic antidepressant overdose: coma, convulsions, and cardiotoxicity.

46. What are monoamine oxidase inhibitors? Describe their side effects.

MAO inhibitors (e.g., selegiline, phenelzine, tranylcypromine) are older medications that are not used as first-line agents for treatment of depression. They may be good for atypical depression (look for hypersomnia and hyperphagia—the opposite of classic depression) that fails to respond to other agents. When patients taking MAO inhibitors eat tyramine-containing foods (especially wine and cheese), they may get a hypertensive crisis. Be sure to discontinue other serotonin-related medications at least 2 weeks before starting an MAO inhibitor due to the risk of serotonin syndrome. Because of its longer half-life, the SSRI fluoxetine must be discontinued at leave 5 weeks before starting an MAO inhibitor.

47. What is the most notorious side effect of trazodone?

Priapism (persistent, painful erection in the absence of sexual desire that may lead to permanent impotence or tissue necrosis if not treated). Consult urology and consider an intracavernosal injection of phenylephrine along with detumescence if it does not resolve after 4 hours.

48. Describe electroconvulsive therapy (ECT). What are the main side effects of ECT? When is ECT used?

ECT is performed by inducing a generalized cerebral seizure under general anesthesia and neuromuscular blockade. Primary side effects of ECT include headache, temporary cognitive impairment, and possible memory loss. ECT is typically used in major depressive disorder that is refractory to antidepressant therapy, but may also be used in refractory bipolar disorder or urgent clinical situations such as acute suicidality, severe psychosis, malignant catatonia, or malnutrition due to a depressive state.

49. True or False: ECT is contraindicated in pregnant patients.

False. There are no absolute contraindications to ECT therapy.

50. How do you distinguish between postpartum blues, postpartum depression, and postpartum psychosis? How is each condition managed?

The main way to distinguish postpartum blues from postpartum depression is the severity and duration of symptoms. Postpartum blues is milder, typically developing within a few days after delivery and resolving within 2 weeks, while postpartum depression lasts longer than 2 weeks and meets the diagnostic criteria for clinical depression (e.g., at least five SIGECAPS symptoms). Postpartum blues should be managed conservatively with reassurance and a scheduled follow-up appointment 2 weeks after delivery, while cognitive-behavioral therapy or antidepressant medical therapy may be used for postpartum depression. Postpartum psychosis is recognized clinically by the rapid onset of delusions, hallucinations, disorganized thought, or other bizarre behavior following delivery. These patients may threaten harm to themselves or their baby. Postpartum psychosis is a medical emergency and typically involves hospitalization.

51. Distinguish between normal grief and pathologic grief (i.e., depression).

Initial grief after a loss (e.g., death of a loved one) may include a state of shock, a feeling of numbness or bewilderment, distress, crying, sleep disturbances, decreased appetite, difficulty in concentrating, weight loss, and guilt (survivor guilt) for up to 1 year—in other words, the same symptoms as depression. It is normal to have an illusion or hallucination about the deceased, but a normal grieving person knows that it is an illusion, whereas a depressed person believes that it is real. Intense yearning (even years after the death) and even searching for the deceased are normal. Feelings of worthlessness, psychomotor retardation, and suicidal ideation are not signs of normal grief; they are signs of depression.

52. How do you recognize and treat panic disorder?

Panic disorder classically affects patients ages 20 to 40 years who have an abrupt surge of intense fear or discomfort that reaches its peak within a few minutes. Patients often think that they are dying or having a heart attack, although in fact they are healthy and have a negative workup for organic disease. Females are more likely to have panic disorder in a 2:1 ratio. Patients often hyperventilate and are extremely anxious. They may experience tingling of the extremities, palpitations, sweating, trembling, sensation of shortness of breath, feelings of choking, chest pain, nausea, and fear of dying. Remember the association between panic disorder and agoraphobia (fear of leaving the house). Treat with SSRIs (e.g., fluoxetine), which are favored over benzodiazepines.

53. What is generalized anxiety disorder? How is it treated?

Patients with generalized anxiety disorder worry about everything (e.g., career, family, future, relationships, and money) at the same time. Symptoms are not as dramatic as in panic disorder; the patient is simply a severe worrier. Patients have difficulty controlling their worries and can have restlessness, fatigue, difficulty concentrating, irritability, muscle tension, and sleep disturbances. Treat with cognitive behavioral therapy and medications: SSRIs (especially if depressive symptoms coexist), buspirone (agonist of 5-hydroxytryptamine 1A serotonin receptor; nonaddictive, nonsedating but slow onset of action), or benzodiazepines (addictive, sedating).

54. Give the classic examples of simple phobias. How are they treated?

Classic examples of simple phobias include fear of needles, blood products, animals, and heights. Treat with behavioral therapy, including flooding (sudden, intense exposure to the feared object without chance for escape), systematic desensitization (gradual increase in intensity and type of exposure until the person is comfortable with intense exposure to the feared object), and biofeedback (learning to control autonomic variables such as heart rate during anxiety-inducing maneuvers).

55. What is social anxiety disorder?

Social anxiety disorder, also known as social phobia, is a specific type of simple phobia (fear of social situations) that is best treated with behavioral therapy. To reduce symptoms, beta-blockers may be used before a public appearance that cannot be avoided, and SSRIs are increasingly being used as a primary treatment. SNRIs and benzodiazepines may also be used.

56. How do you recognize and treat posttraumatic stress disorder (PTSD)? How do you distinguish PTSD from acute stress disorder?

Look for someone who has been through a life-threatening event (e.g., war, severe accident, rape), repeatedly experiences the event (nightmares, flashbacks), exhibits hypervigilant behavior, and cannot stop thinking about the event. Patients may also have dissociative amnesia of the event, irritability, reckless or self-destructive behavior, depression, and poor concentration. Treat with peer group therapy; if you have to choose a medication, use an antidepressant, usually an SSRI. Use the alpha$_1$-antagonist prazosin to treat the sleep disturbance and nightmares. Note that symptoms of posttraumatic stress disorder must be present for at least 1 month. Symptoms that have persisted for less than 1 month indicate acute stress disorder.

57. Explain the concept of somatic symptom disorders (previously called somatoform disorders).

A patient with somatic symptom disorder experiences psychiatric stress and expresses it through physical symptoms. Patients do not do so on purpose.

58. Describe the four major somatic symptom disorders.

Somatization disorder: the patient has multiple different complaints in multiple different organ systems over many years and has had extensive workups in the past. Mnemonic: Patients with **soma**tization disorder have **so many** physical complaints.

Conversion disorder: the patient has an obvious precipitating factor (e.g., fight with boyfriend), then develops unexplainable neurologic symptoms (e.g., blindness, stocking-glove numbness). This is thought to be a physical manifestation of emotional distress. Think of it as the patient has subconsciously *converted* the emotional distress into this physical manifestation. The patient is not malingering and truly believes the symptom is real. However, clinical evidence is incompatible with symptomatology.

Hypochondriasis: the patient continues to believe that he or she has a disease despite extensive negative workup. These patients tend to be excessively worried about a minor symptom and are not reassured by multiple negative workups.

Body dysmorphic disorder: the patient is preoccupied with an imagined physical defect; for example, a teenager who thinks that his or her nose is too big when it is normal in size.

59. How are somatic symptom disorders treated?

Treat all somatic symptom disorders with frequent return visits to the clinic and/or psychotherapy. Screen for and treat any coexisting depression.

60. Distinguish among somatic symptom disorders, factitious disorders, and malingering.

In **somatic symptom disorders**, the patient does not intentionally create symptoms (it is an unconscious process). In **factitious disorders**, patients intentionally create an illness or symptoms (e.g., they inject insulin to create hypoglycemia) and subject themselves to procedures to assume the role of a patient (no financial or other secondary gain). In **malingering**, patients intentionally create their illness for secondary gain (e.g., money, release from work or jail). Think of it as patients with factitious disorders want to **f**eel like a patient, while patients who are **ma**lingering want **m**oney or a similar external motivation.

61. How do you recognize dissociative fugue (also called psychogenic fugue or fugue state)?

Dissociative fugue is a reversible amnesia for personal identity, including the memories, personality, and other identifying characteristics of individuality. It usually involves unplanned travel or wandering. There is complete amnesia for the fugue episode. The classic patient develops amnesia, travels, and assumes a new identity, but does not remember the event upon returning.

62. **What psychiatric disorder is most likely to be associated with childhood sexual abuse?**
Dissociative identity disorder (formerly known as multiple personality disorder)

63. **Define personality disorders.**
Personality disorders are lifelong maladaptive traits that affect the way in which a person interacts with the world. Look for a history dating back to childhood or teenage years. No real treatment is available, although psychotherapy may be attempted.

64. **Give a one- or two-sentence description of each of the following 10 personality disorders.**

Cluster A (Awkward disorders)
- **Paranoid:** patients are paranoid and think that everyone (friends, too) is out to get them; they often initiate lawsuits.
- **Schizoid:** patients are classic loners who have no friends and no interest in having friends. They also have a restricted range of emotions.
- **Schizotypal:** patients have bizarre beliefs (cults, superstition) and a bizarre manner of speaking but no psychosis.

Cluster B (Bad company: dramatic, emotional, or erratic disorders)
- **Histrionic:** patients are overly dramatic, attention-seeking, and inappropriately seductive; they constantly seek the center of attention.
- **Narcissistic:** patients are egocentric, lack empathy, are often envious of others or believe that others are envious of them, and manipulate others for their own gain; they have a sense of entitlement and perceive any criticism as a personal insult.
- **Antisocial:** these patients are antisociety. Patients have long criminal records and may have tortured animals or set fires as children. A history of pediatric conduct disorder is required for this diagnosis. Patients are aggressive and do not pay their bills or support their children. They are liars and have no remorse or conscience. Antisocial personality disorder has a strong association with alcoholism, drug abuse, and somatization disorder. Most antisocial patients are male.
- **Borderline:** patients have unstable moods, behaviors, relationships, and self-image. Look for splitting; that is, these patients consider other individuals to be either all good or all bad and may frequently change categories. Other clues include threats of self-harm, micropsychotic episodes (2 minutes of psychosis), impulsiveness, and constant crisis.

Cluster C (**C**owardly, **c**lingy, and **c**ompulsive)
- **Avoidant:** patients have no friends but want them; they avoid others out of fear of criticism and rejection (inferiority complex). This is distinguished from schizoid personality disorder, in which the patient is isolated but has no desire for social contact.
- **Dependent:** patients cannot be or do anything alone. Generally, they have low self-esteem. A wife may stay with her abusive husband despite continued abuse.
- **Obsessive-compulsive:** patients are obsessed with rules, perfection, and organization. They may seem anal retentive and stubborn. Rules are more important than objectives, and affect is restricted. Money is a frequent concern and is often hoarded. This is distinct from obsessive-compulsive disorder (OCD), as patients with this personality type do not find their obsessions distressful.

65. **Define obsessive-compulsive disorder. How is it treated?**
OCD is marked by recurrent intrusive thoughts (obsessions) that lead to impulsive recurrent behaviors (compulsions) to such a degree that it causes dysfunction in the occupational or interpersonal life of the patient. Look for washing rituals (e.g., washing the hands 30 times per day) or checking rituals (checking to see if the door is locked 40 times per day). Patients may be aware that their behavior is abnormal but are unable to stop themselves. Onset is usually in adolescence or early adulthood. Treat with SSRIs (especially fluvoxamine) or clomipramine (a serotonin-specific tricyclic antidepressant). Therapies such as cognitive behavioral therapy and flooding also may be effective.

66. **Describe the hallmark findings of narcolepsy. How is it treated?**
Narcolepsy is a sleep disorder characterized by daytime sleepiness despite a normal daily sleep regimen. Patients have decreased latency for rapid-eye-movement (REM) sleep (patients go into REM as soon as they fall asleep); sleep paralysis (paralysis upon awakening); cataplexy (random loss of muscle tone that causes patients to fall down); and hallucinations as they awaken (hypnopompic) or fall asleep (hypnagogic). Patients may have a hypocretin deficiency. Treat with **modafinil** (a nonamphetamine stimulant), methylphenidate, or amphetamines.

67. **What is the difference between objective and subjective psychologic tests?**
Objective tests are generally multiple-choice tests that are scored by a computer; the classic example is the IQ test. **Subjective tests** have no "right" answers and are scored by the test-giver (the classic example is the Rorschach test).

68. Characterize each of the following psychologic tests as objective or subjective, and briefly describe its use.

Name of Test	Description
Stanford-Binet	Objective IQ test for adults
Wechsler Intelligence Scale for Children	Objective IQ test for children (age 4–17 yr)
Rorschach test	Subjective test in which patients describe what they see in an inkblot
Thematic Apperception Test	Subjective test in which the patient describes what is going on in a cartoon drawing of people
Beck Depression Inventory	Objective test to look for depression
Minnesota Multiphasic Personality Inventory	Objective test to measure personality type
Halstead-Reitan Battery	Objective test used to determine the location and effects of specific brain lesions
Luria-Nebraska Neuropsychological Battery	Objective test that assesses many cognitive functions as well as cerebral dominance (left or right)

Note: Psychologic tests can be used to aid in a difficult diagnosis; they are not used or needed for a straightforward case.

69. True or False: Roughly 85% of cases of intellectual disabilities are mild.
True. Patients with mild intellectual disability can have a reasonable level of independence, with assistance or guidance during periods of stress.

70. What are the common causes of intellectual disability?
Although intellectual disability is usually idiopathic, look for fetal alcohol syndrome (the leading preventable cause of intellectual disability), Down syndrome (leading overall known cause of intellectual disability), and fragile X syndrome (in males).

71. How do you recognize and diagnose autism spectrum disorder?
Autism symptoms start at a very young age, beginning as early as 6 months and becoming well established by age 2 or 3 years. Look for impaired social interaction (isolative, unaware of surroundings), impaired verbal and nonverbal communication (strange words, babbling, repetition), and restricted activities and interests (head banging, strange movements). Autism is a spectrum of disorders in which patients may range from very highly functioning (previously called Asperger syndrome) to severely intellectually disabled. Most individuals with autism manifest some degree of intellectual disability that is typically moderate in severity.

No single cause has been identified for the development of autism. Genetic origins are suspected on the basis of twin studies and a higher incidence among siblings. Possible contributing factors include fetal alcohol exposure, infections (congenital rubella infection), other perinatal factors, and immunologic causes.

72. What is a learning disorder?
Learning disorders describe isolated impairment in math, reading, writing, speech, language, or coordination. All other skills are normal; no intellectual disability is present (e.g., "Johnny just can't do math").

73. Define conduct disorder. With what adult disorder is it associated?
Conduct disorder is the pediatric form of **antisocial personality disorder**. Look for fire setting, cruelty to animals, lying, stealing, and/or fighting. As adults, patients often have antisocial disorder. **Note:** Evidence of conduct disorder as a child is required for a diagnosis of antisocial personality disorder in adults.

74. Define attention-deficit/hyperactivity disorder (ADHD).
As the name implies, patients are hyperactive and have short attention spans. ADHD is more common in males than in females. Look for a fidgety child who is impulsive and cannot pay attention but is not cruel. These symptoms must be present in two different settings (e.g., at home and school). Treat with stimulants (paradoxic calming effect) such as methylphenidate (Ritalin), an amphetamine, or atomoxetine. Stimulants and amphetamines may cause insomnia, abdominal pain, anorexia, weight loss, and growth suppression. Atomoxetine is an SNRI and alternative to stimulant therapy, but it has serious potential side effects, including cardiovascular events and suicidal thoughts.

75. Describe the behavior of a child who has oppositional-defiant disorder. How is it distinguished from conduct disorder?
The child displays negative, hostile, and defiant behavior toward authority figures (e.g., parents, teachers). The child exhibits such behavior around adults but behaves normally around peers and is not a cruel, lying criminal (unlike patients with conduct disorder).

76. Give the classic description of children with separation anxiety disorder.

Affected children refuse to go to school because they think that something will happen to them or their parents if they separate. They will do anything to avoid separation (e.g., feign stomachache, headache, temper tantrum).

77. How do you recognize anorexia?

The classic patient is a female adolescent who is a good athlete or student with a perfectionistic personality. According to DSM-V, the diagnostic criteria include restriction of energy intake leading to a significant low body weight, intense fear of gaining weight or becoming fat, and disturbance in the way one's body weight or shape is experienced. Patients often have a body mass index (BMI) of 18 or lower. Roughly 10% to 15% of patients die from complications of starvation or coexisting bulimia (electrolyte imbalances, cardiac arrhythmias, infections). Although more positive therapies are preferred, patients sometimes need to be hospitalized against their will for IV nutrition. Patients with anorexia may be of a restrictive type (severely restricted caloric intake) or a binge-purge type (self-induced vomiting or laxative abuse).

78. Define bulimia. What are the classic findings of the mouth and fingers?

Bulimic patients have binge-eating episodes, during which they feel a lack of control and then engage in purging behavior (vomiting, laxatives, exercise, fasting). Those affected are typically normal weight or overweight adolescent females. If these patients ever meet criteria for anorexia, they are diagnosed with the binge-purge type of anorexia (i.e., the anorexia diagnosis trumps the bulimia diagnosis). Patients may require hospitalization for electrolyte disturbances. Classic findings include eroded tooth enamel caused by frequent vomiting and eroded skin over the knuckles from putting the fingers into the throat to induce vomiting.

79. Describe Tourette syndrome. How is it treated?

Tourette syndrome is a motor tic disorder (eye-blinking, grunting, throat-clearing, grimacing, barking, or shoulder shrugging) that is exacerbated by stress and remits during activity or sleep. Although part of the classic description of Tourette syndrome, coprolalia (swearing) affects only 10% to 30% of patients. Males are affected more often than females. Of interest, Tourette syndrome can be caused or unmasked by the use of stimulants (e.g., for presumed ADHD). Antipsychotics (haloperidol) or dopamine receptor blockers (e.g., fluphenazine, pimozide) can be used if the symptoms are severe. Tourette syndrome tends to be a lifelong problem.

80. True or False: Depression in children frequently presents as an irritable rather than a depressed mood.

True

81. What are the three leading causes of death in adolescents?

Accidents, homicide, and suicide together account for about 75% of teenage deaths.

82. What is the most commonly abused illicit drug? Describe its effects on users.

Marijuana. Watch for a teenager who is withdrawn and shows a decline in school performance. Other symptoms include amotivational syndrome (chronic use results in laziness and lack of motivation), time distortion, impaired judgment, conjunctival injection, paranoia, and the so-called munchies (eating binges during intoxication). No physical symptoms have been reported for withdrawal, but psychologic cravings may be present. Marijuana is not dangerous in overdose (although patients may experience temporary dysphoria) and is a controversial teratogen (evidence is weak).

83. What symptoms are associated with cocaine intoxication? Cocaine withdrawal?

Cocaine causes sympathetic stimulation (insomnia, tachycardia, mydriasis, hypertension, sweating) with hyperalertness and possible paranoia, aggressiveness, delirium, psychosis, or formications (so-called cocaine bugs; a type of tactile hallucination in which patients think bugs are crawling on them). Overdose can be fatal as a result of arrhythmia, myocardial infarction, seizure, or stroke. During withdrawal, the patient is sleepy, hungry (vs anorexic with intoxication), and irritable with possible severe depression. Cocaine withdrawal is not dangerous, but psychologic cravings are usually severe. Cocaine is teratogenic, causing vascular disruptions in the fetus.

84. Describe the symptoms of amphetamine intoxication.

Amphetamines are longer acting and associated more commonly with psychotic symptoms (patients may appear to be full-blown schizophrenics), but basically their effects are similar to those of cocaine.

85. Describe the effects of opioids. How are opioid overdoses treated?

Heroin and other opioids cause euphoria, analgesia, drowsiness, miosis, constipation, and CNS depression. Overdoses can be fatal because of respiratory depression, which should be treated with **naloxone**. Because the drug is often taken IV, associated morbidity and mortality include endocarditis, HIV infection, hepatitis, cellulitis, and talc damage.

86. What symptoms are seen in opioid withdrawal? How is opioid withdrawal treated?

Withdrawal is not life threatening, but patients act as though they are going to die. Symptoms of opioid withdrawal include piloerection, diarrhea, insomnia, abdominal cramping, mydriasis, excessive yawning, flulike symptoms, and pain. Methadone or buprenorphine can be used to reduce acute withdrawal symptoms.

87. How do you recognize intoxication with lysergic acid diethylamide (LSD) or hallucinogenic mushrooms?

Symptoms of intoxication with LSD or mushrooms include hallucinations (usually visual, unlike the auditory hallucinations common in schizophrenia), mydriasis, tachycardia, hypertension, diaphoresis, and perception and mood disturbances. Neither is dangerous in overdose—unless patients put themselves in physical danger because of their hallucination (e.g., thinking they can fly, then jumping out a window). No withdrawal symptoms or teratogenic effects have been reported. Users may experience flashbacks (brief feelings of being on the drug again even though none was taken) months to years later or a "bad trip" (acute panic reaction or dysphoria), which should be treated with reassurance, a benzodiazepine, or an antipsychotic, if needed.

88. What about phencyclidine (PCP) intoxication?

PCP intoxication causes LSD/mushroom symptoms plus confusion, agitation, and aggressive behavior. Also look for vertical and/or horizontal nystagmus, possible schizophrenic-like symptoms (e.g., paranoia, auditory hallucinations, disorganized behavior and speech), and combative behavior. Overdose can be fatal because of convulsions, coma, and respiratory arrest. Treat with supportive care and urine acidification to hasten elimination. No withdrawal symptoms have been reported.

89. Describe the signs and symptoms of inhalant intoxication. Who is likely to abuse inhalants?

Inhalant intoxication (e.g., gasoline, glue, varnish remover) causes rapid euphoria, dizziness, slurred speech, a feeling of floating, ataxia, and a sense of heightened power. It is usually seen in younger teenagers (11–15 years old) because these substances are cheap, legal to buy, and readily available. Inhalants can be fatal in overdose as a result of respiratory depression, cardiac arrhythmias, or asphyxiation and may cause severe permanent sequelae (CNS, liver or kidney toxicity, peripheral neuropathy). Chronic abuse may also cause methemoglobinemia, lead toxicity, anemia, muscle weakness, and carbon monoxide poisoning. There is no known withdrawal syndrome associated with inhalants.

90. True or False: Benzodiazepines and barbiturates can be fatal in overdose but not in withdrawal.

False. Both can be fatal in overdose and withdrawal.

91. Describe the signs and symptoms of benzodiazepine or barbiturate intoxication.

Benzodiazepines and barbiturates cause sedation and drowsiness, as well as disinhibition and reduced anxiety. They can be fatal in overdose as a result of respiratory depression; treat acute overdoses of a benzodiazepine with **flumazenil** (although this may precipitate seizures). In withdrawal, death may result from seizures and/or cardiovascular collapse. Treat withdrawal on an inpatient basis with a long-acting benzodiazepine, and gradually taper off the dose over several days. Benzodiazepines and barbiturates are especially dangerous when mixed with alcohol because all three are CNS depressants.

92. What are the symptoms of caffeine withdrawal?

Headaches and fatigue.

93. What is the basic rule of thumb about the difference in symptoms between intoxication and withdrawal for the same drug?

The symptoms are usually the opposite of each other. For example, stimulants (e.g., cocaine, amphetamines) cause insomnia with intoxication and hypersomnolence in withdrawal, whereas depressants (e.g., alcohol, benzodiazepines, and barbiturates) cause sedation with intoxication and insomnia in withdrawal.

CHAPTER 33

PULMONOLOGY

1. Describe the difference between obstructive and restrictive pulmonary disease on pulmonary function testing.

   In chronic obstructive pulmonary disease (COPD), the functional expiratory volume in 1 second divided by the total forced vital capacity (FEV_1/FVC) is less than normal (<0.7). In restrictive lung disease (classically fibrotic lung disease, chest wall deformities, neuromuscular disease, obesity), FEV_1/FVC is often normal or increased. FEV_1 may be equal in both conditions, but the ratio of FEV_1/FVC is always different.

2. What is COPD?

   COPD is a progressive, inflammatory lung disease that causes air flow obstruction. The disease encompasses both chronic bronchitis, which refers to inflammation of the bronchi and bronchioles, and emphysema, which is characterized by destruction of alveoli and poor gas exchange. Patients usually present with chronic productive cough and shortness of breath. Tobacco smoking is the main cause, though air pollution (especially indoor air pollution such as from wood-burning stoves), genetics, and aging contribute to COPD. Typical exam findings include diminished breath sounds, rhonchi, and wheezing. On x-ray, look for hyperinflated, hyperlucent lungs, an elongated and narrow mediastinum, and flattened diaphragms.

3. How is COPD diagnosed and treated?

   COPD is diagnosed by pulmonary function test or spirometry, and severity is graded by the GOLD criteria. The diagnosis is made by an FEV_1/FVC ratio less than 70% predicted, and severity is determined based on degree of limitation in FEV_1.

   Initial treatments include use of an inhaled long-acting beta-agonist (LABA; e.g., salmeterol) or long-acting anticholinergic (e.g., tiotropium). Inhaled corticosteroids are sometimes used in more severe cases or with peripheral eosinophilia. Chronically hypoxic patients with ambulatory oxygen saturations less than 88% or arterial PaO_2 measurements less than 55 may be prescribed home oxygen therapy. Smoking cessation, of course, should be recommended and can significantly slow the progression of the disease. Routine influenza and pneumonia vaccines should be administered.

4. How are COPD exacerbations treated?

   Although COPD is a chronic disease, patients can also present with acute exacerbations. Symptoms of an exacerbation include worsened cough, an increase or change in sputum production, and worsening dyspnea. Exacerbations are typically treated with inhaled bronchodilators, a steroid burst, and, for severe cases, a course of antibiotics. Patients may also need respiratory support ranging from supplemental oxygen to intubation. However, patients should not be overoxygenated because if they are CO_2 retainers, their ventilation-perfusion ratio will be altered, causing increased blood levels of carbon dioxide. Additionally, respiratory drive can be inhibited, further compromising ventilation and precipitating hypercarbic respiratory failure.

5. What is interstitial lung disease (ILD)?

   ILD refers to a broad group of restrictive lung diseases with decreased diffusing capacity (DLCO) and elevated alveolar-arterial gradient in addition to reduced lung volumes (FVC and total lung capacity [TLC]). Many patterns exist on computed tomography (CT) of the chest, including honeycombing, ground glass, and mosaicism. Etiologies include pneumoconiosis/inhalational exposures, connective tissue diseases (CTD), sarcoidosis, hypersensitivity pneumonitis, and drug toxicities. Immunosuppression may be considered for patients with CTD-ILD. Similar to patients with COPD, chronic home oxygen therapy should be considered if patients have ambulatory oxygen saturations less than 88% or arterial blood gas PaO_2 measurements less than 55. Depending on age, comorbidities, and timeline of disease progression, patients with ILD should be considered for lung transplantation. Step 2 questions will center around clinical scenarios:

   • Asbestosis: prior occupational history will include some level of construction, usually with shipyards or plumbing. Patients may have pleural plaques and are at increased risk of bronchogenic carcinoma (more so than mesothelioma).
   • Berylliosis: classically in aerospace industry exposures.
   • Coal miner lung: from coal dust exposure. May have concomitant rheumatoid arthritis in Caplan syndrome.
   • Silicosis: from sandblasting exposures. Silica has an association with increased susceptibility to *M. tuberculosis* from disruption of macrophages.

- CTD-ILD: CTDs include rheumatoid arthritis, systemic lupus erythematosus, Sjögren syndrome, systemic sclerosis, mixed CTD, and myositis. Look out for physical exam hints (digital fissures/ulcerations/ashes, arthropathies, Raynaud phenomenon) and autoimmune serologies.
- Sarcoidosis: classically black females with enlarged lymph nodes with noncaseating granulomas and bilateral hilar adenopathy on chest radiograph.
- Hypersensitivity pneumonitis: look broadly for exposures to molds (farmer's lung) and birds (Bird fancier's lung).
- Drug toxicities: look for use of amiodarone, methotrexate, bleomycin, and nitrofurantoin.

6. How do you recognize and treat asthma?
Watch for chronic wheezing in "allergic" (atopic) children with a family history of asthma, allergies, or eczema. In the acute setting, treat with beta2-agonists. Use steroids if the attack is severe or does not respond to $beta_2$-agonists. Inhaled glucocorticoids (preferred agent), leukotriene modifiers (zafirlukast, montelukast, zileuton), long-acting beta-agonists, omalizumab, and cromolyn sodium are prophylactic agents and are not used for acute attacks. Phosphodiesterase inhibitors (theophylline, aminophylline) are older agents that are now used infrequently. Do not prescribe beta-blockers for asthmatics or patients with COPD; they block the $beta_2$-receptors that are needed to open the airways.

7. What is the concern with the use of long-acting beta-agonists in the treatment of asthma?
The US Food and Drug Administration has recommended that LABAs not be used as solo agents in the treatment of asthma in children or adults due to an increased risk of death. The advisory recommends that LABAs not be used alone as initial therapy for asthma of any severity, that they not be added when asthma control is actively deteriorating, that they only be used long term in patients whose asthma cannot be adequately controlled with other asthma controller medications, and that the LABA be discontinued, if possible, once asthma control is achieved.

8. What is a common cause of wheezing in children under age 2 years?
Reactive airway disease due to viral infection, commonly respiratory syncytial virus infection, which classically occurs in the winter and causes a fever. Asthma may also be the cause but is usually associated with a chronic history.

9. What should you think if a patient with acute asthma stops hyperventilating or has a normal carbon dioxide (CO_2) level?
Beware the asthmatic who is no longer hyperventilating or whose CO_2 is normal or rising. The patient should be hyperventilating, which causes low CO_2. If the patient seems calm or sleepy, do not assume all is okay. Such patients are probably crashing; they need an immediate arterial blood gas analysis and possible intubation. Fatigue alone is sufficient reason to intubate. Remember also that any patient with COPD may normally live with a higher CO_2 and lower oxygen (O_2) level. Treat the patient, not the lab value. If the patient is asymptomatic and talking to you, the lab value should not cause panic.

10. When should you intubate?
As a rough rule of thumb, think about intubation in any patient whose CO_2 is greater than 50 mm Hg or whose O_2 is less than 50 mm Hg, especially if the pH in either situation is less than 7.30 while the patient is breathing room air. Usually, unless the patient is crashing rapidly, a trial of oxygen by nasal cannula, face mask, or biphasic positive airway pressure (Bi-PAP) is given first. If it does not work or if the patient becomes too tired (use of accessory muscles is a good clue to the work of breathing), intubate. Clinical correlation is always required; patients with chronic lung disease may be asymptomatic at lab value levels that seem to defy reason. Alternatively, lab values may look great, but if the patient is becoming tired from increased work of breathing or is significantly altered (e.g., Glasgow Coma Scale <8), intubation may be needed.

11. What should you do if a patient has a solitary pulmonary nodule on chest radiograph?
The first step is to compare the current film with old films (if available). If the lesion has not changed in more than 2 to 3 years, it is very likely to be benign. A nodule that has increased in size on serial imaging should be biopsied or excised. CT scans are used to evaluate and follow a solitary pulmonary nodule. A nodule that has a low probability of being malignant can be followed with serial CT scans. A positron emission tomography scan is used to evaluate intermediate probability nodules. A nodule that has a high probability of being malignant should be excised.

12. What classic clues on the Step 2 exam point to the cause of a solitary pulmonary nodule?
- Immigrant: think of tuberculosis; do a purified protein derivative (PPD) skin test or interferon gamma release assay (IGRA; QuantiFERON) if suspicion is low to moderate. If there is concern that the patient has active pulmonary tuberculosis, the patient should be placed on isolation with acid-fast bacilli smears and *Mycobacterium tuberculosis* polymerase chain reaction tests, as a negative interferon gamma release assay does not rule out active tuberculosis.
- Southwest US exposure: think of *Coccidioides immitis*.
- Cave explorer, exposure to bird droppings or Ohio/Mississippi river valleys (Midwest): think of histoplasmosis.
- Smoker over the age of 50 years: think of lung cancer; order bronchoscopy if central, or biopsy if peripheral.
- Person under age 40 years with none of the previous: think of hamartoma.

13. What should you know about pulmonary function in the setting of surgery?

A baseline chest radiograph is not part of the standard preoperative evaluation but is often used for patients over age 60 or patients with known pulmonary or cardiovascular disease. Preoperative pulmonary function testing is somewhat controversial, and the question probably will not appear on Step 2. Overall, the best indicator of possible postoperative pulmonary complications is preoperative pulmonary function. The best way to reduce pulmonary complications postoperatively is to **stop smoking** preoperatively, especially if it is stopped at least 8 weeks prior to surgery. Aggressive pulmonary toilet, incentive spirometry, adequate but not overly aggressive pain control, and early ambulation help to prevent or minimize postoperative pulmonary complications. Lastly, remember that the most common cause of a postoperative fever in the first 24 hours is atelectasis.

14. How do you recognize and treat adult respiratory distress syndrome (ARDS)?

ARDS results from acute lung injury and causes noncardiogenic pulmonary edema, respiratory distress, and hypoxemia. Common risk factors are sepsis, pneumonia, aspiration of gastric contents, major trauma, pancreatitis, shock, near-drowning, drug overdose, major burns, and blood transfusions. Look for ARDS to develop within 24 to 48 hours of the initial insult. The classic patient has mottled/cyanotic skin, intercostal retractions, rales or rhonchi, and no improvement of hypoxia with oxygen administration. Radiographs show pulmonary edema with a normal cardiac silhouette (no cardiomegaly). Treat with intubation, mechanical ventilation with low tidal volumes (6–8 cc/kg of ideal body weight), and positive end-expiratory pressure, while addressing the underlying cause (if possible). Patients with worsening hypoxemia despite this may be paralyzed with cisatracurium and placed prone, with conservative fluid management to avoid volume overload as an additional contributor to hypoxemia.

15. How is pneumonia diagnosed?

The diagnosis of pneumonia is usually based on clinical findings (fever, rales, or rhonchi) plus elevated white blood cell count and an abnormal chest radiograph consistent with pneumonia. Sputum and blood cultures may be obtained, preferably before empiric antibiotic therapy is begun.

16. What is the difference between typical and atypical pneumonia?

Typical pneumonia is usually caused by bacteria such as *Streptococcus pneumoniae* or *Staphylococcus aureus*, the most common causes of pneumonia. Atypical pneumonia may be caused by viral infection (e.g., influenza or adenovirus), *Mycoplasma*, *Chlamydia* spp., *Legionella*, *Moraxella*, or *Haemophilus*.

	Typical Pneumonia	*Atypical Pneumonia*
Prodrome	Short (<2 days)	Long (>3 days) (headache, malaise, body aches)
Fever	High (>102°F)	Low (<102°F)
Age	>40 yr	<40 yr
Chest radiograph	One distinct lobe involved	Diffuse or multilobe involvement
Bug	*Streptococcus pneumoniae*	Many (*Haemophilus, Mycoplasma, Chlamydia* spp.)
Antibiotic*	Ceftriaxone, broad spectrum	Macrolides (e.g., azithromycin), doxycycline, or certain fluoroquinolones (e.g., levofloxacin, moxifloxacin)

*Avoid the temptation to pull out the "bigger-gun" antibiotics (very wide spectrum, potent) unless the patient is crashing or unstable.

17. What is the difference between aspiration pneumonia and aspiration pneumonitis?

Aspiration pneumonia refers to a bacterial infection in the lung. Polymicrobial infections, including both aerobic and anaerobic, and enteric organisms are common. Aspiration pneumonia should be suspected in a patient who has persistent fever, hypoxia, cough, and abnormal chest x-ray for more than 48 hours following an aspiration event. Such aspiration events are usually precipitated by loss of consciousness from underlying neurologic disease (e.g., dementia or stroke), intoxication, severe illness (e.g., myocardial infarction), or undergoing general anesthesia on a full stomach. Classically, aspiration pneumonia occurs in the right middle and lower lobes in upright patients, as the infection is gravity dependent and the right mainstem bronchus is somewhat more vertically oriented than the left. In supine patients, superior segments of the lower lobes or posterior segments of the upper lobes are commonly affected.

Aspiration pneumonitis very commonly follows an aspiration event and refers to the chemical irritation and inflammation in the lungs caused by aspiration of stomach acid and food. Aspiration pneumonitis can present with cough, dyspnea, hypoxia, low-grade fever, crackles and coarse breath sounds on lung auscultation, and/or infiltrates on chest x-ray. Acute symptoms usually resolve within 48 hours, and treatment is supportive.

17. What are the classic clinical clues for the different causative bugs in pneumonia?

College student: *Mycoplasma* sp. (look for cold agglutinins) or *Chlamydia* sp.
Alcoholic: *Klebsiella* sp. ("currant jelly" sputum), *Staphylococcus aureus,* other enteric bugs (aspiration)
Cystic fibrosis: *Pseudomonas* sp. or *Staphylococcus aureus*
Immigrant: tuberculosis
COPD: *Haemophilus influenzae, Moraxella* sp.
Known tuberculosis with pulmonary cavitation: *Aspergillus* sp.
Silicosis (metal, granite, pottery workers): tuberculosis
Exposure to air conditioner or aerosolized water: *Legionella* sp.
HIV/AIDS: *Pneumocystis jirovecii* or cytomegalovirus (if you are shown koilocytosis and the patient is very immunosuppressed), although *Streptococcus pneumoniae* is still the most common cause of pneumonia in HIV-positive patients
Exposure to bird droppings: *Chlamydia psittaci* or histoplasmosis
Child less than 1 year old: respiratory syncytial virus
Child 2 to 5 years old: parainfluenza (croup)

19. What should you suspect if a child has recurrent pneumonias?
If the pneumonia always occurs in the same spot (especially the right middle and/or right lower lobe), it most likely is due to foreign body aspiration. Remember that a foreign body is most likely to go down the right mainstem bronchus. This diagnosis should be considered especially if the child has no other signs of immunodeficiency (e.g., other types of infections, symptoms of cystic fibrosis) before or during the episodes. If immunodeficiency is the cause of recurrent pneumonias, the child should have a history of chronic bilateral lung problems and other types of infection.

20. What is "round" pneumonia?
Pneumonia may appear round, typically in children, which causes it to simulate a mass. In such cases involving children, assume pneumonia and treat appropriately. A follow-up x-ray can be obtained to confirm resolution, which is not usually required in children, who almost never develop lung malignancies. In an adult, a round pneumonia should be viewed with suspicion (more likely to be a malignancy), and further workup with a CT scan is typically employed.

21. Why should you get a follow-up chest x-ray in all smokers over age 50 who develop pneumonia?
A follow-up chest x-ray is indicated in smokers over 50 who develop pneumonia to make sure it clears after appropriate antibiotic treatment. If pneumonia does not clear by 4 to 6 weeks, suspect something other than bacterial pneumonia. The classic culprit is malignancy—specifically **bronchoalveolar carcinoma**, which is a subtype of adenocarcinoma (Fig. 33.1). In addition, recurrent pneumonias in the same location in an adult may be due to an endobronchial mass, whether benign or malignant.

22. What should you know about infant respiratory distress syndrome?
Infant respiratory distress syndrome is due to atelectasis from a deficiency of surfactant; it is seen almost exclusively in premature infants and infants of diabetic mothers. Look for rapid, labored respirations, substernal retractions, cyanosis, grunting, and/or nasal flaring. Arterial blood gas shows hypoxemia and hypercarbia;

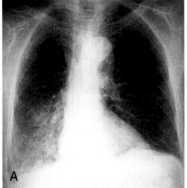
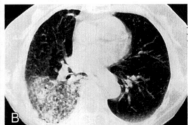

Fig. 33.1 Consolidation in the right lower lobe, seen on front chest radiograph (A) and computed tomography (B), progressed despite antibiotic therapy. Biopsy proved bronchoalveolar carcinoma. (From Katz DS, Math KR, Groskin SA, eds. *Radiology Secrets.* Philadelphia: Hanley & Belfus; 1998:80. With permission.)

radiograph shows diffuse atelectasis (described as diffuse, granular infiltrates). Treat with oxygen, give surfactant, and intubate if necessary. Complications include intraventricular hemorrhage and pneumothorax or bronchopulmonary dysplasia (complications of acute or chronic mechanical ventilation). In contrast, transient tachypnea of the newborn is a benign and common condition characterized by isolated rapid breathing that resolves within 72 hours of life and is treated with supportive care.

23. **What prenatal tests help to determine whether respiratory distress syndrome will occur?**
Measurement of amniotic fluid in the pregnant mother can determine whether the fetus is producing adequate surfactant. A lecithin-to-sphingomyelin ratio greater than 2:1 or the presence of **phosphatidylglycerol** in the amniotic fluid indicates fetal lung maturity and a low likelihood of infant respiratory distress syndrome. The fluorescence polarization test reflects the ratio of surfactant to albumin in amniotic fluid and is a direct measurement of surfactant concentration. An elevated ratio indicates fetal lung maturity. Betamethasone is indicated to encourage fetal lung maturity if a preterm delivery at less than 34 weeks of gestation is suspected.

24. **Define diaphragmatic hernia. How is it recognized clinically?**
A defect in the diaphragm allows bowel to herniate into the chest. Diaphragmatic hernia is mentioned in the pulmonary section because it presents with respiratory difficulty, not gastrointestinal problems. Herniated bowel pushes on the developing lung and causes lung hypoplasia on the affected side. Look for a scaphoid abdomen and bowel sounds in the chest. Herniated bowel can be seen on the chest radiograph; 90% are left sided.

25. **How do you recognize and diagnose a tracheoesophageal fistula? How is it treated?**
The most common type (85% of cases) of tracheoesophageal fistula is an esophagus with a blind pouch proximally and a fistula between a bronchus/carina and the distal esophagus (see Fig. 12.13). Look for a neonate with excessive oral secretions, coughing or cyanosis with attempted feedings, abdominal distention, and aspiration pneumonia. The diagnosis is made by the inability to pass a nasogastric tube; alternatively, an injection of air via a nasogastric tube under x-ray (i.e., fluoroscopy) shows only the proximal esophagus. Treatment is early surgical correction.

26. **What is the most common lethal genetic disease in whites? How do you recognize it?**
Cystic fibrosis, which is an autosomal recessive disease. Always suspect cystic fibrosis in pediatric patients with rectal prolapse, meconium ileus, esophageal varices, recurrent pulmonary infections, or failure to thrive. The classic complaint from the mother is a "salty-tasting" baby. Patients also commonly have pancreatic insufficiency and infertility (98% of affected males and 50% of females); they also may develop cor pulmonale (right-heart failure). Most states now screen for cystic fibrosis in the standard newborn screening.

27. **How is cystic fibrosis diagnosed and treated?**
Diagnosis is made by an abnormal increase in the electrolytes of the patient's sweat (sodium and chloride) and/or DNA testing. Treat with chest physical therapy, annual influenza vaccine, fat-soluble vitamin supplements, pancreatic enzyme replacement, bronchodilators, dornase alfa, and aggressive treatment of infections with antibiotics that cover *Staphylococcus, Haemophilus influenzae,* and *Pseudomonas* spp. *Staphylococcus* is the predominant organism in children and *Pseudomonas* spp. in adults. Eventually these patients will need lung transplantation.

28. **What should you do if a patient has a pleural effusion?**
If you do not know the cause of the effusion (Fig. 33.2), consider thoracocentesis to examine the fluid in an attempt to determine its etiology. Common tests ordered on pleural fluid include Gram stain, culture and sensitivity testing (including tuberculosis culture), cell count with differential, glucose (low with infection), protein (high with infection), cytology (to look for malignancy), amylase (if pancreatitis is a suspected cause of effusion), triglycerides (if a chylous effusion is suspected), albumin, and lactate dehydrogenase (the last two tests help to determine whether the fluid is an exudate or transudate by using Light criteria).

29. **What is pulmonary hypertension?**
Pulmonary hypertension (PHTN) is defined as an elevated mean pulmonary arterial pressure (≥ 20 mm Hg) as assessed on right heart catheterization. PHTN represents increased stress on the right ventricle, leading to dysfunction and potential right ventricular failure. The World Health Organization classifies PHTN into five groups, which assists with understanding diagnostic workup and treatment.

WHO Classification	Workup	Treatment
Group I: Pulmonary arterial hypertension	History of intravenous drug use (methamphetamine), CTD evaluation, HIV	Prostacyclins (epoprostenol); endothelin receptor antagonists (macitentan, bosentan); phosphodiesterase-5 inhibitors (sildenafil, tadalafil)

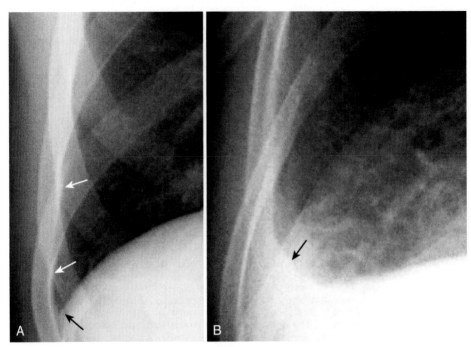

Fig. 33.2 Normal and blunted right lateral costophrenic sulcus. (A) The hemidiaphragm usually makes a sharp and acute angle as it meets the lateral chest wall on the frontal projection to produce the lateral costophrenic sulcus *(black arrow)*. Notice how aerated lung normally extends to the inner margin of each of the ribs *(white arrows)*. (B) When an effusion reaches about 300 mL in volume, the lateral costophrenic sulcus loses its acute angulation and becomes blunted *(black arrow)*. (From Herring W. *Learning Radiology: Recognizing the Basics*. Saunders; 2020:60-69 [fig. 8.5].)

WHO Classification	Workup	Treatment
Group 2: PHTN from left-sided heart disease	Elevated pulmonary capillary wedge pressure on right heart catheterization, transthoracic echo	Optimize heart failure medications, diuresis
Group 3: PHTN from chronic hypoxemic lung disease	Pulmonary function tests; high resolution computed tomography	Oxygen supplementation, smoking cessation
Group 4: Chronic thromboembolic pulmonary hypertension	Ventilation-perfusion lung scanning	Anticoagulation, pulmonary thromboendarterectomy
Group 5: Unclear/miscellaneous	Evaluate for hematologic diseases as well as systemic and metabolic disorders	Treat the underlying disorder

CTD, Connective tissue disease; *HIV*, human immunodeficiency virus; *PHTN*, pulmonary hypertension.

CHAPTER 34

RADIOLOGY

1. Cover the right-hand columns in Table 34.1 and specify what imaging study you should order for each condition

Table 34.1 Screening and/or Confirmatory Radiologic Tests for Different Diseases

CONDITION	SCREENING (OR ONLY) TEST TO ORDER	CONFIRMATORY TEST	COMMENTS
Cardiovascular			
Aortic aneurysm	Abdominal US	CT with contrast	One-time screening for males ages 65–75 yr who have ever smoked (≥100 cigarettes)
Aortic dissection	CT with contrast	MRA or TEE	
Aortic trauma (tear)	CT with contrast	MRA or TEE	
Carotid stenosis	Duplex US	MRA	
Gastrointestinal			
Abdominal abscess	CT scan with contrast		
Abdominal trauma	FAST scan (focused assessment with sonography for trauma) to assess for hemoperitoneum	CT with contrast	Laparotomy is the gold standard if the patient is hemodynamically unstable
Appendicitis	US (particularly in pregnant patients and children)	CT with contrast	Never truly confirmed until surgery
Bowel obstruction	Abdominal x-ray	CT with contrast	
Bowel perforation	Upright abdominal film/CXR	CT with contrast	On x-ray, look for free air under the diaphragm. Left lateral decubitus abdominal film is appropriate if the patient cannot be positioned for upright film
Cholecystitis	US	Nuclear hepatobiliary study (HIDA scan)	Look for gallbladder wall thickening and pericholecystic fluid on US
Choledocholithiasis	US	ERCP or MRCP	
Cholelithiasis	US		
Diverticulitis	CT with contrast		No endoscopy acutely as there is a risk of perforation
Esophageal disease	Gastrografin or barium x-ray	CT with contrast (for rupture)	Endoscopy usually necessary as a follow-up study
GI bleeding	Endoscopy	Tagged red cell scan if unable to visualize on endoscopy	

Continued

Table 34.1 Screening and/or Confirmatory Radiologic Tests for Different Diseases—cont'd

CONDITION	SCREENING (OR ONLY) TEST TO ORDER	CONFIRMATORY TEST	COMMENTS
Hematemesis*	Endoscopy		
Meckel diverticulum	Meckel scan (nuclear medicine)		
Peptic ulcer disease	Endoscopy		
Pyloric stenosis	US	Barium x-ray	
Gynecologic			
Fibroids	US	MRI	
Ovarian disease	US	MRI	Laparoscopy may be needed
Pelvic mass (female)	US	MRI or CT with contrast or laparoscopy	
Pregnancy evaluation	US		Transvaginal US for early pregnancy; transabdominal for the remainder
Neurologic			
Acute stroke	Noncontrast CT	MRI	
Brain tumor	CT with contrast	MRI with contrast	
Head trauma	Noncontrast CT		
Intracranial hemorrhage	Noncontrast CT		
Multiple sclerosis	MRI		
Skull fracture	Noncontrast CT		
Orthopedic			
Arthritis	X-ray	MRI if more detailed evaluation is needed	
Bone metastases	Bone scan	PET scan	Plain x-rays for multiple myeloma
Fracture	X-ray	Noncontrast CT	CT can pick up many fractures not seen on x-ray
Osteomyelitis	X-ray	Bone scan or tagged white blood cell nuclear scan	MRI without contrast can be helpful
Pelvic trauma	X-ray	Noncontrast CT	Consider retrograde urethrogram if there is blood at the meatus
Scaphoid fracture	X-ray	MRI	
Respiratory			
Chest mass	Chest x-ray	CT with contrast	
Chest trauma	Chest x-ray	CT with contrast	
Hemoptysis	Chest x-ray	Bronchoscopy or CT with contrast	
Pneumonia	Chest x-ray	CT with contrast	
Pulmonary embolism	CT with contrast	Pulmonary angiogram	Ventilation/perfusion nuclear scan if unable to tolerate radiation (pregnancy) or contrast
Pulmonary nodule	Chest x-ray	Noncontrast CT	May need PET scan to assess for malignancy

Continued

Table 34.1 Screening and/or Confirmatory Radiologic Tests for Different Diseases—cont'd

CONDITION	SCREENING (OR ONLY) TEST TO ORDER	CONFIRMATORY TEST	COMMENTS
Urologic			
Hematuria (persistent)	CT urogram with contrast (without contrast if painful hematuria)	Cystoscopy	
Hydronephrosis	US	CT with contrast	Renal ultrasound can also identify hydronephrosis
Nephrolithiasis	Noncontrast CT	Intravenous pyelography rarely indicated or used	
Ureteral reflux	Voiding cystourethrogram (VCUG)		
Suspected urethral trauma	Retrograde urethrogram		

Note: With suspected GI perforation, do not use barium (it can cause a chemical peritonitis); use water-soluble contrast (e.g., Gastrografin).

CT, Computed tomography; *CTA,* computed tomographic angiogram; *ERCP,* endoscopic retrograde cholangiopancreatography; *GI,* gastrointestinal; *HIDA,* hepato-iminodiacetic acid; *MRA,* magnetic resonance angiogram (an MRI test); *MRCP,* magnetic resonance cholangiopancreatography; *MRI,* magnetic resonance imaging; *PET,* positron emission tomography; *US,* ultrasound.

*For brisk bleeds, endoscopy is preferred. For occult bleeding, barium study or endoscopy may be used. An "unknown" GI bleed means that initial tests failed to localize the bleed and that the patient is still actively bleeding.

CHAPTER 35

RHEUMATOLOGY

1. **What is the most common form of arthritis?**
   Osteoarthritis (OA) (at least 75% of cases), which is also called degenerative joint disease (Fig. 35.1)

2. **If the cause of arthritis is in doubt, what should you do?**
   When in doubt, or if you suspect something other than OA, perform an x-ray of and aspirate fluid from the affected joint. Examine the fluid for cell count and differential, glucose, bacteria (Gram stain and culture), and crystals.

3. **How do you distinguish among the common causes of arthritis?**

	OA	RA	Gout	Pseudogout	Septic
Usual age/sex	Older adults	Women 20–45 yr	Older men	Older adults	Any age
Classic joints	DIP, PIP, hip, knee	PIP, MCP, wrist	Big toe	Knees, elbows	Knee
Joint fluid WBC	<2000	>2000	>2000	>2000	>50,000
% Neutrophils	<25%	>50%	>50%	>50%	>75%
Appearance	Transparent	Translucent or opaque	Translucent or opaque	Translucent or opaque	Opaque

DIP, Distal interphalangeal joints; *MCP,* metacarpophalangeal joints; *OA,* osteoarthritis; *PIP,* proximal interphalangeal joints; *RA,* rheumatoid arthritis; *WBC,* white blood cells.

4. **What other clues point to a diagnosis of OA?**
   OA typically occurs in those over the age of 40 and has few signs of inflammation on exam; thus the joints are not hot, red, or tender like in the other four types of arthritis listed earlier. Look for Heberden nodes (visible and palpable distal interphalangeal [DIP] joint osteophytes) (Fig. 35.2) and Bouchard nodes (proximal interphalangeal [PIP] joint osteophytes), worsening of symptoms after use and in the evening, bony spurs, and increasing incidence with age. Imaging will show loss of joint space associated with cartilage degeneration, and possibly osteophyte formation. Treat with weight reduction, physical therapy/activity, as-needed nonsteroidal antiinflammatory drugs (NSAIDs) or acetaminophen, corticosteroid injections, and orthopedic referral for joint replacement surgery if severe and not responsive to conservative measures.

5. **What clues point to a diagnosis of rheumatoid arthritis (RA)?**
   RA often causes systemic symptoms (fever, malaise, subcutaneous nodules, pericarditis, pleural effusion, uveitis), prolonged morning stiffness, swan neck and boutonnière deformities, and atlantoaxial instability requiring cervical spine radiographs prior to surgery. The diagnosis is often made by an elevated sedimentation rate or C-reactive protein and positive rheumatoid factor, which is present in most adults but often negative in children. Anticyclic citrullinated peptide antibody (anti-CCP) is more specific for RA. Radiographs and magnetic resonance imaging can also support the diagnosis. General treatment strategies reflect the fact that the destruction of affected joints due to inflammation occurs early in the course of rheumatoid arthritis. The patient should be offered treatment with disease-modifying antirheumatic drugs (DMARDs) as soon as possible after the onset of disease. Escalate the intensity of treatment until synovitis and inflammation have improved.

   There are five general classes of medications used for the treatment of RA, with DMARDs forming the backbone of treatment. Treatment options include the following: analgesics (from acetaminophen to narcotics), NSAIDs, glucocorticoids, nonbiologic DMARDs (methotrexate, sulfasalazine, leflunomide, hydroxychloroquine, and minocycline), and biologic DMARDs. Biologic DMARDs include tumor necrosis factor (TNF) inhibitors (etanercept, infliximab, and adalimumab), an interleukin-1 receptor antagonist (anakinra), a CD20 inhibitor (rituximab), and biologic response modifiers (abatacept).

6. **What clues point to a diagnosis of gout?**
   Gout classically begins with podagra (gout in the big toe). Also look for high uric acid levels (not always present and tend to be lower in an acute attack), tophi (subcutaneous uric acid deposits that look like punched-out lesions on bone radiographs), **needle-shaped monosodium urate crystals with negative birefringence** in the joint fluid, and male gender (more commonly affected than female gender). Alcohol and protein-rich foods

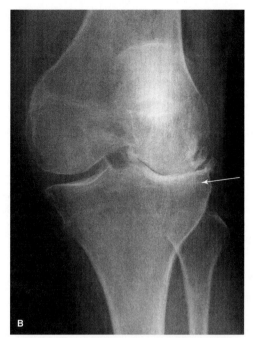

Fig. 35.1 Features of osteoarthritis on x-ray images. Knee showing osteoarthritis within the lateral compartment of the femorotibial joint. (From Aitken MJ, Gibson A. *Crash Course Rheumatology and Orthopaedics.* Elsevier; 2019:67-71.)

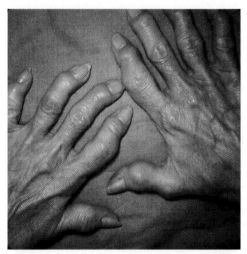

Fig. 35.2 Osteoarthritic hands with Heberden (distal interphalangeal) and Bouchard (proximal interphalangeal) nodes on both index fingers and thumbs. (From Canale ST, Beaty JH. *Campbell's Operative Orthopaedics.* 11th ed. St. Louis: Mosby; 2007 [fig. 70.4].)

(e.g., shellfish, red meats) may precipitate an attack. Colchicine or NSAIDs (but *not* aspirin, which causes decreased excretion of uric acid by the kidney) are used for acute attacks. For scenarios in which colchicine or NSAIDs are contraindicated, steroids can be considered so long as septic arthritis is ruled out. For maintenance therapy, high fluid intake, alkalinization of the urine, and/or allopurinol or probenecid (neither drug is for acute attacks) may be used.

7. **What causes pseudogout? How is it diagnosed?**
   Pseudogout is caused by deposition of calcium pyrophosphate crystals into joints. Look for **rhomboid crystals** with **weakly positive birefringence** (vs negative birefringence with gout crystals in the joint fluid). Radiographs of affected joints can demonstrate chondrocalcinosis (Fig. 35.3). Risk factors include osteoarthritis, hyperparathyroidism, hemochromatosis, and renal diseases causing hypomagnesemia (Gitelman and Bartter syndromes). Acute attacks can be treated with corticosteroid injections, NSAIDs, or colchicine.

8. **What clues point to a diagnosis of septic arthritis? What are the common causes?**
   In septic arthritis, Gram stain usually reveals bacteria in the synovial fluid. *Staphylococcus aureus* is the most common organism except in sexually active young adults, in whom the most common bug is *Neisseria gonorrhoeae*. Do blood cultures in addition to joint cultures, because the bug usually reaches the joint via the hematogenous route. Also do screening for sexually transmitted infection in appropriate patients.

9. **Name some other causes of arthritis.**
   - Prior trauma (posttraumatic arthritis)
   - Lupus and other collagen vascular diseases (e.g., scleroderma)
   - Psoriasis
   - Inflammatory bowel disease
   - Lyme disease
   - Ankylosing spondylitis
   - Reactive arthritis
   - Hemophilia
   - Paget disease
   - Hemochromatosis, Wilson disease
   - Neuropathy (i.e., Charcot joint)

10. **True or False: Psoriasis can cause an arthritis that resembles OA.**
    False. The arthritis more closely resembles rheumatoid arthritis. On the Step 2 exam, look for psoriatic skin lesions to make an easy diagnosis. The arthritis usually affects the hands and feet, and though it resembles rheumatoid arthritis, the rheumatoid factor is negative (seronegative spondyloarthropathy). Along with ankylosing spondylitis, inflammatory bowel disease, and reactive arthritis, psoriatic arthritis is associated with the human leukocyte antigen B27 (HLA-B27) serotype. NSAIDs are first-line therapy. Other treatments include nonbiologic DMARDS (methotrexate, PUVA, retinoic acid derivatives, and cyclosporine) and biologic DMARDS, including TNF inhibitors (etanercept, infliximab, adalimumab, golimumab).

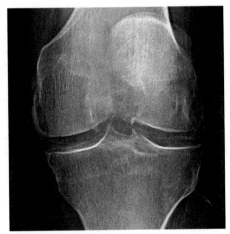

Figure 35.3 Chondrocalcinosis (see medial and lateral meniscal calcifications) on an x-ray of a knee. (From Misra D, et al. CT imaging for evaluation of calcium crystal deposition in the knee: initial experience from the Multicenter Osteoarthritis (MOST) study. *Osteoarthr Cartil.* 2015;23(2):244-248 [fig. 2A].)

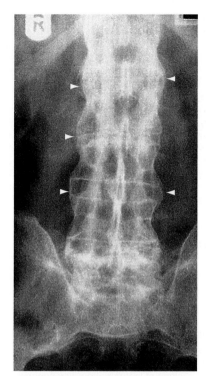

Fig. 35.4 Ankylosing spondylitis. "Bamboo spine" of advanced ankylosing spondylitis. (From Clunie GPR, Ralston SH. *Davidson's Principles and Practice of Medicine.* Churchill Livingstone; 2018:981-1060.)

11. Describe the hallmarks of ankylosing spondylitis

    Ankylosing spondylitis is associated with HLA-B27. Most often a 20- to 40-year-old man with a positive family history presents with back pain and morning stiffness. Patients may assume a bent-over posture. The sacroiliac joints are primarily affected, and radiographs may reveal a **"bamboo" spine** (Fig. 35.4). Patients have other autoimmune type symptoms, such as fever, elevations in erythrocyte sedimentation rate and C-reactive protein, and anemia. Some develop uveitis. Treat with NSAIDs, methotrexate, sulfasalazine, or TNF antagonists (etanercept, infliximab, adalimumab).

12. How do you recognize reactive arthritis as the cause of arthritis?

    Reactive arthritis is also associated with HLA-B27. The classic triad of symptoms consists of **urethritis** (due to chlamydial infection), **conjunctivitis**, and **arthritis** ("can't pee, can't see, can't climb a tree"). Reactive arthritis may also follow enteric bacterial infections. Superficial oral and penile ulcers are common. Diagnose and treat the sexually transmitted disease, and use NSAIDs for arthritis. Also treat the patient's sexual partners.

13. Why do patients with hemophilia get arthritis?

    Recurrent hemarthroses (bleeding into the joints) can cause a debilitating arthritis. Treatment is with acetaminophen. Avoid aspirin and other NSAIDs due to bleeding concern.

14. What clues point to Lyme disease as the cause of arthritis?

    Look for a history of a tick bite or hiking in the woods, **erythema chronicum migrans** rash (Fig. 35.5), and migratory arthritis (later). Treat *Borrelia burgdorferi,* the causative bacteria of Lyme disease, with doxycycline, amoxicillin, or cefuroxime. Avoid doxycycline in children under the age of 8 years and in pregnant or lactating women.

15. True or False: One of the major Jones criteria for the diagnosis of rheumatic fever is arthritis

    True. Migratory polyarthritis is one of the major Jones criteria. Look for a history of strep throat. The other major criteria are carditis, chorea, erythema marginatum, and subcutaneous nodules.

16. Why do patients with sickle cell disease often have arthritis?

    Patients frequently experience arthralgias (pain) from ischemic sickle crises, but the classic cause of arthritis is avascular necrosis (e.g., hip arthritis from avascular necrosis of the femoral head).

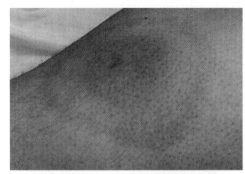

Fig. 35.5 Erythema migrans rash of Lyme disease. Bull's eye lesion on lateral thigh. (From Firestein GS. *Kelley's Textbook of Rheumatology.* 9th ed. Philadelphia: Saunders; 2012 [fig. 110.1]. Courtesy Juan Philadelphia: Salazar, MD, University of Connecticut Health Center.)

17. Define Charcot joint. What clues point to its presence?
A Charcot joint is seen most commonly in diabetes but also occurs in other neuropathies. Somatic sensory and autonomic neuropathy causes autonomic dysfunction and changes in vascularization and causes the patient to overuse or misuse joints, which become deformed and painful. The best treatment is prevention. After even seemingly mild trauma, patients with neuropathy in the area of the trauma need radiographs to rule out fractures.

18. How do hemochromatosis and Wilson disease cause arthritis? How are these diseases radiographically similar to pseudogout?
Via deposition of excessive iron (hemochromatosis) or copper (Wilson disease) into the joints. Radiographically, hemochromatosis and Wilson disease may be notable for chondrocalcinosis (calcium deposition within articular cartilage), which is most commonly associated with pseudogout.

19. What generalized systemic signs of inflammation may suggest an autoimmune disorder?
Systemic signs and symptoms of inflammation include elevations in erythrocyte sedimentation rate and C-reactive protein, fever, anemia of chronic disease, fatigue, and weight loss. If these symptoms are present (especially in a woman of reproductive age), you should consider the possibility of an autoimmune disease.

20. Describe the hallmarks of systemic lupus erythematosus (SLE)
SLE can cause malar rash, discoid rash, photosensitivity, renal insufficiency, arthritis, pericarditis and pleuritis, positive **antinuclear antibody** (**ANA**), positive anti-Smith antibody, positive syphilis results (on the Venereal Disease Research Laboratory and rapid plasmin reagin screening tests, with negative *Treponema pallidum* particle agglutination (TP-PA) assay and direct syphilitic testing), positive lupus anticoagulant, blood disorders (thrombocytopenia, leukopenia, anemia, or pancytopenia), neurologic disturbances (depression, psychosis, seizures), and oral ulcers. Any of these may be presenting symptoms. Use the ANA titer as an initial diagnostic test (high sensitivity, low specificity) and confirm with the **anti-Smith antibody** test (higher specificity). Treat with NSAIDs, hydroxychloroquine, corticosteroids, or immunosuppressive/immunomodulating agents (methotrexate, cyclophosphamide, cyclosporine, azathioprine, mycophenolate, tacrolimus, leflunomide, or belimumab).

21. Describe the hallmarks of scleroderma
Scleroderma (also known as progressive systemic sclerosis) classically presents with **CREST** symptoms (**c**alcinosis, **R**aynaud phenomenon, **e**sophageal dysmotility with dysphagia, **s**clerodactyly, and **t**elangiectasia), heartburn, and masklike leathery facies. Use the ANA test for the initial diagnostic test; confirm the diagnosis with the **anticentromere antibody** test (for CREST symptoms only) and the **antitopoisomerase antibody** (for full-blown scleroderma). Treatment depends on the symptoms. Sclerotic skin lesions can be treated with topical glucocorticoids, calcipotriol, or methotrexate. Systemic therapy depends upon the organs affected.

22. What are the hallmarks of Sjögren syndrome?
Sjögren syndrome causes dry eyes (keratoconjunctivitis sicca) and dry mouth (xerostomia) and is often associated with other autoimmune diseases. Patients tend to have SS-A (Ro) and SS-B (La) antibodies. Treat with eye drops and good oral hygiene. A classic question on the OB-Gyn and pediatrics questions is that SS-A/SS-B antibody positivity in pregnant mothers is associated with congenital heart block.

23. What are the signs and symptoms of dermatomyositis?
Dermatomyositis causes polymyositis (see question 28) plus skin involvement (a **heliotrope rash around the eyes** with associated periorbital edema is classic) (Fig. 35.6). Patients usually have trouble rising from a chair or climbing steps because of the effects on proximal muscles. Muscle enzymes are elevated, and electromyography is irregular. Muscle biopsy establishes the diagnosis. Affected patients have an increased incidence of malignancy.

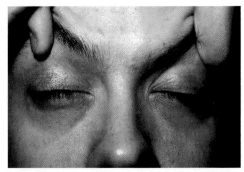

Fig. 35.6 Dermatomyositis. Heliotrope (violaceous) discoloration around the eyes and periorbital edema. (From Habif TP. *Clinical Dermatology.* 5th ed. Mosby; 2009 [fig. 17.19].)

24. **With what is polyarteritis nodosa associated? How is it diagnosed?**
Polyarteritis nodosa is a type of vasculitis classically associated with hepatitis B infection and cryoglobulinemia. Patients present with fever, abdominal pain, weight loss, renal disturbances, and/or peripheral neuropathies. Lab abnormalities include elevations in erythrocyte sedimentation rate and C-reactive protein, leukocytosis, anemia, and hematuria or proteinuria. Patients often have a positive **antineutrophil cytoplasmic antibody** titer. The vasculitis involves medium-sized vessels. Biopsy of an affected organ is the gold standard for diagnosis.

25. **Describe the usual presentation of Kawasaki disease. How is it treated?**
Kawasaki disease usually affects children younger than 5 years; it is more common in Japanese and female children. Patients present with truncal rash, high fever (which lasts >5 days), conjunctival injection, cervical lymphadenopathy, strawberry tongue, late skin desquamation of palms and soles, and/or arthritis. Patients may develop coronary vessel vasculitis and subsequent aneurysms, which may thrombose and cause a myocardial infarction. Kawasaki disease should be suspected in any child who has a heart attack. Treat during the acute stage with aspirin and intravenous immunoglobulins within 10 days of symptom onset to reduce the risk of coronary aneurysm.

26. **How does Takayasu arteritis present?**
Takayasu arteritis tends to affect Asian women between the ages of 15 and 30 years. It is called the "pulseless disease" because you may not be able to feel the pulse or measure blood pressure on the affected side. The vasculitis affects large vessels, typically the aortic arch and its branches. Carotid involvement may cause neurologic signs or stroke, and congestive heart failure is not uncommon. Angiogram shows the characteristic lesions. Treat with steroids.

27. **How do you recognize Behçet syndrome on the Step 2 exam?**
Behçet syndrome classically presents in young men in their 20s with painful oral and genital ulcers. Patients may also have uveitis, arthritis, and other skin lesions (especially erythema nodosum). Steroids are the mainstay of therapy.

28. **How do you distinguish among fibromyalgia, polymyositis, and polymyalgia rheumatica?**

	Fibromyalgia	Polymyositis	Polymyalgia Rheumatica
Classic age/sex	Young adult women	Female aged 40–60 yr	Female age >50 yr
Location	Various	Proximal muscles	Pectoral and pelvic girdles, neck
ESR	Normal	Elevated	Markedly elevated (often >100)
EMG/biopsy	Normal	Abnormal	Normal
Classic findings	Anxiety, stress, insomnia, point tenderness over affected muscles	Elevated CPK, abnormal EMG/ biopsy, higher risk of cancer	Temporal arteritis, great response to steroids, very high ESR, elderly patients

	Fibromyalgia	Polymyositis	Polymyalgia Rheumatica
Treatment	Antidepressants, NSAIDs, trigger point injections, pregabalin, physical activity	Steroids	Steroids

CPK, Creatine phosphokinase; *EMG,* electromyography; *ESR,* erythrocyte sedimentation rate; *NSAIDs,* nonsteroidal antiinflammatory drugs.

29. Give the basic facts of Paget disease. How is it linked with cancer?

    In Paget disease, bone is broken down and regenerated, often simultaneously. It is usually seen in persons over 40 years old and is more common in men. It is often discovered in an asymptomatic patient through a radiograph. Classic cases involve the pelvis and skull; watch for a person who has had to buy larger-sized hats. Patients may complain of bone pain, arthritis, or hearing loss. **Alkaline phosphatase** is markedly elevated in the presence of normal calcium and phosphorus levels. The risk of osteosarcoma is increased in affected bones. The main treatment is the antiresorptive agents (e.g., zoledronic acid, alendronate, risedronate, pamidronate).

30. If a pediatric patient has uveitis and an inflammatory arthritis, but the rheumatoid factor is negative, what disease should you suspect?

    Rheumatoid arthritis. The rheumatoid factor is often negative in the pauciarticular variant. Affected patients commonly develop uveitis.

CHAPTER 36

SHOCK

1. **Define shock**
   Shock is a state of life-threatening circulatory insufficiency in which blood flow to and perfusion of peripheral tissues are inadequate to sustain proper organ or cellular function. Initial effects of shock are reversible, but as it progresses both in duration and severity, rapid organ failure and death may result. Although they are not explicitly mentioned in a rigid definition of shock, for USMLE purposes you may consider hypotension with either oliguria or anuria to be associated findings. Reflex tachycardia is also often present.

2. **List the four primary classifications of shock**
   The four primary classifications of shock are:
   1. Distributive
   2. Hypovolemic
   3. Cardiogenic
   4. Obstructive

3. **Which four hemodynamic factors are used to distinguish the four types of shock from one another?**
   Cardiac output, preload, afterload, and tissue perfusion are used to distinguish the four types of shock from one another.

4. **Describe how cardiac output (CO), preload, afterload, and tissue perfusion are measured or estimated in a clinical setting**
   In a clinical setting, CO is measured by cardiac index; preload is measured by pulmonary capillary wedge pressure (PCWP); afterload is measured by systemic vascular resistance (SVR); and tissue perfusion is estimated by systemic venous oxygen saturation (SVO_2).

5. **What are the normal physiologic ranges for CO, PCWP, SVR, and SVO_2 in a healthy recumbent adult?**
   - **CO**: 2.8–4.2 L/min/m^2
   - **PCWP**: 9–23 mm Hg
   - **SVR**: 900–1400 dyn × s/cm^5 or 11.3×17.5 Wood units
   - **SVO_2**: ~65%

6. **List the characteristic hemodynamic changes that occur in each type of shock**

Type of Shock	CO	PCWP	SVR	SVO_2
Distributive	Increased	Early: WNL Late: Low	Low	Increased
Hypovolemic	Early: WNL Late: Low	Early: WNL Late: Low	Increased	Early: Increased Late: Low
Cardiogenic	Low	Increased	Increased	Low
Obstructive	Early: WNL Late: Low*	Early: WNL Late: Low	Increased	Increased*

CO, Cardiac output; *PCWP*, pulmonary capillary wedge pressure; *SVR*, systemic vascular resistance; *SVO_2*, systemic venous oxygen saturation; *WNL*, within normal limits.
*In obstructive shock due to **cardiac tamponade**, cardiac output is *increased* and SVO_2 is *low*. This can be used to distinguish cardiac tamponade from other potential etiologies of obstructive shock.

7. **List three examples of distributive shock**
   Neurogenic, septic, and anaphylactic shock

8. **How do you recognize neurogenic shock?**
   Patients experiencing neurogenic shock typically have a history of severe central nervous system trauma or hemorrhage and often present with flushed skin because the loss of sympathetic tone causes extensive vasodilation. The lack of sympathetic tone may also cause the heart rate to remain normal in a hypotensive patient (because of the impaired sympathetic tone, reflex tachycardia cannot occur).

9. **How do you recognize septic shock?**
   Look for fever, tachycardia, tachypnea, skin that is flushed and warm to the touch, extremes of age, and leukocytosis. (*Note:* Leukocytosis may be absent if the patient is immunosuppressed.) Start broad-spectrum antibiotics after "pan-culturing" the patient's blood, sputum, and urine.

10. **What clues suggest anaphylactic shock?**
    Look for a history of recent exposure to the common culprits: bee stings, peanuts, shellfish, penicillins, sulfa drugs, or any new medication. Anaphylactic shock is mediated by IgE. Treat with **epinephrine** (typically administered intramuscularly) and fluids. Administer oxygen and intubate if necessary. A tracheostomy or cricothyroidotomy should be performed if laryngeal edema or another contraindication prevents intubation. Bronchodilators, corticosteroids, and antihistamines are all second-line agents in anaphylaxis. Monitor all patients for at least 6 hours after the initial reaction.

11. **List six potential etiologies of hypovolemic shock**
    Hemorrhage, burns, heat-related dehydration, profuse vomiting or diarrhea, salt-wasting renal dysfunction, and third-spacing

12. **How do you recognize hypovolemic shock?**
    Look for a history of fluid loss as described previously. Patients usually have orthostatic hypotension, tachycardia, sunken eyes, and tenting of the skin, with infants additionally having a sunken fontanelle. Patients in hypovolemic shock may also present with cold, clammy, pale skin.

13. **List three potential etiologies of cardiogenic shock. Give three examples of each etiology**
    Arrhythmias, cardiomyopathies, and mechanical dysfunction are three potential etiologies of cardiogenic shock. Arrythmias that may lead to cardiogenic shock include atrial fibrillation or flutter, ventricular fibrillation, and heart block. Cardiomyopathies include myocardial infarction, myocarditis, and heart failure. Examples of mechanical dysfunction include valvular stenosis or rupture, ventricular septal defect, and atrial myxoma.

14. **What clues on physical exam suggest cardiogenic shock?**
    Most patients in cardiogenic shock have cold, clammy skin and look pale due to the lack of tissue perfusion. Distended neck veins and pulmonary congestion (e.g., crackles heard when auscultating lung bases) are usually present on physical exam.

15. **List five potential etiologies of obstructive shock**
    Pulmonary embolism, pulmonary hypertension, tension pneumothorax, hemothorax, and cardiac tamponade

16. **What clues suggest pulmonary embolus as a cause of obstructive shock?**
    Look for deep venous thrombosis (positive **Homan sign** with painful, swollen leg) or risk factors for deep venous thrombosis. Remember the **Virchow triad**: endothelial damage, stasis, and hypercoagulable state. Watch for common risk factors, including postoperative status (especially after orthopedic or pelvic surgery), recent delivery (amniotic fluid embolus), traumatic long bone fractures (fat emboli), or malignancy. Patients classically have acute onset of chest pain, tachypnea, shortness of breath, right-axis shift on electrocardiography (as a sign of right-heart strain), and positive computed tomography pulmonary angiography or ventilation/perfusion scan.

17. **How do you recognize pericardial tamponade as a cause of shock?**
    Look for a history of a stab wound or significant blunt trauma to the left chest, often presenting with distended neck veins. Bedside cardiac ultrasound is a quick way to assess for tamponade. Perform pericardiocentesis emergently if obstructive shock begins.

18. **Explain toxic shock syndrome**
    Toxic shock syndrome usually presents in a woman of reproductive age who leaves her tampon in place too long or in a patient with wound packing that has been in for too long. Look for skin desquamation. Toxic shock syndrome may be caused by the *Staphylococcus aureus* toxin TSST-1 or by an invasive group A *Streptococcus pyogenes* infection.

19. **What clues suggest Addison disease as a cause of shock?**
    Patients with Addison disease usually have a history of therapeutic corticosteroid use and/or autoimmune disease and typically have lab results indicating hyperkalemia and hyponatremia. These patients may present with advanced neurologic symptoms, including confusion, delirium, or coma. Treat with glucocorticoids such as hydrocortisone plus aggressive normal saline fluid resuscitation.

20. **What is the most important point to remember when managing a patient in shock? In addition to vital signs, which additional physiologic parameters should you monitor?**
    The most important point to remember is to monitor the ABCs (airway, breathing, circulation). Patients in shock often need immediate lifesaving intervention. Do not hesitate to intubate, do not feed the patient, and (if possible) do not give narcotics. Treat the underlying condition. Mental status changes are often an important clue indicating clinical deterioration. Also monitor by electrocardiogram, urine output, arterial blood gas, hemoglobin/hematocrit, and Swan-Ganz parameters. (Swan-Ganz is not commonly used in clinical practice but may still be tested on the USMLE.)

21. After ABCs are secured, what should you do for a patient in shock?
After establishing the ABCs, quickly give oxygen and begin fluid resuscitation unless the patient is in congestive heart failure. If congestive heart failure is present, avoid fluids, or you will worsen the volume overload that your patient is already experiencing. Once you have administered oxygen and started fluid resuscitation, you may proceed to treating the underlying condition.

22. How should fluids be given if a patient is in shock?
"Two large-bore IVs" is the phrase you will commonly hear on the wards and see on your exams. "Large bore" typically means either 14 or 16 gauge. Infuse 1 to 2 L as fast as it will go (the standard bolus is 10–20 mL of normal saline or lactated Ringer solution per kg body weight). After the bolus, reassess the patient to determine if the bolus helped; this is called a fluid challenge. Positive signs include increases in blood pressure and urine output after the bolus. Do not be afraid to give a second (or third) bolus if your patient does not improve after the first one. Remember to watch for fluid overload so you do not cause or exacerbate congestive heart failure. Consider placing a Foley catheter to ensure accurate monitoring of urine output.

23. What should you do if multiple fluid challenges fail to resolve your patient's hypotension?
Use invasive hemodynamic monitoring (i.e., central line placement or Swan-Ganz catheter) to help determine the cause of the shock and to guide therapeutic decisions. The patient may require vasopressor medications to elevate the blood pressure.

24. Discuss the use of dobutamine, dopamine, norepinephrine, and isoproterenol to support blood pressure in the setting of shock
Dobutamine is a beta$_1$-agonist used to increase cardiac output by increasing cardiac contractility; it also has mild beta$_2$ activity that may result in peripheral vasodilation.
Dopamine activates dopamine receptors at low doses, which results in selective vasodilation (the traditional use for renal perfusion is questionable). At moderate doses, its beta$_1$-agonist effects dominate, which increases contractility. At the highest doses, dopamine has alpha$_1$-agonist effects and therefore may cause vasoconstriction. Note that these dose-dependent effects are hotly debated in clinical practice but may still be tested on the USMLE.
Norepinephrine is used for its vasoconstrictive alpha$_1$-agonist effects, but it also has inotropic beta$_1$ effects. It is primarily given to patients with hypotension to increase peripheral resistance and improve perfusion of vital organs.
Isoproterenol is primarily an inotropic and chronotropic agent rather than a vasopressive agent. It is used for hypotension caused by bradycardia and is effective due to its beta$_1$. and beta$_2$.adrenergic effects.

25. What about the use of phenylephrine, epinephrine, and phosphodiesterase inhibitors in the setting of shock?
Phenylephrine is used for its vasoconstrictive alpha$_1$-agonist effects. It is similar to norepinephrine in this way, except phenylephrine has no beta-adrenergic effects.
Epinephrine is a strong beta$_1$-agonist with moderate beta$_2$- and alpha$_1$-agonist activity. It is typically used in patients experiencing cardiac arrest or anaphylactic shock.
Milrinone and **inamrinone** are phosphodiesterase inhibitors. They are used in patients with refractory heart failure (they are not first-line agents) because they have a positive inotropic effect by reducing the metabolism of cyclic adenosine monophosphate (cAMP) and therefore increasing cAMP concentration. They cannot be used in hypotensive patients, however, as they may exacerbate fluid overload and precipitate cardiogenic shock.

CHAPTER 37

SMOKING

1. **Does smoking really deserve its own chapter in this book?**
   Smoking is the single most significant source of preventable morbidity and premature death in the United States. This is a recurrent theme on the boards, so whenever you are not sure which risk factor to choose to reduce morbidity or mortality, smoking is a safe guess.

2. **How is smoking related to heart disease?**
   Smoking is the best risk factor to eliminate for prevention of deaths related to heart disease; it is responsible for 30% to 45% of such deaths in the United States. This risk is decreased by 50% within 1 year of quitting; by 15 years after quitting, the risk is the same as someone who has never smoked.

3. **What cancers are more likely in smokers?**
   Smoking increases the risk for cancers of the lung (smoking causes 85%–90% of cases), oral cavity (90% of cases), esophagus (70%–80% of cases), larynx, pharynx, bladder (30%–50% of cases), kidney (20%–30%), pancreas (20%–25%), cervix, stomach, colon, and rectum.

4. **Describe the effect of smoking on the lung.**
   Lung cancer and chronic obstructive pulmonary disease (emphysema, chronic bronchitis, and bronchiectasis) are due to smoking. Emphysema almost always results from smoking; if the patient is very young or has no smoking history, you should consider **alpha$_1$-antitrypsin deficiency**. Although the changes of emphysema are irreversible, the risk of death still decreases if the patient stops smoking.

5. **What about secondhand smoke?**
   Secondhand smoke has been proven to be a risk factor for lung cancer and other lung disease. The risk increases linearly with increasing exposure. When parents smoke, their exposed children are at an increased risk for asthma and upper respiratory infections, including otitis media.

6. **What other bad things does smoking do?**
   Smoking retards the healing of peptic ulcer disease, and cessation stops the development of **Buerger disease** (Raynaud symptoms in a young male smoker). Smoking by a pregnant woman increases the risk of low birth weight, prematurity, spontaneous abortion, stillbirth, and infant mortality. Cessation of smoking preoperatively is the best way to decrease the risk of postoperative pulmonary complications, especially if it is stopped at least 8 weeks before surgery.

7. **True or False: Women who smoke should not take birth control pills.**
   True, if the woman is over the age of 35 years and smokes or is younger than 35 and smokes 15 or more cigarettes per day. The risk of thromboembolism is increased sharply in women who smoke and take birth control pills. Postmenopausal women, however, can take estrogen therapy regardless of smoking status.

8. **How does smoking affect drug metabolism by the liver?**
   Smoke generated by burning tobacco or cannabis leaves induces cytochrome P450 1A1 and 1A2 enzymes, which lead to increased clearance of certain medications, including caffeine, chlorpromazine, clozapine, haloperidol, olanzapine, and propranolol. It is important to understand that smokers will require larger therapeutic doses of these medications compared to patients who do not smoke.

CHAPTER 38

UROLOGY

1. Cover the right-hand columns and specify the classic differences between testicular torsion and epididymitis. What imaging test can diagnose and distinguish these two conditions?

	Testicular Torsion	Epididymitis
Age	<20 yr (usually prepubertal)	>20 yr
Appearance	Testis may be elevated into the inguinal canal; swelling	Swollen testis, overlying erythema, urethral discharge/urethritis, prostatitis
Prehn sign	Pain stays the same or worsens	Pain decreases with testicular elevation
Cremasteric reflex	Abnormal	Normal, present
Treatment	Attempt to reduce, but ultimately most go to immediate surgery to salvage testis; surgical orchiopexy for both testes	Antibiotics*

*In men age <50 years, epididymitis is commonly due to sexually transmitted disease (e.g., chlamydial infection and gonorrhea). Treat with ceftriaxone and doxycycline. In men age >50 years, epididymitis is commonly due to urinary tract infection (e.g., *Escherichia coli*). Treat with trimethoprim-sulfamethoxazole or ciprofloxacin.

Ultrasound is the diagnostic test of choice in the setting of testicular/scrotal pain. It can easily differentiate between these two conditions as well as visualize testicular tumors (which sometimes present with pain, although they are classically painless).

2. How does testicular cancer usually present? Describe the major risk factors, histology, and treatment.

Testicular cancer usually presents as a painless testicular mass or enlargement of the testes in a young man (15–35 years old). The main risk factor is cryptorchidism. Roughly 90% are germ cell tumors; the most common type is **seminoma**. The nonseminoma germ cell tumors include yolk sac tumors, choriocarcinomas, embryonal carcinomas, and teratomas. Stromal tumors (non germ cell) include Leydig cell and Sertoli cell tumors. Testicular cancer is generally treated with orchiectomy and radiation; if disease is widespread, use chemotherapy. Alpha-fetoprotein is a marker for yolk sac tumors; human chorionic gonadotropin (hCG) is a marker for choriocarcinoma. Leydig cell tumors may secrete androgens and cause precocious puberty.

3. How is renal cell carcinoma diagnosed and treated?

Painless hematuria (gross or microscopic) is the most typical presenting sign. Patients rarely present with the classic triad of hematuria, flank pain, and a palpable flank mass. Males may also have a left-sided varicocele secondary to tumor blockage of the left gonadal vein that drains into the left renal vein. Computed tomography (CT) scan is a good initial diagnostic test (Fig. 38.1). Treatment for disease confined to the kidney or with extension limited to renal vein invasion (classic) is surgical resection. With other organ invasion or distant metastatic disease (usually to lung or bone), immunotherapy (e.g., interleukin-2 [IL-2]) is the preferred treatment.

4. How is bladder cancer diagnosed and treated?

The most common presenting symptom is gross hematuria. Diagnosis is made with cystoscopy and biopsy; CT and magnetic resonance imaging (MRI) can help define invasion and metastatic disease. Treatment can include intravesicular chemotherapy, transurethral resection, and radical cystectomy depending upon the extent of the malignancy.

5. What is the classic cause of orchitis? How is it treated? Does it usually cause infertility?

Mumps can cause orchitis, which classically presents with a painful, swollen testis in a postpubertal male. The best treatment is prevention (immunization against the mumps virus). Mumps orchitis rarely causes sterility because it is usually unilateral. Bacterial orchitis is typically due to spread from adjacent bacterial epididymitis and is termed epididymoorchitis.

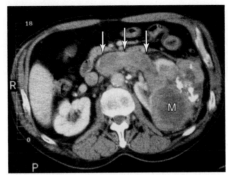

Fig. 38.1 Renal cell carcinoma. A computed tomography scan at the midportion of the kidneys demonstrates a large left renal mass *(M)* that extends into the renal vein and into the inferior vena cava *(arrows). P,* posterior; *R,* right. (From Mettler F. *Essentials of Radiology.* 2nd ed. Philadelphia: Saunders; 2004 [fig. 7.25].)

6. What are the symptoms and sequelae of benign prostatic hyperplasia (BPH)?

   BPH can cause urinary hesitancy, intermittency, terminal dribbling, decreased size and force of the urinary stream, sensation of incomplete emptying, nocturia, urgency, dysuria, and frequency. It may result in acute urinary retention, urinary tract infections, hydronephrosis, and even kidney damage or failure in severe cases.

7. How is BPH treated?

   Medical therapy, which is started when the patient becomes symptomatic, includes long-acting alpha$_1$-blockers (e.g., terazosin, doxazosin, tamsulosin, alfuzosin, and silodosin) and 5-alpha-reductase inhibitors (finasteride, dutasteride). Transurethral resection of the prostate (TURP) is used for more advanced cases, especially with repeated urinary tract infections, urosepsis, urinary retention, and/or hydronephrosis or kidney damage due to reflux. Surgical prostatectomy is used in some patients but is associated with a higher complication rate.

8. How do you recognize and manage acute urinary retention?

   Acute urinary retention generally presents with abdominal pain; palpation of a full, distended bladder on abdominal exam; enlarged prostate on exam and/or a history of BPH in men; and a lack of urination in the past 24 hours or longer. A volume less than 50 mL is a normal postvoid residual volume on bladder scan in patients under 65 years old, and a volume less than 100 mL is normal in patients over age 65 years. The first step is to empty the bladder. If you cannot pass a regular Foley catheter, consider the use of a larger catheter with a firm Coude tip, or alternatively do a suprapubic tap to drain the bladder. Then address the underlying cause—usually BPH, which in this setting is generally treated with TURP.

9. What are the common causes of erectile dysfunction?

   Erectile dysfunction is caused most commonly by vascular problems and atherosclerosis. Medications are also a common culprit (especially antihypertensive and antidepressant agents). Diabetes can cause impotence through vascular (increased atherosclerosis) or neurogenic (diabetic autonomic neuropathy) compromise. Hypogonadism can also cause impotence (look for small testes and loss of secondary sexual characteristics). Patients undergoing dialysis are often impotent. Remember "**p**oint and **s**hoot": **p**arasympathetics mediate erection; **s**ympathetics mediate ejaculation.

   The history often gives you a clue if the cause of impotence is psychogenic. Look for a normal pattern of nocturnal erections, selective dysfunction (the patient has normal erections when masturbating but not with his partner), and a history of stress, anxiety, or fear.

10. What are the signs of urethral injury?

    Usually urethral injury occurs in the context of pelvic trauma. The four classic findings are an absent or abnormally positioned prostate on exam (i.e., "high-riding prostate"), difficulty or inability to urinate, blood at the urethral meatus, and scrotal/perineal ecchymosis.

11. True or False: Urethral injury is a contraindication to passing a Foley catheter.

    True. Always look for the four warning signs of urethral injury. If even one of these signs is present, do not attempt to pass a Foley catheter. Order a retrograde urethrogram to rule out urethral injury in this setting (Fig. 38.2).

12. Distinguish between hydrocele and varicocele.

    A **hydrocele** represents a remnant of the processus vaginalis (remember embryology?) and transilluminates. It generally causes no symptoms and needs no treatment. A **varicocele** is a dilatation of the pampiniform venous plexus ("bag of worms," usually on the left). It does not transilluminate, disappears in the supine position, and becomes prominent with standing or the Valsalva maneuver. Varicoceles may cause infertility or pain and can be treated surgically.

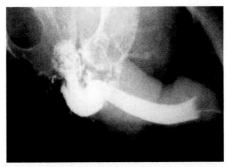

Fig. 38.2 Retrograde urethrogram in pelvic fracture patient demonstrates complete disruption of posterior urethra. (From Wein A, et al. *Campbell-Walsh Urology.* 9th ed. Philadelphia: Saunders; 2007 [fig. 83.10].)

13. Describe the classic findings of nephrolithiasis.

Nephrolithiasis (kidney stones) can cause acute severe colicky flank pain that often radiates to the groin. Patients typically cannot find a position of comfort and shift positions frequently. Nephrolithiasis may cause hematuria (gross or microscopic, though the absence of hematuria does not rule out nephrolithiasis), and often an abdominal radiograph reveals the stone (85% of stones are radiopaque). A noncontrast helical CT scan is the diagnostic test of choice.

14. What are the different types of stones? What causes them?

Roughly 75% to 85% of stones contain calcium. Look for hypercalcemia (usually due to hyperparathyroidism) or small bowel bypass, which increases oxalate absorption and thus calcium stone (envelope-shaped crystals) formation. Roughly 10% to 15% of stones are struvite (magnesium-ammonium-phosphate) stones (coffin-lid crystal), which are caused by urinary tract infection (usually with *Proteus* species). The classic example is the staghorn calculus (a stone that fills the entire calyceal system). About 5% to 10% of stones are uric acid (rhomboid crystal). Look for gout or leukemia. The remaining 1% to 3% are cystine stones (hexagonal crystal), which suggest hereditary cystinuria.

15. How is nephrolithiasis treated?

The cornerstones of nephrolithiasis treatment are large amounts of fluid hydration, narcotics for pain, an alpha-blocker (tamsulosin) to reduce ureteral spasm, and observation because most stones pass spontaneously. Most stones less than or equal to 4 mm in diameter pass spontaneously. Stones 4 to 10 mm in diameter may or may not pass. Spontaneous passage is unlikely with stones greater than or equal to 10 mm in diameter. If a stone does not pass, treat with lithotripsy, ureteroscopy with stone retrieval, or open surgery (last resort).

16. Define cryptorchidism. When does it occur?

Cryptorchidism is arrested descent of the testicle(s) between the renal area and the scrotum. The more premature the infant, the greater the likelihood of cryptorchidism. Many arrested testes eventually descend on their own within the first year. Intramuscular hCG may be used to induce testicular descent. After 1 year, surgical intervention (orchiopexy) is warranted in an attempt to preserve fertility as well as to facilitate future testicular exams. Affected testes have an increased risk for testicular cancer.

17. True or False: It is important to place abdominal testes in the scrotum surgically to decrease the risk of cancer.

False. Cryptorchidism is a major risk factor for testicular cancer (40 times increased risk), but bringing the testis into the scrotum probably does not alter the increased risk. It does make cancer easier to detect via testicular exam. The higher the testicle is found (the further away from the scrotum), the higher the risk of developing testicular cancer and the lower the likelihood of retaining fertility.

18. Where do the left and right ovarian/testicular veins drain?

The right ovarian/testicular vein drains into the inferior vena cava, whereas the left ovarian/testicular vein drains into the left renal vein.

19. When is kidney transplantation considered for patients with renal disease?

Kidney transplant is an option for patients with end-stage renal disease (glomerular filtration rate <10–15 mg/min), unless they have active infections or other life-threatening conditions (e.g., AIDS, malignancy). Lupus erythematosus and diabetes are not contraindications to transplantation.

20. Who makes the best donor for patients who need a kidney transplant?

Living, related donors are best (siblings or parents), especially when human leukocyte antigens (HLA) are similar, but cadaveric kidneys are more commonly used because of availability. Before transplant, perform ABO blood typing and lymphocytotoxic (HLA) cross-matching to ensure a reasonable chance at success.

21. Describe unacceptable kidney donors

Unacceptable kidney donors include newborns (most centers set an age <18 years as an exclusion criterion) and patients with a history of generalized or intraabdominal sepsis, malignancy, or any disease with possible renal involvement (e.g., diabetes, hypertension, lupus erythematosus).

22. Where is the transplanted kidney placed? What happens to the native kidneys?

A transplanted kidney is placed in the iliac fossa or pelvis (for easy biopsy access in case of later problems as well as for technical reasons). Usually the recipient's kidneys are left in place to reduce the morbidity of the surgery.

23. What are the three basic types of rejection with kidney transplantation?

Hyperacute, acute, and chronic.

24. What causes hyperacute rejection? What is the classic clinical description?

Hyperacute rejection is due to preformed cytotoxic antibodies against the donor kidney; it occurs with ABO blood type mismatch as well as other preformed antibodies. In the classic clinical description, the surgery is completed, the vascular clamps are released to allow blood flow, and the transplanted kidney quickly turns bluish-black. Treat by removing the kidney.

25. What causes acute rejection? How does it present? How is it treated?

Acute rejection is T-cell mediated. It presents days to weeks after the transplant with fever, oliguria, weight gain, tenderness and enlargement of the graft, hypertension, and/or laboratory derangements. Increases in creatinine are more reliable than increases in blood urea nitrogen. Treatment involves pulse corticosteroids, anti–T-cell antibody therapies (polyclonal antibodies, OKT3), other antibody therapies (basiliximab, daclizumab), and other immunosuppressants (tacrolimus, mycophenolate, cyclosporine). **Accelerated rejection** occurs over the first few days and is thought to reflect reactivation of previously sensitized T cells.

26. What causes chronic rejection? How does it present? How is it treated?

Chronic rejection can be T-cell or antibody mediated. This late cause (months to years after transplant) of renal deterioration presents with gradual decline in kidney function, proteinuria, and hypertension. Treatment is supportive and not effective, but the graft may last several years before it gives out completely. A new kidney can be transplanted if this occurs.

27. Discuss the mechanism of action of the commonly used immunosuppressant drugs in transplant medicine

- Steroids inhibit the production of IL-1, IL-2, and IL-6 as well as tumor necrosis factor-alpha and interferon-gamma. Prednisone is most commonly used.
- Methotrexate is a folic acid antagonist, but the precise mechanism in immunosuppression is unclear.
- Cyclosporine is a calcineurin inhibitor that inhibits IL-2 production.
- Tacrolimus is another calcineurin inhibitor that inhibits signaling through the T-cell receptor and production of IL-2.
- Mycophenolate prevents T-cell activation.
- Azathioprine is an antineoplastic that is cleaved into mercaptopurine and inhibits DNA/RNA synthesis (which causes decreased production of B and T cells).
- Antithymocyte globulin is an antibody against T cells.
- OKT3 is an antibody to the CD3 receptor on T cells.
- Hydroxychloroquine interferes with antigen presentation.
- Basiliximab is a monoclonal antibody against the IL-2 receptor.
- Daclizumab is a monoclonal antibody against the IL-2 receptor.

28. How do you distinguish the nephrotoxicity of cyclosporine from rejection?

Cyclosporine is a well-known cause of nephrotoxicity that can be difficult to distinguish from graft rejection clinically. When in doubt, a percutaneous needle biopsy of the graft should be done if the patient is taking cyclosporine because in most cases the two can be distinguished histologically. Diffuse mononuclear cell infiltrate will more likely be observed in the setting of rejection, while vascular lesions and thrombi are expected in the setting of nephrotoxicity. Renal ultrasound also helps. Practically speaking, if you increase the immunosuppressive dose, acute rejection should decrease, whereas cyclosporine toxicity stays the same or worsens.

29. What risks are associated with immunosuppression?

Immunosuppression carries the risk of infection (with common as well as rare bugs that infect patients with AIDS) and an increased risk of cancer (especially lymphomas and epithelial cell cancers).

30. Define epispadias and hypospadias. How are they treated?

Both are congenital penile anomalies. In **hypospadias**, the urethra opens on the ventral (under) side of the penis. In **epispadias**, the urethra opens on the dorsal (top) side of the penis. Epispadias is associated with exstrophy of the bladder. Both are treated with surgical correction.

31. Define Potter syndrome. With what is it associated?

Potter syndrome is bilateral renal agenesis, which causes oligohydramnios in utero (because the fetus swallows fluid but cannot excrete it). It is also associated with limb deformities, abnormal facies, and hypoplasia of the lungs. It can occur with autosomal recessive polycystic kidney disease, chronic placental insufficiency, and posterior urethral valves. It is incompatible with life because of the severe associated lung hypoplasia.

CHAPTER 39

VASCULAR SURGERY

1. **What clues suggest carotid stenosis? How is it diagnosed?**
   The classic presentation of carotid stenosis is a transient ischemic attack (TIA)—especially amaurosis fugax, which is the sudden onset of transient, unilateral blindness, sometimes described as a "shade pulled over one eye." Physical exam may reveal a carotid bruit. Ultrasound of the carotid arteries (duplex scan of the carotids) is used to diagnose and quantify the degree of stenosis.

2. **How is carotid stenosis managed?**
   In symptomatic patients, if the stenosis is **70% to 99%**, patients usually are advised to undergo carotid endarterectomy (CEA) for the best long-term prognosis—if their state of health allows them to tolerate the surgery. If stenosis is 50% to 69%, the data are less clear, and patient factors affect the decision. CEA is generally recommended for men, patients ages 75 or older, patients with recent stroke (not TIA), and patients with hemispheric symptoms other than transient monocular blindness (amaurosis fugax). Female patients, patients younger than 75 years, and those with mild symptoms generally do better with medical management if stenosis is 50% to 69%. If stenosis is less than 50%, medical management is indicated.

   Patients should not undergo carotid endarterectomy after a stroke that leaves them severely disabled, but small, nondisabling strokes are not contraindications to surgery. Carotid endarterectomy should not be performed during a TIA or stroke in evolution. Surgery is always done electively, not on an emergent basis.

   In asymptomatic patients, if the stenosis is 60% to 99%, CEA is indicated. If stenosis is less than 60%, medical management is indicated. Medical management includes antihypertensive agents, statins, and antiplatelet therapy.

   The role of carotid angioplasty and carotid stenting in carotid stenosis is not yet clearly defined. Carotid endarterectomy remains the treatment of choice for suitable carotid stenosis.

   Because medical therapy has improved since the initial studies comparing CEA with medical management were performed, medical management of lower-grade carotid stenosis and asymptomatic carotid stenosis is gaining favor. This is an area that is still being clarified in the medical literature and likely won't be tested on the USMLE.

3. **What is the most common cause of death during vascular surgery?**
   Myocardial infarction (MI), regardless of the procedure performed. Peripheral vascular and aortic disease are generalized markers for atherosclerosis, and almost all patients have significant coronary artery disease. Always evaluate patients for modifiable and treatable atherosclerosis risk factors (i.e., cholesterol, hypertension, smoking, diabetes).

4. **What are the classic findings in a patient with an abdominal aortic aneurysm? How is it evaluated?**
   Abdominal aortic aneurysm (AAA) (Fig. 39.1) classically presents as a pulsatile abdominal mass that may cause abdominal pain or back pain. If pain is present, rupture/leak of the aneurysm should be suspected, although an unruptured aneurysm may cause some degree of pain. Presumed ruptured AAA is a surgical emergency. Ultrasound or computed tomography (CT) scan is used for initial evaluation and diagnostic confirmation in stable patients, as well as for serial monitoring.

5. **How is an abdominal aortic aneurysm managed? What clues indicate that the aneurysm has ruptured?**
   If the aneurysm is smaller than 5 cm, you can follow it with serial ultrasound examinations to ensure that it is not enlarging. These smaller aneurysms should be managed with risk factor reduction (smoking cessation and treatment of hypertension and dyslipidemia). If the aneurysm is larger than 5 cm (or if you are told that it is enlarging rapidly), surgical correction should be advised if the patient can tolerate the surgery.

   A **pulsatile abdominal mass plus hypotension** requires emergent laparotomy for a presumed ruptured aneurysm, which carries a mortality rate of roughly 80%. The management of an abdominal aortic aneurysm dissection depends upon the location of the dissection. Patients who survive the initial tear typically present with

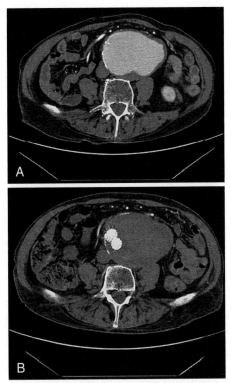

Fig. 39.1 Cross-sectional computed tomography (CT) image (A) of an 11-cm abdominal aortic aneurysm. (B) CT image 3 months after endovascular repair. Note the thrombosed aneurysm and patent limbs of the stent graft. (From Townsend Jr CM, Beauchamp RD, Evers BM, et al. *Sabiston Textbook of Surgery.* 18th ed. Philadelphia: Saunders; 2008 [fig. 65.4].)

a severe sharp or tearing sensation in the back or chest. Acute dissections involving the ascending aorta are considered surgical emergencies. Dissections confined to the descending aorta are treated medically unless the dissection progresses or continues to bleed.

6. Define Leriche syndrome. What pathology does it indicate?
Leriche syndrome is the combination of claudication in the buttocks, buttock atrophy, and impotence in men due to aortoiliac occlusive disease. Most patients need an aortoiliac bypass graft.

7. Define claudication. What are the associated physical findings?
Claudication is pain, usually in the lower extremity, brought on by exercise and relieved by rest. It occurs with severe atherosclerotic disease and is the equivalent of angina for the extremities. Associated physical findings include cyanosis (with dependent rubor), atrophic changes (thickened nails, loss of hair, shiny skin), decreased temperature, and decreased (or absent) distal pulses.

8. How are patients with claudication managed?
The best treatment is conservative: cessation of smoking, exercise, and good control of cholesterol, diabetes, and hypertension. Antiplatelet agents are warranted in patients with claudication. Aspirin is preferred, but clopidogrel may be used for patients who cannot tolerate aspirin. Cilostazol may be used for the treatment of intermittent claudication. Beta-blockers may worsen claudication (as a result of beta$_2$-receptor blockade), but benefits may outweigh the risks in some patients (e.g., prior myocardial infarction). If claudication progresses to rest pain (forefoot pain, generally at night, which is classically relieved by hanging the foot over the edge of the bed) or interferes with lifestyle or work obligations, perform an arterial duplex for diagnosis and use angioplasty or surgical revascularization procedure for treatment. Because claudication and peripheral vascular disease are generalized markers for atherosclerosis, check for other atherosclerosis risk factors.

9. What is the probable cause of severe, sudden onset of foot pain in patients with no previous history of foot pain, trauma, or associated chronic physical findings?

This scenario may indicate an embolus (look for atrial fibrillation; the pulse may be absent in the affected area) or compartment syndrome (common after revascularization procedures).

10. Describe the classic presentation of aortic dissection.

The classic presentation is a tearing or ripping pain in the chest or back. Always think of aortic dissection if a patient presents with chest pain and focal neurologic deficit. On physical exam, look for a systolic blood pressure difference of greater than 20 mm Hg in the upper extremities, hypertension, and acute aortic regurgitation on exam (diastolic heart murmur). Look for a widened mediastinum on x-ray (only present in 63% of cases) or an isolated new pleural effusion. Diagnose with CT angiogram. Risk factors include smoking, hypertension, drug use, and connective tissue disorders.

There are two types of dissection: type A, which involves the ascending aorta; and type B, which involves the descending aorta. Generally, type A is treated with surgery and type B is treated with medical management. Medical treatment includes blood pressure control (systolic blood pressure of 100–120 mm Hg) and heart rate control (60–80 beats per minute).

11. Describe the classic presentation of chronic mesenteric ischemia.

The classic patient has a long history of postprandial abdominal pain (also known as intestinal angina; eating is "exercise" for the intestines), which causes "fear" of food and extensive weight loss. This diagnosis is difficult because, like all atherosclerotic disease, it presents in patients over 40 who have other conditions that may cause the same problem (e.g., peptic ulcer disease, pancreatic cancer, stomach cancer). Look for a history of extensive atherosclerosis (known coronary artery disease, peripheral vascular disease, stroke, or multiple risk factors), abdominal bruit, hemoccult-positive stool, and lack of jaundice (jaundice suggests pancreatic cancer). Most patients get a CT scan of the abdomen; negative results raise the suspicion of ischemia. Diagnosis can be made with selective angiography of the superior mesenteric artery. Magnetic resonance angiography and CT angiography are emerging tools, but angiography is still the preferred modality. Patients are treated with surgical revascularization because of the risks of bowel infarction and malnutrition.

12. How does an acute bowel infarction present?

Classically, a patient with a history of extensive atherosclerosis, multiple atherosclerosis risk factors, or atrial fibrillation presents with abdominal pain or tenderness (the classic presentation is "pain out of proportion to the exam"), bloody diarrhea, and possibly peritoneal signs (e.g., rebound tenderness, guarding). Watch for thumbprinting (thickened bowel walls that resemble thumbprints) on abdominal radiographs. Patients may also have tachycardia, hypotension, and/or shock.

13. What causes arteriovenous fistulas and pseudoaneurysms in the extremities? How do you recognize them?

Penetrating trauma in an extremity or iatrogenic catheter damage may be followed by the development of an arteriovenous fistula or pseudoaneurysm. Watch for bruits over the area or a palpable pulsatile mass. Small fistulas can be left alone, but other patients require surgical or angiographic intervention.

14. What are the signs and symptoms of venous insufficiency? How is it treated?

Venous insufficiency generally occurs in the lower extremities. Patients may have a history of deep venous thrombosis, varicose veins, and/or swelling in the extremity with pain, fatigability, or heaviness. Symptoms are relieved by elevating the extremity. Patients may also have increased skin pigmentation around the ankles with possible skin breakdown and ulceration.

Treatment is at first conservative, including elastic compression stockings, elevation with minimal standing, and treatment of ulcers with cleaning, wet-to-dry dressings, and antibiotics, if cellulitis occurs.

15. True or False: A superficial palpable cord is a fairly specific sign of deep venous thrombosis.

False. A superficial palpable cord usually represents superficial thrombophlebitis.

16. Describe the usual history of a patient with superficial thrombophlebitis. How is it treated?

Patients often have a history of varicose veins and present with localized leg pain with superficial cordlike induration, reddish discoloration, and mild fever. Superficial thrombophlebitis is not a significant risk factor for pulmonary embolus, and patients do not need anticoagulation. Treatment is usually conservative, including nonsteroidal antiinflammatory drugs and warm compresses. The condition generally subsides on its own within a few days. A thrombectomy under local anesthesia can be done for severe or nonresolving symptoms.

17. Define subclavian steal syndrome. What symptoms does it cause? How is it treated?

Subclavian steal syndrome is usually due to left subclavian artery obstruction proximal to the vertebral artery origin. To perfuse an exercising arm, blood is "stolen" from the vertebrobasilar system; that is, the flow of the vertebral artery is retrograde into the distal subclavian artery instead of forward into the brainstem. Patients present with central nervous system (CNS) symptoms (e.g., syncope, vertigo, confusion, ataxia, dysarthria) and upper extremity claudication during exercise. Treat with surgical bypass.

18. What are the symptoms of thoracic outlet obstruction? How is it treated?

Thoracic outlet obstruction refers to symptoms caused by obstruction of the nerves or blood vessels that serve the arm as the neurovascular bundle passes from the thoracocervical region to the axilla. Affected patients have upper extremity paresthesias (nerve impingement), weakness, cold temperature (arterial compromise), edema, and/or venous distention (venous compromise). The absence of CNS symptoms helps to differentiate this condition from subclavian steal syndrome. Causes include trauma, pregnancy, cervical ribs (ribs arising from a cervical vertebra that are usually asymptomatic but may compromise subclavian blood flow) or muscular hypertrophy (classic in young male weightlifters). Treat with surgical intervention (e.g., cervical rib resection).

CHAPTER 40

VITAMINS AND MINERALS

1. Specify the signs and symptoms of the various vitamin deficiencies and toxicities

Vitamin	Deficiency	Toxicity
A	Nyctalopia (night blindness), xerosis cutis (dry skin) and scaly rash, xerophthalmia (dry eyes), Bitot spots (debris on conjunctiva); increased infections	Pseudotumor cerebri, bone thickening, teratogenic (craniofacial and heart defects)
C (ascorbic acid)	Scurvy (hemorrhages, skin petechiae, gingivitis, loose teeth), poor wound healing, hyperkeratotic hair follicles, bone pain (from periosteal hemorrhages)	Nephrolithiasis; can worsen hemochromatosis by promoting iron absorption
D	Rickets, osteomalacia, hypocalcemia	Hypercalcemia, nausea, renal toxicity
E	Anemia, peripheral neuropathy, ataxia	Necrotizing enterocolitis (infants)
K	Hemorrhage, prolonged prothrombin time	Hemolysis (can lead to kernicterus)
B_1 (thiamine)	Wet beriberi (high-output cardiac failure), dry beriberi, (peripheral neuropathy), Wernicke and Korsakoff syndromes	
B_2 (riboflavin)	Angular stomatitis, dermatitis	
B_3 (niacin)	Pellagra (dementia, dermatitis, diarrhea), stomatitis	
B_6 (pyridoxine)	Peripheral neuropathy, stomatitis, convulsions in infants, microcytic anemia, seborrheic dermatitis	Peripheral neuropathy (only B vitamin with toxicity)
B_{12} (cobalamin)	Megaloblastic anemia *plus* neurologic symptoms (subacute combined degeneration, dementia, ataxia)	
Folic acid	Megaloblastic anemia *without* neurologic symptoms	

2. Specify the signs and symptoms of the various mineral deficiencies and toxicities

Mineral	Deficiency	Toxicity
Iron	Microcytic anemia, koilonychia (spoon-shaped fingernails)	Hemochromatosis
Iodine	Goiter, cretinism, hypothyroidism	Myxedema
Fluoride	Dental caries (cavities)	Fluorosis with mottling of teeth and bone exostoses
Zinc	Hypogeusia (decreased taste), rash, slow wound healing	
Copper	Menkes syndrome (X-linked; kinky hair, intellectual disability)	Wilson disease

Mineral	Deficiency	Toxicity
Selenium	Cardiomyopathy and muscle pain	Loss of hair and nails
Manganese	Dermatitis	"Manganese madness" in miners of ore (behavioral changes/psychosis)
Chromium	Impaired glucose tolerance	

3. **What are the fat-soluble vitamins? In what general category of patients are they deficient?**
Vitamins A, D, E, and K are fat soluble. Deficiency of any of these vitamins may be due to malabsorption (e.g., cystic fibrosis, cirrhosis, celiac disease, duodenal bypass, bile-duct obstruction, pancreatic insufficiency, chronic giardiasis). In such patients, parenteral supplements are required if high-dose oral supplements fail.

4. **What vitamin, mineral, and electrolyte deficiencies are classically seen in alcoholics?**
Any can be seen, but watch especially for folate, thiamine, phosphorus, and magnesium deficiencies.

5. **What is the most common cause of vitamin B_{12} deficiency?**
Pernicious anemia, in which antiparietal cell antibodies destroy the ability to secrete intrinsic factor. Conditions associated with pernicious anemia include autoimmune disease such as hypothyroidism, type I diabetes, and vitiligo (Fig. 40.1). Removal of the ileum and the tapeworm *Diphyllobothrium latum* are exotic causes of B_{12} deficiency. Diagnosis of pernicious anemia is clinched by a low serum B_{12} level. The presence of antiintrinsic factor antibodies is highly confirmatory for pernicious anemia. There is emerging evidence that medications such as proton-pump inhibitors, H_2-receptor blockers, and metformin increase the risk of B_{12} deficiency. Diagnosis of B_{12} deficiency can be confirmed by elevated levels of methylmalonic acid (MMA), especially in cases of borderline levels of B_{12}. Of note, increased levels of MMA also help to distinguish B_{12} deficiency from folate deficiency, both of which can present as megaloblastic anemia. The Schilling test is of historical interest but is no longer commonly employed in the diagnosis of B_{12} deficiency.

6. **What is the classic iatrogenic cause of vitamin B_6 deficiency?**
Prolonged therapy with isoniazid (especially in young people). Pyridoxine supplementation is recommended for patients on isoniazid therapy for tuberculosis.

7. **Which medications may cause folate deficiency?**
Anticonvulsants (especially phenytoin), methotrexate, and trimethoprim.

8. **Which vitamin is a known teratogen?**
Vitamin A. Female patients taking one of the oral vitamin A analogs as treatment for acne must have a negative pregnancy test before the medication is started and should be counseled about the risks of teratogenicity. Some form of birth control should be used with vitamin A therapy, and periodic pregnancy tests should be offered.
   Isotretinoin is such a significant teratogen that access to this medication is very restricted. All patients and prescribers must be in a special program designed to eliminate fetal exposure to isotretinoin. There are strict qualification criteria, including monthly pregnancy testing, and two forms of contraception are recommended.

9. **Which vitamin should be taken by all sexually active women of reproductive age?**
Folate, which reduces the risk of neural tube defects in the fetus. The maximal benefit occurs before the woman knows that she is pregnant.

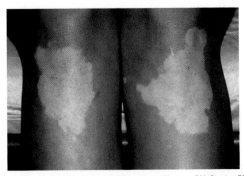

Fig. 40.1 Sharply demarcated, symmetric, depigmented areas of vitiligo. (From Kliegman RM, Stanton BF, St. Geme JW, et al. *Nelson Textbook of Pediatrics.* 19th ed. Philadelphia: Elsevier; 2011 [fig. 645.4])

10. **What are the physical findings of rickets (vitamin D deficiency) in children?**
    - Craniotabes (poorly mineralized skull; bones feel like a ping-pong ball)
    - Rachitic rosary (costochondral beading; small round masses on anterior rib cage)
    - Delayed fontanelle closure
    - Bossing of the skull
    - Kyphoscoliosis
    - Bow-legs and knock-knees
    Bone changes appear first at the lower ends of the radius and ulna.

11. **Which vitamin is given to all newborns?**
    Vitamin K is given as prophylaxis against hemorrhagic disease of the newborn.

12. **Which clotting factors are affected by vitamin K? What is the interaction of vitamin K and the liver?**
    Vitamin K is needed for hepatic synthesis of factors II, VII, IX, and X as well as proteins C and S. Chronic liver disease (cirrhosis) can cause prolongation of the prothrombin time and international normalized ratio because of the liver's inability to synthesize clotting factors even in the presence of adequate vitamin K levels. This problem should be corrected with fresh frozen plasma or prothrombin complex concentrate; vitamin K is ineffective in the setting of severe liver disease.

13. **Describe the relationship between vitamin K and broad-spectrum antibiotics.**
    Prolonged therapy with broad-spectrum antibiotics is a potential cause of vitamin K deficiency. These medications can eliminate the normal gut bacteria that synthesize much of the vitamin K required daily.

14. **What is the classic Step 2 description of a vitamin C–deficient patient?**
    An elderly person with a diet of "hot dogs and soda" or "tea and toast" who presents with bleeding gums and bone pain.

15. **What is the interaction of vitamin C and iron?**
    Vitamin C increases iron absorption.

INDEX

A

ABCs, in shock management, 294–295
ABCDE characteristics, of mole, 54
ABCDEs, of trauma, 107
Abdominal abscess, radiologic tests for, 283t–285t
Abdominal aortic aneurysm (AAA)
    findings in, 302, 303f
    management of, 302–303
Abdominal testes, cancer and, 299
Abdominal trauma, 108, 108f
    radiologic tests for, 283t–285t
Abdominal x-ray, newborns, 248–249
Abducens (cranial nerve VI) lesion, 237
Abetalipoproteinemia, 129, 133f
Abnormal uterine bleeding (AUB), 121–122
ABO blood group incompatibility, in hemolytic disease of the newborn, 209
Abortion, 204
Abruptio placentae, 207, 211
Abscess, 125
    breast, 166
    tuboovarian, 119
Absence seizure, 184
Acanthocytes, 133f
Accelerated rejection, 300
Accidents, adolescents in, death of, 275
Acetaminophen, 71
    differentiation with aspirin and other NSAIDs, 260
    overdose of, 260
        antidote for, 259t
    side effects of, 257t–258t
Acetazolamide, side effects of, 257t–258t
N-Acetylcysteine, 260
Achalasia, 94–95, 95f
Achlorhydria, 84
Achondroplasia, inheritance pattern of, 111t–112t
Acid-base, electrolytes and, 13–18
    causes of, 13
Acid burns, 68
Acidosis
    bicarbonate for, 14
    effect on potassium and calcium levels, 168
Acne, 49
Acne vulgaris, 49
Acoustic neuroma, 183, 224, 225f
Actinic keratoses, 56, 57f
Actinomyces sp., Gram stain result for, 153t–154t
Actinomyces israelii, 126
Active euthanasia, 81
Acute abdomen, 102–110, 102t
Acute bowel infarction, 304
Acute dystonia, 267
Acute fatty liver, of pregnancy, 211
Acute ischemic stroke, 144
Acute kidney injury (AKI), 172–177
    categories of, 172
    causes of, 172
    intrarenal, 172

Acute kidney injury (AKI) *(Continued)*
    intravenous contrast and, 172
    medications causing, 172
    muscle breakdown and, 172
    and myoglobinuria, 172
    postrenal, 172
    prerenal, 172
    and rhabdomyolysis, 172
    signs and symptoms, 172–177
Acute laryngotracheitis (croup), 162, 163f
Acute rejection, 300
Acute tubular necrosis, 172
Acute urinary retention, 298
Acyclovir, for chickenpox, 159
Addison disease (hypoadrenalism), 74
    shock and, 294
Adenomyosis, 121
Adenosine deaminase deficiency, 149
Adhesions, small bowel obstruction and, 105
Adjustment disorder, 270
Admission rate bias, 26–27
Adolescent
    anorexia in, 275
    causes of death in, 275
Adrenal mass, 78, 79f
Adrenal tumors, significance of, 226
Adrenocorticotropic hormone (ACTH), 73
Adrenogenital syndrome (congenital adrenal hyperplasia), 111t–112t, 126
Adult polycystic kidney disease, inheritance pattern of, 111t–112t
Adult respiratory distress syndrome (ARDS), 279
Advance directives, 82, 118
AFP. *See* Alpha-fetoprotein (AFP)
Afterload, 293
Age group, rapidly growing segment, 116
Aging. *See also* Older adults
    hearing loss and, 64
AIDS-defining illnesses, 149t–151t. *See also* Human immunodeficiency virus (HIV) infection
Airway
    obstruction, 109
    securing of, in anaphylaxis, 146
    in trauma protocol, 107
Akathisia, 267
Alanine aminotransferase (ALT), in alcoholic hepatitis, 20
Albinism, cancer in, 214t–215t
Alcohol, 198t–199t
    pregnancy and, 20
Alcohol abuse, 19–21
    cancer and, 19–21
    epidemiology of, 21
Alcoholic hallucinosis, 19
Alcoholic hepatitis, 90
Alcoholics, vitamin, mineral and electrolyte deficiencies in, 307
Alcoholism
    inheritance pattern of, 111t–112t
    treatment of, 20

Note: Pages followed by *b*, *t*, or *f* refer to boxes, tables, or figures, respectively.